PRINCIPLES OF EXERCISE TESTING AND INTERPRETATION

Principles
of Exercise Testing
and Interpretation

KARLMAN WASSERMAN, M.D., Ph.D.

Professor of Medicine, UCLA School of Medicine
Chief, Division of Respiratory Physiology and Medicine
Harbor-UCLA Medical Center

JAMES E. HANSEN, M.D.

Professor of Medicine, UCLA School of Medicine
Director, Clinical Respiratory Physiology Laboratory
Harbor-UCLA Medical Center

DARRYL Y. SUE, M.D.

Associate Professor of Medicine, UCLA School of Medicine
Medical Director, Department of Respiratory Therapy
Harbor-UCLA Medical Center

BRIAN J. WHIPP, Ph.D., D.Sc.

Professor of Physiology and Medicine
UCLA School of Medicine
Associate Chief, Division of Respiratory Physiology and Medicine
Harbor-UCLA Medical Center

Division of Respiratory Physiology and Medicine
Department of Medicine
Harbor-UCLA Medical Center
Torrance, California

LEA & FEBIGER   PHILADELPHIA

Lea & Febiger
600 South Washington Square
Philadelphia, Pa. 19106
U.S.A.
(215) 922-1330

Library of Congress Cataloging-in-Publication Data

Principles of exercise testing and interpretation.

Bibliography: p.
Includes index.
1. Exercise tests.   2. Heart function tests.
3. Pulmonary function tests.   4. Exercise — Physiological
aspects.   I. Wasserman, Karlman,   II. Harbor-UCLA Medical
Center. Division of Respiratory Physiology and Medicine.

RC71.8.P75 1986   616.07'54   86-86

PRINTED IN THE UNITED STATES OF AMERICA

Print Number: 5 4 3

Dedicated to our families

Preface

WHEN subjects complain of exercise intolerance, it is usually because they are unable to perform a physical task that they expect to accomplish without unusual effort, and undue feelings of fatigue, shortness of breath, or pain. Isolating the cause or causes of this exercise intolerance is the major objective of clinical exercise testing. This book addresses the problem of evaluating the patient with exercise limitation from the viewpoint of physiology, pathophysiology, and differential diagnosis.

Exercise testing laboratories for detection of coronary artery disease are well established at most hospitals. The requirements for such laboratories have been provided by the American Heart Association, and the practice and pitfalls of using the electrocardiogram to diagnose coronary artery disease have been described in a number of monographs. Although this book does not exclude considerations of coronary artery disease, its focus is more comprehensive and includes most conditions that lead to exertional dyspnea, including primary heart diseases (coronary artery, valvular, congenital and cardiomyopathic), disorders of the pulmonary and peripheral circulations, abnormalities in lung function, and obesity.

Why write a book on exercise testing and interpretation? Advances in both measurement and computational technology in recent years have resulted in an expansion of knowledge in exercise physiology, particularly with regard to the most essential elements in energy generation and cellular respiration and the coupling of circulation and ventilation to support these vital functions. This book is designed to help physicians and exercise physiologists keep pace with this expanding knowledge, and to help them use these new techniques in diagnosis and reporting results from exercise tests.

Exercise testing is valuable for: 1) diagnosing the many causes of exertional dyspnea; 2) evaluating the severity of the impairment of exercise performance and; 3) evaluating the effect of medical, surgical or physical rehabilitative therapy. This book is designed to provide a guide for exercise physiologists and physicians wishing to set up a laboratory for the purpose of any of the above objectives. Chapters 1 and 2 present the essential physiological concepts needed to provide an infrastructure of understanding for the later chapters. Chapters 3 and 4 deal with the measurement of exercise performance and the pathophysiology of the cardiovascular and respiratory disorders limiting exercise. Chapters 5, 6 and 7 in turn, provide a rationale for the selection of efficient testing protocols, the choice of normal values, and a logical scheme for interpretation of the abnormalities of test results. Finally, clinical examples are provided in Chapter 8, in the form of actual cases, for the purpose of teaching the principles of interpretation and also to demonstrate the spectrum of disorders that cause exercise limitation. Thus, this book attempts to span the field of "exercise" from basic concepts in exercise physiology to the practical aspects of delivering a meaningful report for the medical record on the mechanism and degree of a subject's exercise limitation.

Torrance, California

KARLMAN WASSERMAN
JAMES E. HANSEN
DARRYL Y. SUE
BRIAN J. WHIPP

Acknowledgments

THE AUTHORS are extremely grateful to Leah Coone for her editorial skill and dedication, and to Carol Brandon, Barbara Young, and Shirley Zagala for their accomplished secretarial support in the preparation of this book.

The authors are also indebted to their current and former colleagues in the Division of Respiratory Physiology and Medicine at the Harbor-UCLA Medical Center for their many stimulating discussions and collaborations over the years.

K.W. is also indebted to his wife Gail for affectionately tolerating the writing and editing of this book during innumerable nights and weekends.

K.W.
J.E.H.
D.Y.S.
B.J.W.

Contents

Appendix

Index   269

Exercise Testing and Interpretation: An Overview

CHAPTER 1

PHYSICAL EXERCISE requires the interaction of physiological mechanisms that enable the cardiovascular and respiratory systems to support the increased metabolic rate and gas exchange of contracting muscles. Both the ventilatory and cardiovascular systems are stressed during exercise and the ability to respond adequately to this stress is a measure of their physiological health. It is well recognized that ventilation and cardiac output increase as the metabolic rate increases. An appreciation of the normal responses of the gas transport systems supporting cell respiration is essential in order to recognize the pathophysiology of the many disease states that affect them.

The large metabolic rate increase during exercise requires a great increase of O_2 flow into the muscles. Simultaneously, the large quantity of CO_2 produced by the muscles must be removed to avoid severe tissue acidosis with its adverse effects on cellular function. To satisfy the increased gas exchange needs of the muscle cell during exercise, a close coupling of physiological mechanisms involving the lungs, the pulmonary circulation, the heart, and the peripheral circulation is required (Fig. 1-1). The coupling must efficiently follow the metabolic rate in order to maintain tissue O_2 supply and CO_2 elimination as well as arterial blood gas homeostasis. Exercise testing offers the examiner the possibility of studying both the cardiovascular and respiratory systems simultaneously under stress and allows evaluation of their ability to perform their common major function, i.e., gas exchange.

Because of the increased number of therapeutic modalities for conditions that cause exercise limitation, exercise testing has become increasingly important in medicine. We need to document and correctly diagnose the pathophysiology of the cardiovascular

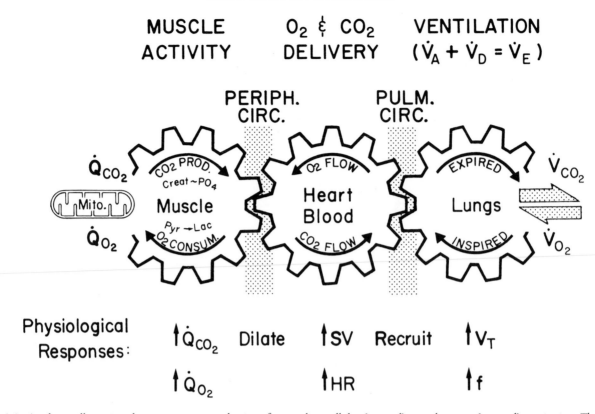

FIG. 1-1. A scheme illustrating the gas transport mechanisms for coupling cellular (internal) to pulmonary (external) respiration. The gears represent the functional interdependence of the physiological components of the system. The large increase in O_2 utilization by the muscles ($\dot{Q}_{O_2}$) is achieved by increased extraction of O_2 from the blood perfusing the muscles, the dilatation of selected peripheral vascular beds, an increase in cardiac output (stroke volume and heart rate), an increase in pulmonary blood flow by recruitment and vasodilatation of pulmonary blood vessels, and finally, an increase in ventilation. O_2 is taken up ($\dot{V}_{O_2}$) from the alveoli in proportion to the pulmonary blood flow and degree of O_2 desaturation of hemoglobin in the pulmonary blood. In the steady-state, $\dot{V}_{O_2} = \dot{Q}_{O_2}$. Ventilation (tidal volume (V_T) and breathing frequency (f)) increase in relation to the newly produced CO_2 ($\dot{Q}_{CO_2}$) arriving at the lungs and the drive to achieve arterial CO_2 and hydrogen ion homeostasis. These variables are related in the following way:

$$\dot{V}_{CO_2} = \dot{V}_A \cdot P_{a_{CO_2}}/P_B.$$

Where: $\dot{V}_{CO_2}$ = minute CO_2 output, $\dot{V}_A$ = minute alveolar ventilation, $P_{a_{CO_2}}$ = arterial CO_2 tension, and P_B = barometric pressure.
The representation of gears uniformly sized is not intended to imply equal changes in each of the components of the coupling. For instance, the increase in cardiac output is proportionally smaller than the increase in metabolic rate. This results in an increased extraction of O_2 from, and CO_2 loading into, the blood by the muscles. In contrast, at moderate work intensities, minute ventilation increases in approximate proportion to the new CO_2 brought to the lungs by the venous return. The development of metabolic acidosis, at heavy and very heavy work intensities, results in an increased ventilation to provide respiratory compensation for the metabolic acidosis.

and respiratory systems to treat and assess treatment of exercise limitation. For example, it is important to determine whether new medical, surgical, and rehabilitative procedures are effective interventions. Also, an individual patient may have mixed defects, e.g., cardiac and respiratory, and it is often necessary to determine the relative contribution of each to the patient's symptoms before embarking on major therapeutic procedures directed at either one. Exercise testing, because it allows an assessment of the circulatory and ventilatory reserves under stress, may also provide useful information prior to surgery or other therapy. Finally, because dyspnea is accompanied by abnormal breathing and gas exchange patterns during work, exercise testing might help isolate the mechanism of this symptom.

The authors would like to dispel a concept that has developed in American medicine, i.e., that there is cardiac stress testing and pulmonary stress testing. It is impossible to stress only the heart or only the lungs. Rather, all exercise requires the coordinated function of both the heart and lungs as well as the peripheral and pulmonary circulations to achieve the cellular gas exchange required to live and work. Diseases of the heart can cause both abnormal breathing and gas exchange responses, which can be used to help identify heart disease. Similarly, abnormal cardiac responses can occur secondary to pulmonary disorders. To interpret exercise tests, physiologists and physicians must appreciate the inseparable interactive roles of the cardiovascular and respiratory systems in supporting cellular respiration for generating energy for muscle contraction.

Physiology of Exercise

THE PERFORMANCE of muscular work requires the responses of the physiological system to be integrated to minimize the stress to the component mechanisms supporting the energetics. The conversion of stored energy into work during exercise is the function of the skeletal muscles. The muscles have inherent capabilities to perform work in a range of rates and durations, using a variety of substrates and operating under different conditions. A thorough understanding of these characteristics is essential for identifying the needs of cellular (internal) respiration of muscles during exercise. These needs of internal respiration can only be met by complex interactive systems that provide gas exchange between the muscle cells and the atmosphere (external respiration) (see Fig. 1-1).

Normal gas exchange between the cells and the environment requires: 1) efficiently operating lungs and chest bellows, 2) an effective pulmonary circulation through which the regional blood flow is matched to the appropriate ventilation, 3) a heart capable of pumping the quantity of oxygenated blood necessary to sustain tissue energy exchange processes, 4) an effective system of blood vessels that can selectively distribute blood flow to match tissue gas exchange requirements, 5) blood with an adequate hemoglobin concentration, and 6) respiratory control mechanisms capable of regulating arterial blood gas tensions and pH. The response of each of the coupling links in the gas exchange process is normally quite predictable and can be used as a frame of reference for evidence of impaired responses.

In this chapter we will review the essentials of skeletal muscle physiology, including the relationship of structure and function, cellular respiration, substrate metabolism, and the effect of an inadequate O_2 supply. After considering internal respiration, we will examine the linkage between internal and external respiration, including the factors that determine the magnitude and time course of the cardiovascular and ventilatory responses and how these are coupled with the metabolic stress of exercise.

Skeletal Muscle

MECHANICAL PROPERTIES

Human skeletal muscles consist of two basic fiber types (Types I and II) which are classified on the basis of both their contractile and biochemical properties.[1] Type I slow-twitch fibers take a relatively long time to develop peak tension following their activation, i.e., some 80 msec, compared to the 30 msec average for Type II fast-twitch fibers. The slow contractile properties of Type I fibers appear to result largely from the relatively low activity of the myosin ATPase, the lower Ca^{++} activity of the regulatory protein troponin, and the slower rate of Ca^{++} uptake by sarcoplasmic reticulum. These same properties appear to confer a relatively high resistance to fatigue on the Type I fibers.

Biochemical differences between the two basic fiber types center chiefly on their capacity for oxidative and glycolytic activities. The Type I fibers, being especially rich in myoglobin, are classified as red fibers, while the Type II fibers, which contain considerably less myoglobin, are classified as white fibers. The Type I slow-twitch fibers tend to have significantly higher levels of oxidative enzymes than the Type II fast-twitch fibers that typically have a high glycolytic activity and enzyme profile. The Type II fibers are further classified into Type IIa and Type IIb, based on the greater oxidative and lesser glycolytic potential of the Type IIa fibers compared with the Type IIb fibers. With respect to substrate stores, muscle glycogen concentration is, in fact, similar in both Type I and Type II fibers, but the triglyceride content is two to three times greater in the Type I slow-twitch fibers. Evidence suggests that the Type I slow-twitch fibers are more efficient than the Type II fast-twitch fibers, generating more work or developing more tension per unit of substrate energy.[2]

There is considerable potential for change in the enzyme concentrations of a particular fiber by specific training. For example, a fast-twitch fiber in an endurance-trained athlete could have higher concentrations of oxidative enzymes than slow-twitch fibers in a chronically sedentary subject (the enzyme concentrations increasing only in the "trained" muscle).[3]

These structural and functional differences between fiber types depend to a large extent on the neural innervation of the fibers. A single motor neuron supplies numerous individual muscle fibers; this functional assembly is termed a "motor unit." These fibers are distributed throughout the muscle, rather than being spatially contiguous. Fibers comprising a motor unit are characteristically of the same "Type,"

and substrate depletion occurs within each fiber of the contracting unit.

Fiber type distribution within human skeletal muscle varies from muscle to muscle. For example, the soleus muscle typically has a much higher density of slow-twitch fibers (greater than 80%) than the gastrocnemius muscle (about 50%) or the triceps brachii (about 20 to 50%). The vastus lateralis muscle (approximately 50% slow-twitch fibers) has been widely used for analysis of fiber type characteristics in man. The basic fiber type pattern for this muscle appears highly variable in different subjects. Endurance-trained athletes typically have a high percentage of slow-twitch fibers in this muscle (greater than 90% not being uncommon) compared with untrained, control subjects (about 50%) or trained sprinters (20 to 30%).

The basic fiber type pattern appears to be genetically determined, but is greatly influenced by the neural characteristics of the efferent motor neuron. When the motor nerves innervating the fast flexor digitorum longus and the slow soleus muscles of the cat are cut and cross-spliced, thereby switching the nerve from a "fast" to a "slow" muscle, and vice versa, the contractile and biochemical characteristics of the muscle begin to resemble the features of the muscle originally innervated by the nerve.[4] Thus an important trophic influence on muscle function is conferred by its nerve supply. Training, however, does not cause significant interchanges between Type I and Type II fibers, but can cause changes within Type II fibers (i.e., from a Type a to a Type b, and vice versa).[5]

The pattern of activation of these fiber types depends on the form of exercise. For low-intensity exercise, the Type I slow-twitch fibers tend to be recruited predominantly, while the Type II fast-twitch fibers are recruited at higher work rates, especially at or above some 70 to 80% of the maximal aerobic power.[6]

ENERGETICS

Skeletal muscle may be considered a machine that is fueled by the chemical energy of substrates derived from ingested food stored as carbohydrates and lipids in the body. Although protein is a perfectly viable energy source, it is not used to fuel the energy needs of the body to any appreciable extent, except under conditions of starvation.

The substrate chemical energy is not used directly for muscle contraction. It must first be stored in the bond energy of adenosine triphosphate (ATP). The terminal phosphate bonds of this compound have a high free energy of hydrolysis (ΔG) and are designated as "high energy" phosphate bonds ($\sim P$). Current estimates of ΔG per $\sim P$, for physiological conditions such as those occurring in contracting muscle, are as high as 12 to 14 Kcal/mole. Muscle is ultimately, therefore, a digital device operating in discrete multiple units of $\sim P$ energy, with one $\sim P$ thought to be utilized per myosin cross-bridge linkage to and subsequent release from actin. The muscle uses this energy for the conformational changes externally manifested by shortening or increasing tension.

Thus muscular exercise depends on the intrinsic structural characteristics of muscle and on the body's systems which maintain an appropriate physicochemical milieu for adequate ATP generation.

Cell Respiration

Energy for muscular contraction is obtained predominantly by the oxidation of fuel in the mitochondrion with a small additional amount from biochemical mechanisms in the cell cytoplasm (Fig. 2-1). This energy is used to form high-energy compounds, pre-

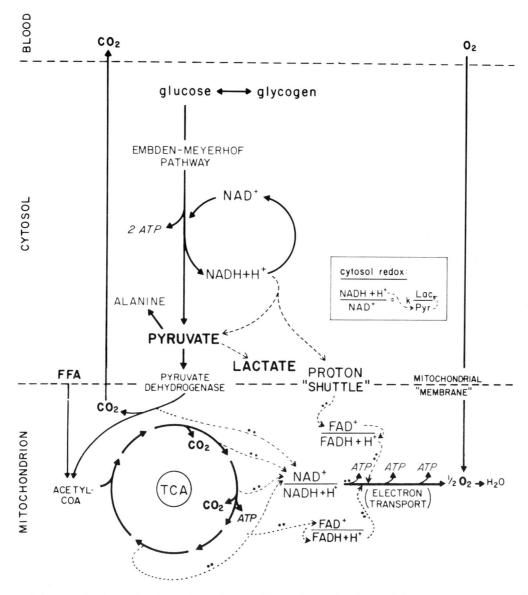

FIG. 2-1. Scheme of the major biochemical pathways for production of ATP. The transfer of H^+ and electrons to O_2 in the mitochondrion and the "shuttle" of protons from the cytosol to the mitochondrion are illustrated as important components in the efficient utilization of substrate for ATP generation. Also illustrated is the important O_2 flow from the blood to the mitochondrion without which the entire energy generating mechanisms would come to a halt.

dominantly creatine phosphate and ATP, from which energy in the terminal phosphate bond can be made available for cellular reactions involved in synthesis, active transport, and muscle contraction. Exercise entails an acceleration of the energy-yielding reactions in the muscles in order to produce ~P at an increased rate for muscle contraction. This requires an increased utilization of O_2, to be matched by increased delivery of O_2 from the atmosphere to the mitochondrion and the simultaneous removal of CO_2, the major catabolic end-product of exercise.

Acetate, produced from the catabolism of carbohydrates, fatty acids, or occasionally amino acids, after esterification with coenzyme-A (acetyl-CoA), reacts with oxaloacetate in the mitochondrion to form citrate in the Krebs or tricarboxylic acid (TCA) cycle (see Fig. 2-1). Here the catabolic reactions result in CO_2 release and the transfer of hydrogen ions or protons and their associated electrons down the mitochondrial electron transport chain to cytochrome oxidase where they react with O_2 to form water. For each pair of electrons transferred, sufficient energy is released to form approximately three ATP molecules.

Six ATP molecules are gained during the catabolism of glucose to pyruvate if the reduced nicotinamide adenine dinucleotide ($[NADH + H^+]$) in the cytosol, formed during glycolysis, is reoxidized by the proton shuttle in the mitochondrial membrane (see Fig. 2-1).[7] The shuttle accepts hydrogen ions from the cytosolic $[NADH + H^+]$ and transfers them to mitochondrial coenzymes, as illustrated in Figure 2-1. This method of regenerating oxidized $[NAD^+]$ in the cytosol maintains the cytosolic redox state and enables glycolysis to continue. Of the six ATP molecules generated from glucose by this mechanism, two are formed in the cytosol by the Embden-Meyerhof (glycolytic) pathway and four in the mitochondrion during the coupled reoxidation of cytosolic $[NADH + H^+]$ by the mitochondrion, i.e., the mitochondrial membrane proton shuttle, flavin adenine dinucleotide (FAD), and the cytochrome electron transport chain.[7]

The formation of acetyl-CoA from pyruvate and its subsequent entry into the TCA cycle yields a total of five reduced NAD molecules. Since the reoxidation process of each mitochondrial $[NADH + H^+]$ by the electron transport chain yields 3 ATP molecules, there is a net gain of 15 ATP. However, two molecules of acetyl-CoA are formed from each glucose molecule so that the total gain is 30 ATP from these reactions. When added to the 2 ATP gained from glycolysis and the 4 others obtained from reoxidation of cytosolic $[NADH + H^+]$, the total gain in

ATP from the complete oxidation of glucose is 36. Because 6 molecules of O_2 are used for the oxidation steps and 36 high energy phosphate bonds are formed, the $\sim P : O_2 = 6$. Six molecules of CO_2 and H_2O are catabolic end-products of these reactions.

Under conditions in which the mitochondrial FAD fails to reoxidize the proton shuttle of the mitochondrial membrane at a rate sufficient to keep cytosolic $[NADH + H^+]/[NAD^+]$ normal, the redox state of the cytosol becomes reduced. As $[NADH + H^+]$ accumulates in the cytosol at the expense of $[NAD^+]$, glycolysis would become inhibited if it were not for an alternate pathway capable of reoxidizing cytosolic $[NADH + H^+]$. Pyruvate can reoxidize the $[NADH + H^+]$ to $[NAD^+]$ but is reduced to lactic acid in the process. This pyruvate oxidation of $[NADH + H^+]$ occurs without immediate use of oxygen and is thus termed anaerobic. This is an expensive substrate price to pay for energy compared to the complete oxidation of a glucose molecule to CO_2 and H_2O, because the net gain in ATP is only 2 instead of 36. This pathway causes glucose and glycogen to be used at a considerably faster rate than in the aerobic state for the same energy production. Also, the two lactic acid molecules formed from each glucose molecule cause a disturbance of acid-base balance in the cell and blood (Fig. 2-2) with unfavorable consequences, such as muscle fatigue and a further stimulus to breathing.

That the turn-on of anaerobic ATP production does not signal the turn-off of aerobic ATP production deserves emphasis. Both aerobic and anaerobic mechanisms share in energy generation at high work rates with the anaerobic mechanism providing an increasing proportion of energy as the work rate is increased. The rate of anaerobic glycolysis is affected by blood oxygenation. For example, increasing blood O_2 content during exercise reduces arterial blood lactate.[8,9]

SUBSTRATE UTILIZATION AND REGULATION

At this point, several terms need to be clarified for precision and to avoid possible confusion (see Fig. 1-1). The symbol $\dot{V}O_2$ indicates O_2 uptake by the lungs. It is distinguished from O_2 consumption by the cells, which is symbolized by $\dot{Q}O_2$. The symbol $\dot{V}CO_2$ indicates CO_2 output by the lungs to distinguish it from CO_2 production by the cells, symbolized by $\dot{Q}CO_2$. Thus the substrate mixture undergoing oxidation is characterized by the net rates of CO_2 yield or production ($\dot{Q}CO_2$), and oxygen utilization or consumption ($\dot{Q}O_2$). The ratio $\dot{V}CO_2/\dot{V}O_2$ as measured at the mouth (i.e., the gas exchange ratio, R),

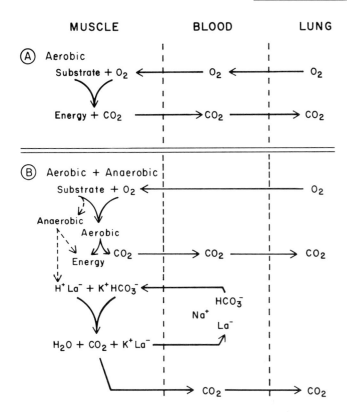

MUSCLE　　　　BLOOD　　　　LUNG

FIG. 2-2. Gas exchange during aerobic (A) and aerobic-plus-anaerobic (B) exercise. The acid-base consequence of the latter is an increase in cell lactic acid production. The buffering of the newly formed lactic acid takes place in the cell at the site of formation, predominantly by bicarbonate. The latter mechanism will increase the CO_2 production of the cell by approximately 22 ml per mEq of bicarbonate buffering of lactic acid. The increase in cell lactate and decrease in cell bicarbonate will result in chemical concentration gradients causing lactate to diffuse out of and bicarbonate to diffuse into the cell.

reflects the metabolic respiratory quotient (RQ) or $\dot{Q}CO_2/\dot{Q}O_2$ accurately *only* when there is a steady-state condition, i.e., CO_2 is not being added to or removed from the body CO_2 stores and the O_2 stores are constant, i.e., $\dot{Q}CO_2 = \dot{V}CO_2$ and $\dot{Q}O_2 = \dot{V}O_2$.

During acute hyperventilation (resulting, for example, from acute hypoxia, pain, anxiety, or of volitional origin), considerably more CO_2 is unloaded from the body CO_2 stores than O_2 is loaded into the O_2 stores. This is because hemoglobin is almost completely saturated with O_2 at the end of the pulmonary capillaries at sea level; in contrast, CO_2 can be unloaded in proportion to the increased ventilation and level of PCO_2. Thus, the gas exchange ratio, R, will exceed the metabolic RQ until a steady state is again attained at the new level of ventilation. Similarly, during the acute metabolic acidosis of exercise, "extra" CO_2 is evolved in the buffering of lactic acid (see Fig. 2-2). This, too, will result in R exceeding RQ until a new steady state is attained (CO_2 pool

size is again constant although depleted) and R again equals RQ. Differences between R and RQ will also occur with acute hypoventilation and during recovery from metabolic acidosis, but in the opposite direction.

When a steady state of gas exchange exists, R provides an accurate reflection of RQ. During exercise under these conditions, R is an index of the mixture of substrates used by the working muscles.

As seen in the following equations, carbohydrate (e.g., glucose) is oxidized with RQ = 1.0 (i.e., 6/6) and has a $\sim P{:}O_2 = 6.0$ (i.e., 36/6):

1) $C_6H_{12}O_6 + 6\,O_2 \rightarrow 6\,CO_2 + 6\,H_2O + 36\,ATP$

and lipid (e.g., palmitate) is oxidized with RQ = 0.71 (i.e., 16/23) and has a $\sim P{:}O_2 = 5.65$ (i.e., 130/23):

2) $C_{16}H_{32}O_2 + 23\,O_2 \rightarrow$
$$16\,CO_2 + 16\,H_2O + 130\,ATP$$

Intermediate steady-state RQ values reflect different proportions of carbohydrate and fat being utilized in the metabolic process (Fig. 2-3). For storage economy, fat is more efficient energy but for economy of O_2 utilization, carbohydrate is more efficient.

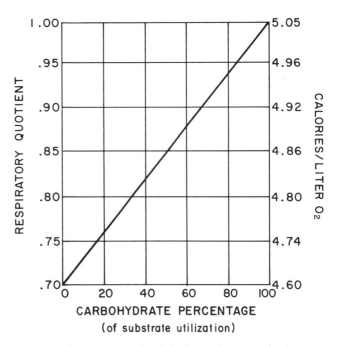

FIG. 2-3. The percentage of carbohydrate substrate in the diet estimated from the respiratory quotient measurement. The calories of energy obtained per liter of oxygen consumed for each combination is given on the right ordinate (See also p. 22) (Modified from Karpovich, P.V: The fuel for muscular work. *In* Physiology of Muscular Activity. Philadelphia, W.B. Saunders, 1982.)

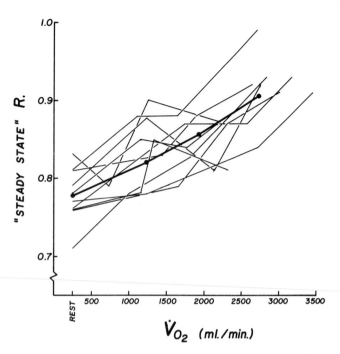

FIG. 2-4. The steady-state R (RQ) at various levels of exercise $\dot{V}_{O_2}$.

muscle glycogen becomes depleted, the exercising subject senses exhaustion.[10] Acute ingestion of glucose allows the work to continue.[11]

The rate of decrease in muscle glycogen during exercise can be slowed by raising blood glucose levels with a continued infusion of glucose.[12] The importance of muscle glycogen in work tolerance is well described by the experiments of Bergstrom et al.,[13] who demonstrated a high positive correlation between the tolerable duration of high intensity work and the muscle glycogen content before the exercise.

Physical fitness has been shown to affect the substrate utilization pattern by allowing a fitter subject to use a greater proportion of energy from fatty acids to perform a given level of work than an unfit one.[14] This glycogen-conserving consequence of fitness presumably allows more work to be performed before glycogen depletion and consequent exhaustion. The specific regulation of different substrates is considered below.

It is apparent from gas exchange measurements that a greater proportion of carbohydrate is used for energy during muscular work than at rest. During exercise, RQ increases from a resting value of approximately 0.8 (on an average "Western diet") toward 1.0, depending on the work rate (Fig. 2-4). While the fuel mixture derives proportionally more from carbohydrate than from lipid stores as work intensity increases, RQ decreases slowly over time during prolonged constant load exercise, reflecting reduction of the glycogen stores (Fig. 2-5). When

Carbohydrates

Skeletal muscle in man contains, on average, 80 to 100 mM (15 to 18 g) glucose per kilogram of wet weight stored as glycogen. For the "standard" 70 kg man, this amounts to approximately 400 g of muscle glycogen. Note that this represents an estimate of the total skeletal muscle pool, whereas a contracting muscle can draw only on its own glycogen reserves and not on the pools in noncontracting muscles.

Normally, there are 5 to 6 g of glucose available in the blood (100 mg/100 ml). Although muscle uptake of blood glucose increases considerably during exercise, the blood concentration does not fall ex-

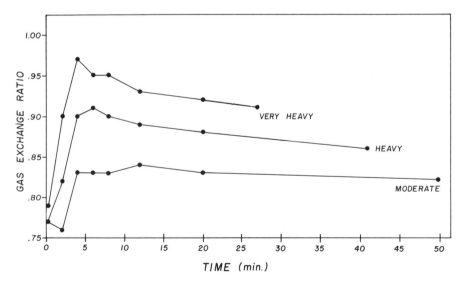

FIG. 2-5. Effect of exercise duration on the gas exchange ratio (R) for moderate, heavy, and very heavy work. Note that the gas exchange ratio declines with time after the initial increase, the latter being greater for the higher work intensity.

cept during prolonged work because of increased rate of glucose release from the liver.

The liver represents a highly labile source of some 50 to 90 g of reserve glycogen. This glycogen is broken down into glucose and released into the blood by glycogenolysis. Glucose can also be produced in the liver (gluconeogenesis) from lactate, pyruvate, glycerol, and alanine precursors when their concentrations are appropriately elevated. The rate of glucose release into the circulation depends upon both the blood glucose concentration and a complex interaction of hormones such as insulin, glucagon, and the catecholamines, epinephrine and norepinephrine.[15] As exercise intensity and duration increase the circulating levels of catecholamines and glucagon increase and insulin decreases. The increase in hepatic glucose production may serve to spare muscle glycogen[15] and thereby delay the onset of fatigue. Gluconeogenesis becomes more important with prolonged exercise, compensating for diminishing hepatic glycogen levels, thereby limiting the fall in blood glucose concentrations. These regulatory processes maintain physiologically adequate concentrations of glucose except when muscle and liver glycogen stores become greatly depleted.

Lipids

Skeletal muscles have access to their own intramuscular store of lipids, averaging 20 mg of triglycerides per g wet weight. This source has been shown to account for a considerable proportion of the total energy required by the muscles.

Extramuscular lipid sources are also utilized during exercise. These derive from adipose tissue where triglycerides undergo hydrolysis to glycerol and free fatty acids (mainly palmitic, stearic, oleic, and linoleic acids). The fatty acids are transported in the blood, bound predominantly to albumin. The store of extramuscular lipid is large. Even in the "standard" 70 kg man, fat accounts for approximately 15 kg of triglycerides, equivalent to 140,000 Kcal of energy.

The sympathetic nervous system and also catecholamines from the adrenal medulla regulate adipose tissue lipolysis. Epinephrine and norepinephrine increase the local concentration of cyclic 3',5'—AMP through activation of adenyl cyclase. This leads to increased rates of hydrolysis of the stored adipose tissue triglycerides. Other factors reduce the rate of adipose tissue lipolysis during exercise, including increased blood lactate and exogenous glucose loads.

The plasma free fatty acids account for only a small proportion (usually less than 5%) of the total plasma fatty acid pool; the remainder are triglycerides. Resting plasma free fatty acid concentrations are approximately 0.5 mM/L, rising during exercise to approximately 2 mM/L. The turnover rate of the plasma free fatty acid pool is high, with a half-time of 2 to 3 minutes at rest and less during exercise. As a consequence, the flux of free fatty acids to the exercising muscle (i.e., plasma flow × plasma FFA concentration) is an important determinant of skeletal muscle uptake.

The plasma concentration of free fatty acids does not increase, and may even decrease slightly, with physical training. Therefore, the increased proportional contribution of free fatty acid oxidation to exercise energetics, which is noted after training at a specific work rate, may reflect increased utilization from intramuscular sources. Adipose tissue lipolysis does not appear to be enhanced by training and may even be depressed.

Amino acid metabolism

There is a slow turnover of muscle protein in resting man as evidenced by the small net release of amino acids into the bloodstream. During exercise, the rate of release of intramuscular alanine increases appreciably but with little or no change in other amino acids.[16] The arterial concentration increases by as much as two-fold during severe exercise.[17] The source of the alanine released from muscle is predominantly from the transamination of pyruvate (derived from increased rates of carbohydrate metabolism), the amino groups provided largely by the branch-chain amino acids valine, leucine, and isoleucine.

A highly linear relationship exists between the plasma concentrations of alanine and pyruvate at rest and during exercise. A decreased muscle release of alanine is observed in phosphorylase-deficient muscle (McArdle's syndrome) associated with the decreased output of pyruvate.[18] The alanine formed by transamination in muscle is transported in the blood to the liver where it serves as a precursor for gluconeogenesis. Thus an alanine-glucose cycle is established between muscle and liver, with the carbon skeleton of alanine supporting hepatic glucose synthesis. The increased plasma alanine concentration is thought to provide a stimulus for increased glucagon secretion from the pancreatic cells,[19] further stimulating hepatic glucose output.

PATTERN OF BLOOD LACTATE INCREASE AND THE ANAEROBIC THRESHOLD

Exercise requires an increase in O_2 flow to the mitochondria of exercising muscles so that ATP needed

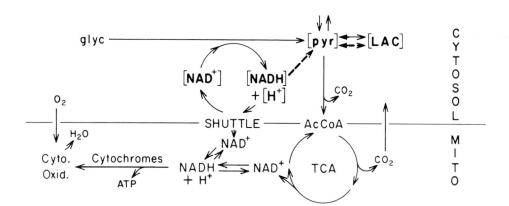

FIG. 2-6. Mechanisms (schematized) by which cell lactate can be increased. Lactate can increase due to accelerated glycolytic formation of pyruvate at a rate faster than mitochondrial utilization. This increase in lactate would be the result of mass action. Lactate can also increase as a consequence of pyruvate reoxidation of cytosolic [NADH + H+] as the latter increases in concentration. This mechanism buffers the rate of depletion of NAD+.

for muscle contraction can be generated. The muscles' O_2 flow must increase approximately 20× for walking, 40× for "jogging," and 60× or more for running. Since approximately 25% of the O_2 is ordinarily removed from the arterial blood by the muscle to support its resting metabolism, the increased O_2 requirement of exercise can only be met when blood flow to the active muscles is increased along with greater O_2 extraction. When the oxygen required by the exercising muscles cannot be totally supported by oxygen delivery, it may be necessary to supplement the aerobic oxidative mechanism with anaerobic mechanisms. This is accomplished by the conversion of pyruvate to lactate in the muscle cells, as described earlier.

Lactic acid is the predominant fixed acid produced during exercise. It has a pK of approximately 3.9 and therefore is essentially totally dissociated at the pH of the muscle cell (approximately 7.0). Because the [H+] associated with lactate production must react immediately with [HCO_3^-] within the cell, CO_2 production by the cell must increase at a rate commensurate with the [HCO_3^-] decrease (22 ml CO_2 for each mEq of bicarbonate buffering lactic acid) (see Fig. 2-2). The increase in cell lactate and decrease in cell [HCO_3^-] is quickly balanced by the transmembrane exchange of these ions, with [HCO_3^-] decreasing in the blood almost mEq for mEq with the increase in lactate concentration. The rapid efflux of CO_2 from the cell generated by the buffering reaction will be evident quickly in the lung gas exchange.

Lactate can accumulate in the blood during exercise if: 1) Glycolysis proceeds at a rate faster than pyruvate can be utilized by the mitochondria, or 2) reduced cytosolic nicotinamide adenine dinucleotide [NADH + H+] cannot be reoxidized rapidly enough by the mitochondrial membrane proton shuttle (Fig. 2-6). The first mechanism is a mass action effect, dependent on pyruvate increase. This results in a quantitatively minor and barely evident lactate in-

crease, at mild and moderate work rates.[20] The second mechanism depends on the change in the cell redox state in response to the rising concentration of [NADH + H+]. The major increase in lactate accumulation typically starts at a work rate ($\dot{V}O_2$) of about 50% of the normal subject's maximum (Fig. 2-7). It is not accompanied by a comparable rise in pyruvate (Fig. 2-8); therefore, this rise in lactate is associated with an increase in lactate/pyruvate ratio. The production of lactate from pyruvate allows reoxidation of cytosolic [NADH + H+], even in a relatively oxygen-deficient state.

The work rate at which lactic acid and the lactate/pyruvate ratio increase is usually distinct in a particular subject and occurs at a consistent $\dot{V}O_2$ for a given form of work. This $\dot{V}O_2$ threshold, above which the anaerobic mechanisms supplement the aerobic ones, has been termed the anaerobic threshold (AT).[21]

The conceptual basis for the anaerobic threshold is: 1) The O_2 required by the metabolically active

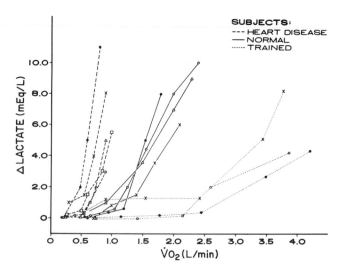

FIG. 2-7. Lactate concentration in arterial blood as related to oxygen consumption for trained normal subjects, normal sedentary subjects, and patients with primary heart disease (From Wasserman, K., and Whipp, B.J.: Exercise physiology in health and disease. Am. Rev. Resp. Dis., *112*:219–249, 1975.)

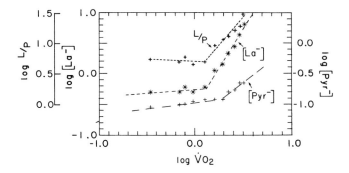

FIG. 2-8. Log lactate [La⁻], log pyruvate [Pyr⁻], and log lactate/pyruvate (L/P) ratio plotted against log $\dot{V}_{O_2}$. The log-log transform of the lactate-$\dot{V}_{O_2}$ and pyruvate-$\dot{V}_{O_2}$ relationships allows easy detection of the lactate and pyruvate inflection points. The pyruvate inflection point generally is at a higher $\dot{V}_{O_2}$ than the lactate inflection point. Because the prethreshold pyruvate slope is the same as (or slightly steeper than) the lactate slope, the L/P ratio does not increase until the lactate inflection point. (*From* Wasserman, K., Beaver, W. L., Davis, J. A., Pu, J-Z, Heber, D., and Whipp, B. J.: Lactate, pyruvate, and lactate-to-pyruvate ratio during exercise and recovery. J. Appl. Physiol., *59*:935-940, 1985.)

muscles can exceed the O_2 supply to the mitochondria when the work rate is sufficiently high; 2) the imbalance between the O_2 supply and O_2 requirement causes the proton scavenging mitochondrial membrane shuttle to lose pace with the rate of [NADH + H⁺] production in the cytosol, resulting in a more-reduced cytosol redox state; 3) pyruvate reacts with the increased [NADH + H⁺], and is reduced to lactate while regenerating NAD⁺ and allowing glycolysis to continue; 4) the new lactic acid formed is buffered in the cell primarily by [HCO₃⁻] (see Fig. 2-2), generating additional CO_2; while 5) [HCO₃⁻] exchanges for lactate across the muscle cell membrane, causing blood HCO₃⁻ to decrease as lactate increases (Fig. 2-9); and 6) the buffering and acid-base disturbances produce predictable changes in gas exchange (Fig. 2-10).

Important functional adaptations affecting mitochondrial O_2 supply occur when cell acidity is increased. These include: 1) vasodilatation in the vascular bed of the muscle in which lactate production is increased, and 2) a shift of the oxyhemoglobin dissociation curve to the right in the more acidic capillary bed thereby allowing O_2 to unload more readily from hemoglobin and O_2 extraction to increase. Both mechanisms act locally to compensate for the O_2 availability-requirement imbalance and partially correct the reduced redox state. They will be discussed again within the context of O_2 supply (see Metabolic-Cardiovascular-Ventilatory Coupling, Oxygen Supply section, p. 15, in this chapter).

Subjects with a high degree of endurance fitness typically do not have increased blood lactate levels until $\dot{V}_{O_2}$ is quite high (> 10× resting $\dot{V}_{O_2}$) (see Fig.

2-7). In contrast, in sedentary individuals, lactate often starts to increase at work rates generally just exceeding the $\dot{V}_{O_2}$ required for ordinary paced walking (approximately 4× rest). Patients with heart disease, classified as Class III by New York Heart Association criteria, have increased lactate levels with minimal activity ($\dot{V}_{O_2}$ < 2× rest).

While lactate production benefits the subject by allowing him to perform at work rates greater than those for which the cardiovascular system is ordinarily capable of supplying the total oxidative need, it has disturbing effects on breathing in two ways: 1) the CO_2 produced from the buffering of lactic acid by bicarbonate provides an additional CO_2 load to the respiratory system that must be eliminated in order to prevent arterial P_{CO_2} from rising, and 2) the increased hydrogen ion concentration caused by arterial bicarbonate decrease stimulates the carotid bodies, predominantly, to increase ventilatory drive; this reduces arterial P_{CO_2} and provides respiratory compensation for the metabolic acidosis.[22] With an incremental exercise test, it is possible to use these effects of lactate production on gas exchange to identify, noninvasively, the $\dot{V}_{O_2}$ at which arterial lactate starts to increase.

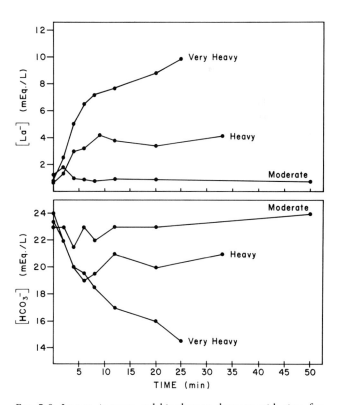

FIG. 2-9. Lactate increase and bicarbonate decrease with time for moderate, heavy, and very heavy work intensities for a normal subject. Bicarbonate changes in opposite direction to lactate and in a quantitatively similar manner. While the target work duration was 50 minutes for each work rate, the endurance time was reduced for the heavy and very heavy work rates.

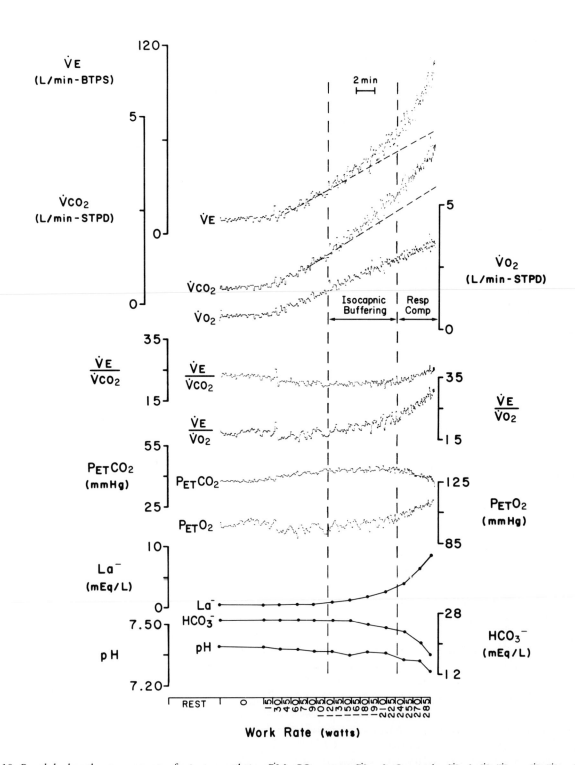

FIG. 2-10. Breath-by-breath measurements of minute ventilation ($\dot{V}E$), CO_2 output ($\dot{V}CO_2$), O_2 uptake ($\dot{V}O_2$), $\dot{V}E/\dot{V}CO_2$, $\dot{V}E/\dot{V}O_2$, $P_{ET_{CO_2}}$, $P_{ET_{O_2}}$, arterial lactate and bicarbonate, and pH for a one-minute incremental work test on a cycle ergometer. The *AT* occurs when lactate increases. This is accompanied by a fall in HCO_3^- and generally an increase in $\dot{V}E/\dot{V}O_2$. "Isocapnic buffering" refers to the period when $\dot{V}E$ and $\dot{V}CO_2$ increase curvilinearly at the same rate without an increase in $\dot{V}E/\dot{V}CO_2$, thus retaining a constant $P_{ET_{CO_2}}$. After the period of isocapnic buffering, $P_{ET_{CO_2}}$ decreases, reflecting respiratory compensation for the metabolic acidosis of exercise.

TABLE 2-1. *Effect of the anaerobic threshold (AT) on exercise responses*

MEASUREMENT	BELOW *AT*	ABOVE *AT*
Exercise duration	Prolonged; limited by muscular and skeletal trauma or substrate	Reduced; limited by "fatigue" or dyspnea
$\dot{V}O_2$ time to steady-state	<3 min	>3 min; steady-state may not occur
$\dot{V}E$, $\dot{V}CO_2$ time to steady-state	<4 min	>4 min; steady-state may not occur
pH	approx. 7.4	metabolic acidosis
$Paco_2$	constant	decreasing

Figure 2-10 shows the effect of an increasing work rate on ventilation and gas exchange for a cycle ergometer exercise test in which the work rate was incremented at one-minute intervals, after a 4-minute warm-up period of pedalling without load. As the work rate is increased, $\dot{V}O_2$, $\dot{V}CO_2$, and $\dot{V}E$ rapidly enter a region in which they increase linearly until the *AT* is reached. At work rates above the *AT*, CO_2 output increases more rapidly than O_2 uptake because CO_2 generated by the bicarbonate buffering of lactic acid is added to the metabolic CO_2 production. Initially, $\dot{V}E$ increases proportionally with the increased CO_2 output (isocapnic buffering). Thus, $\dot{V}E$ retains a constant relationship to $\dot{V}CO_2$ ($\dot{V}E/\dot{V}CO_2$ appears constant or decreases slightly) while it increases relative to $\dot{V}O_2$ ($\dot{V}E/\dot{V}O_2$ increases) just above the *AT* (see Fig. 2-10). As the work rate is incremented further, $\dot{V}E$ starts to increase even more rapidly than CO_2 output, causing Pa_{CO_2} and PET_{CO_2} to decrease and thereby provides respiratory compensation for the exercise-induced lactic acidosis. As seen in Figure 2-10, the metabolic acidosis contributes a major additional ventilatory drive (the nonlinear component of the $\dot{V}E$ increase).

Table 2-1 contrasts the exercise responses for work above and below the *AT*. We believe the *AT* to be the best determinant available to demarcate the upper limit of work rate which can be endured for a prolonged period. Thus, a task performed below the *AT* can be sustained. A task performed above the *AT* cannot be sustained as long; the higher the work rate above the *AT*, the less is its tolerable duration (Fig. 2-11).

We use a classification of work intensity based on the lactate elevation engendered by the work rate, similar to that described by Wells et al.[23] Mild and moderate work intensities are below the anaerobic threshold, i.e., there is no sustained increase in lac-

tate (see Fig. 2-9); heavy and higher intensities are above the anaerobic threshold. For heavy exercise, blood lactate is elevated but can reach a constant level. Work rates at which the blood lactate continues to climb are considered very heavy or severe, and lead to rapid exhaustion.

Metabolic-Cardiovascular-Ventilatory Coupling

During exercise, muscle bioenergetics are stressed while both the cardiovascular and the pulmonary systems respond to support the increased gas exchange requirements. Therefore, transfer of CO_2 and O_2

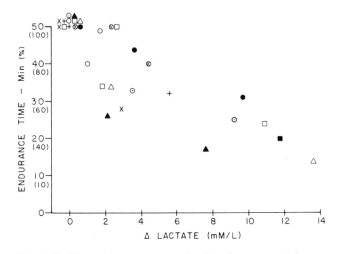

FIG. 2-11. The endurance time as related to the increase in lactate (above the pre-exercise resting value) during the last minute of constant work rate cycle ergometer exercise. Data are from thirty experiments on ten male subjects studied at three work rates, each for a target time of 50 minutes. Endurance is reduced when lactate is increased (From Wasserman, K.: The anaerobic threshold measurement to evaluate exercise performance. Am. Rev. Respir. Dis. (Suppl.), *129*:S35–S40, 1984.)

between the mitochondria and the air requires a finely coordinated interaction of cardiovascular and respiratory mechanisms geared to cellular metabolic activity.

A scheme describing the gas transport mechanisms for coupling cellular (internal) to pulmonary (external) respiration is shown in Figure 1-1. When exercise is initiated, high-energy bonds of pre-existing ATP split to support the immediate energy requirements of muscle contraction. ATP is rapidly regenerated by utilization of creatine phosphate stores. However, as creatine phosphate bond energy is depleted, increasing creatine and inorganic phosphate stimulate oxidation of substrates replenishing muscle ATP.[24] The mitochondrial P_{O_2} decreases consequent to the increased utilization of O_2, providing the necessary diffusion gradient for enhanced O_2 flow from capillaries to mitochondria.

The large increase in muscle O_2 requirements during exercise demands that O_2 flow to the muscle increases, to sustain muscular contractions. The simultaneously increased muscle CO_2 production requires its removal to avoid tissue acidosis which can have adverse effects on cellular function. To accomplish the increased rates of gas exchange needed for exercise, an efficient coupling of cardiovascular and respiratory mechanisms involved in gas transport is required to accommodate the increased cellular respiration.

In response to the increased extraction of O_2 from and addition of CO_2 to the capillary blood by the muscles, muscular blood flow increases. The initial vasodilatation appears to be centrally induced. Subsequent dilatation is predominantly under local humoral control, enabling blood flow to increase to the muscle units having the highest metabolic activity.[25]

Cardiac output is increased at the start of exercise by increasing stroke volume and heart rate. For a given work rate, stroke volume appears to increase to its maximal value almost immediately. This is accomplished by a combination of increased cardiac inotropy and increased venous return secondary to external compression of veins by contracting muscles, leading to right ventricular pressure increase. As exercise continues, further increases in cardiac output at a given work rate are accomplished almost exclusively by increasing heart rate.

In concert with the increase in right ventricular output and pulmonary artery pressure, the pulmonary vascular bed dilates. This dilatation results in the perfusion of previously unperfused lung units and increased perfusion to those lung units underperfused at rest. A lowering of pulmonary vascular resistance is essential for the normal exercise response of the left ventricle since, without it, the weakly muscled right ventricle could not readily pump the increased venous return through the lungs to the left atrium to effect a normal cardiac output increase.

The CO_2 added to the blood by the tissues reaches the lungs in the form of an increased pulmonary blood flow and CO_2 content and must be eliminated by the lungs to achieve arterial blood gas and pH homeostasis. Minute ventilation ($\dot{V}_E$) normally increases at a rate required to remove the added CO_2. In fact, the $\dot{V}_E$ increase is generally so precise that arterial P_{CO_2} and pH are usually regulated at close-to-resting values throughout moderate exercise levels. Above the *AT*, a metabolic acidosis occurs that further increases ventilation. The ventilatory increase is usually accomplished at low and moderate work rates primarily by an increase in tidal volume and, to a lesser degree, breathing frequency. The latter increases more significantly at work rates above the *AT*.

OXYGEN COST OF WORK

The oxygen cost of performing work depends on the work rate. Figure 2-12 shows the time course of oxygen uptake ($\dot{V}_{O_2}$) for various levels of cycle ergometer exercise in a normal individual. Note that a steady-state is reached by 3 minutes at moderate intensity work rates. At heavy and very heavy intensity work rates, $\dot{V}_{O_2}$ continues to increase beyond the initial 3 minutes.

The upward drift in $\dot{V}_{O_2}$ observed after 3 minutes during constant work rate exercise is only seen for work rates above the anaerobic threshold.[26,27] The rate of rise is greater the higher the work rate above

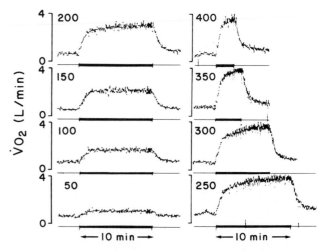

FIG. 2-12. Oxygen uptake related to time for eight levels of constant work rate cycle ergometer exercise, starting from unloaded cycling. The work rate (watts) for each study is shown in the respective panel. The bar on the X-axis indicates the period of the imposed work rate. The $\dot{V}_{O_2}$ asymptote (steady-state) is significantly delayed for work above the anaerobic threshold. (From Whipp, B. J. and Mahler, M.: Dynamics of pulmonary gas exchange dynamics. In Pulmonary Gas Exchange. New York, Academic Press, 1980)

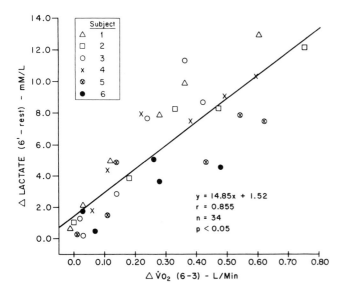

FIG. 2-13. Increase in blood lactate (above resting value) as related to the increase in oxygen consumption between 3 and 6 minutes of constant work rate exercise in six subjects. Normally, $\dot{V}O_2$ does not increase after 3 minutes when the work is performed below the anaerobic threshold ($\Delta\dot{V}O_2(6-3) = 0$). While the drift in $\dot{V}O_2$ after 3 minutes and the lactate increase are correlative, they are not necessarily causative. (From Roston, W.L., Whipp, B.J., Davis, J.A., Effros, R.M., and Wasserman, K.: Oxygen uptake kinetics and lactate concentration during exercise in man (to be published).

the anaerobic threshold.[8] The increase in $\dot{V}O_2$ between 3 and 6 minutes of constant work rate exercise has been shown to correlate well with the increase in arterial lactate (Fig. 2-13).

The rise in $\dot{V}O_2$ after 3 minutes is probably due to at least three mechanisms: 1) progressive vasodilation to the local muscle units by metabolic vasodilators produced in response to relative O_2 lack, e.g., $[H^+]$, thereby increasing O_2 flow to the deficient site; 2) acidemia shifting the oxyhemoglobin dissociation curve to the right thereby facilitating O_2 unloading from hemoglobin; and 3) the O_2 cost of conversion of lactate to glycogen in the liver, and possibly muscle, as the lactate concentration rises. Other mechanisms, such as increased catecholamine levels, increased body temperature at high work rates, and high ventilatory rates, could also add to the O_2 cost of above *AT* work rates.

If the steady-state $\dot{V}O_2$ is measured for a range of moderate work rates on the cycle ergometer, such as shown for 50, 100, and 150 watts in Figure 2-12, a linear relationship between $\dot{V}O_2$ and work rate is obtained (Fig. 2-14). The slope of this relationship is approximately the same for all normal people (approximately 10.1 ml/watt). This means that work efficiency in man is relatively fixed for a given work task (see Work Efficiency section in this chapter). However, while the slope of the $\dot{V}O_2$-work rate relationship is not affected by training, age, or gender,

the position of the relationship depends upon body weight. Obese subjects exhibit an upward displacement of approximately 5.8 ml/min/kg body weight.[28] On the cycle ergometer, this reflects the added work of moving heavier limbs. The effect of body weight on $\dot{V}O_2$ would be more pronounced on the treadmill since more work must be done to move the entire body.

OXYGEN SUPPLY

The oxygen supply to the cells with increased metabolic activity is dependent upon five factors: 1) the partial pressure of O_2 in the arterial blood 2) the hemoglobin concentration and arterial O_2 content; 3) the cardiac output; 4) the distribution of perfusion to the tissues in need of O_2; and 5) the hemoglobin's affinity for O_2. All affect the diffusion gradient of O_2 from the blood to the muscle mitochondria. These factors will each be discussed separately.

Arterial PO2

Mean arterial PO_2 (Pa_{O_2}) is a function of mean alveolar PO_2 (PA_{O_2}). For an idealized lung (all lung units having the same ventilation/perfusion ratio) where the gas exchange ratio is 0.8 and Pa_{CO_2} is equal to 40, PA_{O_2} would equal approximately 100 at sea level. Reductions in Pa_{O_2} relative to the ideal PA_{O_2} are due to one or more of the following mechanisms: 1) a

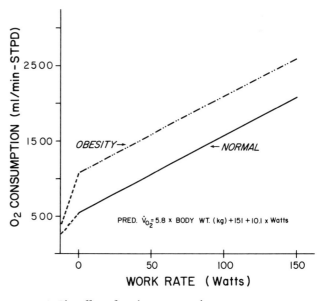

FIG. 2-14. The effect of work rate on steady-state oxygen consumption during cycle ergometer work. The oxygen consumption response in normal subjects is quite predictable for cycle ergometer work regardless of age, gender, or training. The predicting equation is given in the figure. The oxygen requirement to perform work by obese subjects is displaced upward, the displacement dependent on body weight. (From Wasserman, K.: Dyspnea on Exertion. JAMA, *248*:2039-2043, 1982.

right to left shunt; 2) O_2 diffusion disequilibrium at the alveolar-capillary interface; or 3) maldistribution of alveolar ventilation ($\dot{V}A$) with respect to lung perfusion ($\dot{Q}$). Normally, Pa_{O_2} is about 90 mm Hg and the $P(A-a)_{O_2}$ is approximately 10 mm Hg. This is because of a small physiological right-to-left shunt (primarily the Thebesian blood vessels in the heart and the bronchial circulation) and the lack of uniformity of $\dot{V}A/\dot{Q}$ within the lung.

Hemoglobin and Arterial O_2 Content

The arterial O_2 content depends on the arterial P_{O_2} and hemoglobin concentration. Thus anemia, resulting in a decreased blood O_2 content, can compromise the supply of O_2 to the tissues during exercise. Any hemoglobin that is inactive (methemoglobin) or has carbon monoxide on the O_2-binding sites (as in cigarette smokers) will also result in a reduction in O_2 content. Note that under normal sea level conditions ventilatory increases do not significantly elevate the O_2 content. In normal subjects at sea level, only relatively large decreases in ventilation, which cannot be sustained, appreciably reduce O_2 content.

Cardiac Output

The cardiac output obviously must play a key role in the O_2 supply to the cells. At the start of exercise in the upright posture, stroke volume increases rapidly, the magnitude being dependent upon the relative degree of the individual's fitness, age, and size. In the exceptionally fit young person, the stroke volume can increase by as much as 100%; whereas, the increase is much smaller in the less fit elderly person. Further increases in cardiac output come about predominantly by increasing heart rate, i.e., heart rate usually increases linearly with $\dot{V}_{O_2}$. Thus as the stroke volume does not change after its initial increase or changes by only a small amount, the pattern of change of cardiac output between work rates can be inferred from the pattern of changing heart rate. The wide variation of absolute stroke volume between subjects of different fitness levels, however, precludes estimations of the magnitude of the cardiac output change from heart rate measurements.

Distribution of Peripheral Blood Flow

During exercise, the fraction of the cardiac output diverted to the skeletal muscles increases, while the fraction perfusing organs such as the kidney, liver, and gastrointestinal tract decreases. There is an increased O_2 extraction from and addition of CO_2 to the capillary blood of exercising muscle (decreased P_{O_2} and increased P_{CO_2}). As the work rate is in-

creased, the perfusion of the exercising muscles increases further, allowing a still larger fraction of the cardiac output to go to the exercising muscles. This redistribution in perfusion is apparently accomplished by responses to both autonomic nervous system changes as well as by local tissue metabolic factors such as increased $[H^+]$, P_{CO_2}, $[K^+]$, osmolarity, adenosine, temperature, and reduced P_{O_2}.

A useful noninvasive measurement for monitoring perfusion redistribution and increased O_2 extraction resulting in the widening of arterial-mixed venous O_2 content difference ($C(a - \bar{v})O_2$) is the $\dot{V}_{O_2}$/heart rate ratio (O_2 pulse). The O_2 pulse, calculated by dividing $\dot{V}_{O_2}$ by heart rate (HR) (both noninvasive measurements) is equal to the product of stroke volume and arterial-mixed venous O_2 difference (SV $\times$ $C(a - \bar{v})O_2$ as shown below):

$$\text{cardiac output} = \dot{V}_{O_2}/C(a - \bar{v})O_2$$

If HR $\times$ SV is substituted for cardiac output in the above equation, then:

$$HR \times SV = \dot{V}_{O_2}/C(a - \bar{v})O_2$$

or, rearranging:

$$\dot{V}_{O_2}/HR = SV \times C(a - \bar{v})O_2$$

The O_2 pulse is the amount of O_2 removed from each stroke volume. When both stroke volume and the arterial-venous O_2 difference reach their maxima, the O_2 pulse will reach its maximum.

Hemoglobin Affinity for O_2

Altered hemoglobin affinity for O_2, seen with abnormal hemoglobins or with altered acid-base balance, has little effect on arterial blood O_2 content in the patient with normal lungs at sea level. However, the position of the steep part of the oxyhemoglobin dissociation curve, commonly quantified by the P_{O_2} at which the O_2 saturation of hemoglobin is 50% (P_{50}), affects the P_{O_2} for a given oxyhemoglobin saturation in the tissue capillaries. A shift of the oxyhemoglobin dissociation curve to the left (low P_{50}) can impair O_2 extraction by the exercising muscle, whereas a shift to the right (high P_{50}) allows O_2 to unload from hemoglobin more readily. Thus a rightward shift resulting from acidosis, increased temperature, or high levels of 2,3-diphosphoglycerate (2,3-DPG) favors diffusion of O_2 from the capillaries into the mitochondria. This contrasts with the leftward shift resulting from alkalosis, carbon monoxide poisoning, or low 2,3-DPG concentration, where the O_2 diffusion gradient is reduced.

CARBON DIOXIDE CLEARANCE

Like O_2 consumption, CO_2 production increases during exercise because of increasing metabolic activity in the exercising muscles. The amount of CO_2 generated by this process is related to O_2 consumption by the RQ. Additional CO_2 is derived from bicarbonate buffering of lactic acid at high work rates.

In contrast to tissue oxygen supply, the actual cardiac output needed for CO_2 elimination is not critical. Rather, the quantity of ventilation relative to the $\dot{V}CO_2$ determines arterial PCO_2. The tissue PCO_2 is defined by the arterial PCO_2, blood flow, and metabolic activity.

DETERMINANTS OF THE VENTILATORY REQUIREMENT

The quantity of ventilation required to clear a given amount of CO_2 from the blood ($\dot{V}CO_2$) depends on the CO_2 concentration in the alveolar gas ($FA_{CO_2} = PA_{CO_2}/PB$), where PA_{CO_2} is the ideal alveolar PCO_2 — essentially equal to the arterial PCO_2 (Pa_{CO_2}) — and PB is the barometric pressure. Mass balance considerations dictate that, in an idealized lung (where gas concentrations are the same in all alveolar spaces because of uniform $\dot{V}A/\dot{Q}$), $\dot{V}CO_2 = \dot{V}A \times Pa_{CO_2}/PB$. Thus $\dot{V}A$ represents the theoretical alveolar ventilation required for maximally efficient lungs to regulate Pa_{CO_2} at a given input of $\dot{V}CO_2$. This important relationship is plotted in Figure 2-15.

Not all respired air effectively ventilates the lung since some must go to the conducting airways unin-

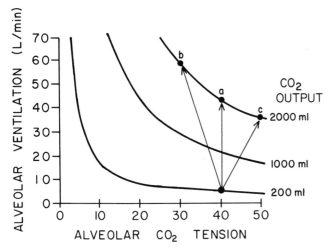

FIG. 2-15. Effect of changing arterial (ideal alveolar) PCO_2 during exercise on alveolar ventilation. The point on the CO_2 output isopleth of 200 ml/min represents the normal resting value. Points a, b, and c illustrate the alveolar ventilation for isocapnia and hypocapnia (−10 mm Hg), and hypercapnia (+10 mm Hg) for an exercise CO_2 output of 2000 ml/min. (From Wasserman, K.: Breathing during exercise. N. Engl. J. Med., *298*:780–785, 1978.

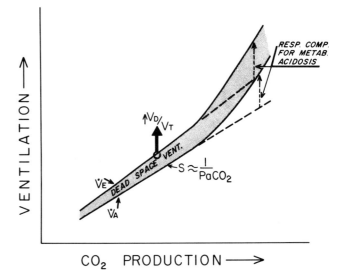

FIG. 2-16. Factors that determine alveolar and minute ventilation during exercise ($\dot{V}A$ and $\dot{V}E$, respectively). VD/VT is the physiological dead space/tidal volume ratio and "S" is the slope. (See "Determinants of the ventilatory requirement" for interpretation of this figure.) (Modified from Wasserman, K.: Breathing during exercise. N. Engl. J. Med., *298*:780–785, 1978.)

volved in gas exchange and to the nonperfused alveoli. The wasted fraction of the tidal volume from the point of view of gas exchange (VD/VT) determines the difference between the actual volume of air respired during breathing ($\dot{V}E$) and the theoretical alveolar ventilation, i.e., $\dot{V}A = \dot{V}E (1 - VD/VT)$. To determine the $\dot{V}E$ needed to eliminate a given quantity or CO_2, substitute $\dot{V}E (1 - VD/VT)$ for $\dot{V}A$ in the alveolar ventilation equation given in the preceding paragraph. The resulting equation is:

$$\dot{V}E \ (BTPS) = \frac{863 \ \dot{V}CO_2 \ (STPD)}{Pa_{CO_2} \ (1 - VD/VT)}$$

where 863 is the product of the barometric pressure, temperature, and water vapor correction factors needed to express $\dot{V}E$ at BTPS and Pa_{CO_2} in mm Hg. From this equation it is evident that the quantity of breathing required for exercise is defined by three factors: 1) the $\dot{V}CO_2$; 2) the level at which Pa_{CO_2} is regulated by the respiratory control mechanisms; and 3) the physiological dead space/tidal volume ratio. The influences of these three factors on $\dot{V}E$ are illustrated in Figure 2-16. At work rates above the *AT*, $\dot{V}E$ and $\dot{V}A$ increase nonlinearly and progress more steeply as $\dot{V}CO_2$ increases because of the added ventilatory drive caused by metabolic acidosis.

CONTROL OF BREATHING

Despite a manifold increase in CO_2 production and O_2 utilization during exercise, the ventilatory control mechanisms normally keep arterial P_{CO_2} and $[H^+]$ remarkably constant over a wide range of metabolic rates.

Ventilation appears to be coupled to CO_2 exchange during exercise. If $\dot{V}_E$ did not increase in appropriate proportion to the increased rate of CO_2 production, a respiratory acidosis with associated disturbances in cellular function would result. Likewise, if ventilation increases proportionally more than the rate of CO_2 production, respiratory alkalosis would result and this would also impair cellular function and O_2 unloading in the muscles. However, exercise usually is an isocapnic, isohydric, hypermetabolic state for moderate work intensities (Fig. 2-17). A metabolic acidosis is normally present only for heavy, or higher, work intensities, due to increased blood lactate accumulation (see Figs. 2-2, 2-7, 2-8, 2-9, and 2-10). Respiratory acidosis is present only in patients

with abnormal respiratory mechanics or impaired chemoreceptor function or in normal subjects breathing through an apparatus that imparts a high resistive load. In contrast, respiratory alkalosis does not typically develop during exercise in normal subjects and is rarely seen in pathophysiological states.

The $\dot{V}_E$, $\dot{V}_{O_2}$, or $\dot{V}_{CO_2}$ responses following the onset of constant work rate exercise can be characterized by three time phases, as evidenced by the experimental data in Figure 2-18, the mechanisms of which are schematized in Figure 2-19: Phase I) the

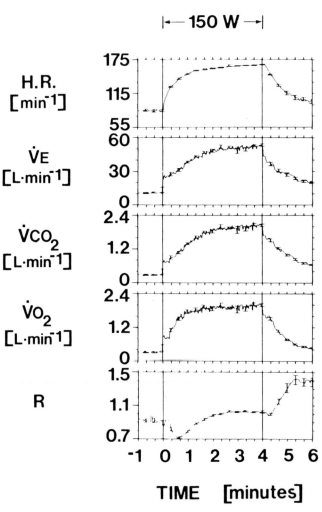

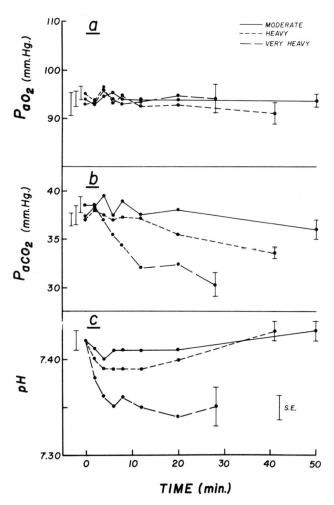

Fig. 2-17. Effect of prolonged constant work rate exercise of moderate, heavy, and very heavy work intensity on arterial blood gases and pH. Each point is the average of ten subjects. (From Wasserman, K., VanKessel, A.L., and Burton, G.G.: Interaction of physiological mechanisms during exercise. J. Appl. Physiol., 22:71–85, 1967.)

Fig. 2-18. Changes in ventilation and gas exchange during constant cycle ergometer work rate exercise starting from rest ("0" time) and ending at four minutes in a normal subject. This study is the average of six similar repetitions in which gas exchange was measured breath-by-breath. The vertical bars are the standard errors of the data. The abrupt increase in $\dot{V}_E$, $\dot{V}_{CO_2}$, and $\dot{V}_{O_2}$ at the start of exercise is termed Phase I and thought to be related, mechanistically, to the abrupt increase in cardiac output at the start of exercise. R is usually unchanged from rest for about 15 sec. The start of Phase II is signalled by a decrease in R and is the period of exponential-like increase in $\dot{V}_E$, $\dot{V}_{CO_2}$, and $\dot{V}_{O_2}$ to its asymptote (Phase III). This is the period when cellular respiration is reflected in lung gas exchange. R decreases transiently during Phase II because $\dot{V}_{O_2}$ increases faster than $\dot{V}_{CO_2}$ due to gas solubility differences in tissues.

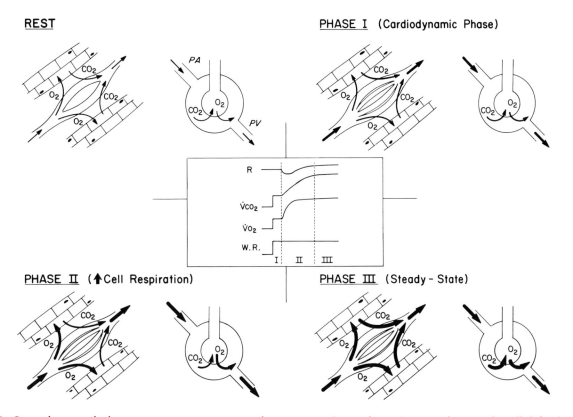

FIG. 2-19. Gas exchange at the lungs in response to constant work rate exercise (center diagram). Gas exchange at the cell (left side of each quadrant) couples to cardiorespiratory gas exchange (right side of each quadrant) through cardiovascular adjustments in the lungs and tissues. Phase I gas exchange is postulated to be caused by the immediate increase in cardiac output (pulmonary blood flow) at the start of exercise (cardiodynamic gas exchange). Phase II gas exchange reflects the decreased O_2 content and increased CO_2 content of the venous blood secondary to increased cell respiration as well as a further increase in cardiac output. (See text for explanation of decrease in R during Phase II). Eventually a steady-state is reached between internal and external respiration (Phase III). PA = pulmonary artery, PV = pulmonary vein, W.R. = work rate. (From Wasserman, K.: Coupling of external to internal respiration. Am. Rev. Respir. Dis. (Suppl.), 129:S21–S24, 1984.)

immediate increase at the start of exercise lasting about 15 seconds during which R generally does not change; Phase II) the subsequent slower increase to steady-state lasting 2 to 3 minutes during which R changes biphasically, initially decreasing and then increasing to the steady-state or asymptotic value; and Phase III) the steady state level if below the AT, or slow drift phase if above the AT. Phase III starts at approximately 3 minutes for $\dot{V}O_2$, and 4 minutes for $\dot{V}CO_2$ and $\dot{V}E$ (Phase II kinetics are slower for $\dot{V}E$ and $\dot{V}CO_2$ than for $\dot{V}O_2$).

The magnitude of the Phase I $\dot{V}E$ response varies somewhat from individual to individual. However, high work rates generally result in only small further increases in Phase I over that observed for the lightest loads. Consequently, for a mild work rate, the increase in $\dot{V}E$ during Phase I is a larger *fraction* of the total ventilatory response than that for a heavy work rate (Fig. 2-20). The ventilatory pattern increase after Phase I is greatly influenced by the work rate in relation to the AT (Fig. 2-21). If the work rate is below the AT, the $\dot{V}E$, f, and VT reach a steady-state

generally by 4 to 5 minutes. In contrast, at work rates above the AT, $\dot{V}E$ and f continue to drift upward and PET_{CO_2} drifts downward until the subject fatigues or achieves a delayed steady-state.

Despite intensive research, there is no general agreement on the mechanisms of respiratory control during exercise. The observation that arterial pH, P_{CO_2}, and P_{O_2} are essentially unchanged during exercise of moderate work intensity (see Fig. 2-17) has been difficult to explain mechanistically. Repeated efforts to discover chemoreceptors in locations where potential stimuli are available (e.g., pulmonary circulation or exercising limbs), possibly explaining the exercise hyperpnea, have been largely unsuccessful. The only receptors clearly demonstrated to play a role in the hyperpnea of exercise are the carotid bodies.

The following is a brief review of the mechanisms proposed to have a role in exercise hyperpnea. See the reviews by Whipp[29] and Wasserman, Whipp, and Casaburi[30] for a more detailed discussion of this subject.

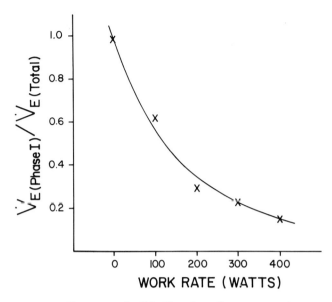

FIG. 2-20. The magnitude of the Phase I ventilatory response to exercise (from rest) as related to steady-state ventilation for various work rates. The higher the work rate, the smaller the fraction of the total ventilatory response attributable to Phase I.

Corticogenic or Conditioned Reflexes

Anxiety might account for part of the rapid ventilatory increase at the start of exercise (Phase I) in some subjects. Krogh and Lindhard[31] suggested that the rapid $\dot{V}E$ increase at the start of exercise might origi-

nate from the cerebral cortex as a conditioned reflex. Recently, Eldridge et al.[32] and DiMarco et al.[33] obtained evidence from studies in cats suggesting that the ventilatory stimulus might involve hypothalamic mediation. However, the patterns of ventilatory and gas exchange responses in man suggest that the sustained ventilatory response is metabolically coupled and that the initial ventilatory response might be linked to the increase in cardiac output.[34,35]

Respiratory Center and Central Medullary Chemoreceptors

The respiratory center includes collections of neurons in the brain stem which discharge rhythmically to stimulate motor neurons to the respiratory muscles. Medullary lesions associated with tumors, primary hypoventilation syndromes, or central respiratory depression associated with hypoxia-inducing pulmonary diseases can cause the respiratory pacemaker mechanisms to depend upon peripheral chemoreceptor input for providing a controlled rhythmic output. Evidence that these pacemaker mechanisms may lose the required rhythmic discharge properties is the apnea produced by O_2 administration in some hypoxic patients.

Although the medullary chemoreceptors are clearly important for ventilatory control at rest, their role in exercise hyperpnea is unclear. Though these

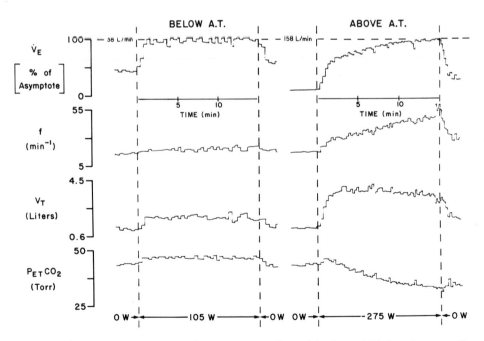

FIG. 2-21. Minute ventilation ($\dot{V}E$) plotted as percentage of its asymptotic value, tidal volume (V_T), breathing rate (f), and end tidal P_{CO_2} (PET_{CO_2}) for work below and above the anaerobic threshold in the same subject. The absolute values of minute ventilation are shown to the left of the vertical dash line at the transition from unloaded cycling (O W) to the indicated work rate. For the work rate below the anaerobic threshold $\dot{V}E$, f, V_T, and PET_{CO_2} reach a constant value after several minutes. For the work rate above the anaerobic threshold, $\dot{V}E$ and f continue to drift upwards and PET_{CO_2} downwards (without a significant change or slight decrease in V_T) signifying the lack of ventilatory steady-state.

chemoreceptors respond to changes in pH and possibly molecular CO_2, cerebrospinal fluid hypercapnia and acidosis do not occur during exercise. Also, the central chemoreceptors do not appear to respond to the acute exercise-induced metabolic acidosis.[22]

In patients with primary alveolar hypoventilation syndrome (patients with hypercapnia and a corresponding degree of hypoxemia with normal respiratory function who have a markedly diminished or absent ventilatory response to hypercapnia), the ventilatory response to exercise is diminished not only because they have rest and exercise hypercapnia (high CO_2 set-point), but also because their arterial P_{CO_2} increases further with exercise (e.g., by 10 mm Hg) (see Fig. 2-15). However, it is difficult to know if this occurs secondary to the central insensitivity to CO_2 or if it is due to a failure of the respiratory center to integrate effectively the afferent stimuli to give an appropriate output.

Carotid Bodies

Much has been learned about the role of carotid bodies during muscular exercise from studies on selected asthmatic patients who had both carotid bodies resected, but whose baroreceptors were left intact.[36] The ventilatory response to exercise was studied in these subjects when they: 1) were asymptomatic; 2) had normal, or near normal, respiratory function; and 3) had normal exercise tolerance. They manifested three major differences from normal subjects in their ventilatory responses to exercise:

1. The subjects without carotid bodies did not increase their ventilatory drive in response to hypoxia[37] nor did they decrease their ventilatory drive in response to hyperoxia.[38]
2. They failed to develop respiratory compensation for the metabolic acidosis[22] and consequently evidenced a greater acidemia during high intensity exercise.
3. Their ventilatory increase during exercise was slow causing a transient hypercapnia during Phase II. Demonstration that carotid bodies have an important role in Phase II ventilatory kinetics in normal subjects has also been demonstrated by Oren et al.[39]

Thus there is good evidence that the carotid bodies have an important role in the normal ventilatory response to exercise.

Aortic Bodies

The aortic bodies seem to be unimportant as ventilatory chemoreceptors in man, in contrast to some other animal species (cats and dogs). Removal of the carotid bodies alone has been shown to eliminate the ventilatory response to hypoxia and the acute metabolic acidosis of exercise.[37]

Vagal Reflexes

The lungs are richly innervated by branches of the vagus nerve. While investigators have postulated that the vagus nerve might contribute importantly to exercise hyperpnea, studies on the ventilatory response to exercise in awake dogs by Phillipson et al.[40] showed that vagal blockade, induced by bilateral cooling of the cervical vagus nerves, did not change the ventilatory response to exercise, although the breathing pattern was altered. The authors concluded that the vagus nerves were not important in the overall ventilatory response to exercise at the work levels studied (up to $4 \times$ resting $\dot{V}O_2$), in dogs.

Mechanoreceptors in Extremities

To explain the exercise hyperpnea, it had been widely assumed that proprioceptors or muscle spindles in the exercising muscle must play a major role in the genesis of exercise hyperpnea.[41] The principal argument in favor of an appreciable role for the neural afferents from exercising muscles stems from the observation of a rapid increase in $\dot{V}E$ at the start of exercise (Phase I), in advance of the arrival of the products of exercise metabolism in the central circulation.

Some neurophysiological studies have helped clarify the possible role of afferents from the exercising limb in exercise hyperpnea. Studies in which the transmission of stimuli from proprioceptors were interrupted[42] demonstrate that these receptors must play only a small role, if any. Both Hornbein et al.[43] and Hodgson and Mathews,[44] using different approaches to stimulate the muscle spindles, demonstrated no significant role for these organs in exercise hyperpnea. Only by interfering with the transmission of impulses from the unmyelinated or small-myelinated neurons, which are indistinguishable from the type that carry the sensation of pain, can the hyperpnea associated with muscle stimulation in anesthetized experimental animals be markedly attenuated.[45] But even if ventilatory stimuli originating in the exercising muscles are active during exercise, the respiratory center is not stimulated with enough intensity by these signals to override the mechanisms that regulate Pa_{CO_2} and arterial pH.

Cardiodynamic Hyperpnea

An alternative explanation of the rapid onset of Phase I hyperpnea to that of mechanoreceptors in the extremities is an abrupt increase in cardiac output at the start of exercise. This increase would deliver increased quantities of blood to receptor sites downstream from the pulmonary capillaries, resulting in an increased P_{CO_2} and $[H^+]$, and decreased P_{O_2} at these sites. These changes could provide a feedback stimulus to ventilation in less than the circulation time between the muscles and arterial chemoreceptors.[35] An alternate cardiac-linked explanation of an increase in $\dot{V}E$ to account for Phase I would be the stimulation of pressure sensitive receptors in the pulmonary artery, right ventricle, or right atrium which are known to be capable of stimulating ventilation (feed-forward).[46]

The reason for linking the Phase I increase in $\dot{V}E$ to the abrupt increase in cardiac output rather than involving nonmetabolic neurogenic mechanisms is that two unlinked neurogenic mechanisms, one for blood flow and one for ventilation, would unlikely produce the isocapnic hyperpnea usually observed from the start through the steady-state of moderate exercise.

Oxygen Uptake Kinetics, Oxygen Deficit, and Oxygen Debt

During exercise, oxygen uptake from the lungs ($\dot{V}O_2$) reflects the oxygen consumed by the cells, excluding that transiently available from: 1) Oxygen in the O_2 stores (oxyhemoglobin of the venous blood, physically dissolved O_2, and possibly oxymyoglobin in the muscles); 2) the O_2 equivalents of high energy compounds (creatine-phosphate) already formed and stored in the muscles; and 3) any pyruvate conversion to lactate reflected by an increase in lactate concentration. At the onset of moderate work, oxygen uptake from the lungs normally increases abruptly (50 to 100% resting $\dot{V}O_2$) and remains relatively unchanged for the first 15 seconds (Phase I). Then the $\dot{V}O_2$ increases as a single exponential with a time constant of approximately 30 seconds (Phase II) (see Fig. 2-18).

The terms O_2 deficit and O_2 debt describe characteristics of the O_2 uptake pattern for constant work rate exercise. The difference between the total oxygen uptake and the product of the steady-state oxygen uptake and the exercise duration is referred to as the oxygen deficit. The total oxygen uptake in excess of the resting oxygen uptake during the recovery period is the oxygen debt. Once the steady-state is reached, the oxygen debt no longer increases, regardless of the exercise duration.[47] However, if the work intensity is very heavy for a normal subject, or if the subject is so impaired that his cardiorespiratory system cannot supply the total oxygen need, a steady-state is not achieved and lactate continues to increase until the subject is forced to stop exercise because of fatigue or breathlessness (see Fig. 2-9). A steady-state in $\dot{V}O_2$ is achieved only when all of the cellular energy requirements are obtained by reactions using oxygen transferred from the atmosphere. As long as the oxygen uptake fails to reach a steady-state for constant work rate exercise, the oxygen deficit and debt continue to enlarge. For work levels at which a steady-state can be achieved, the size of the O_2 debt approximates that of the O_2 deficit.[48]

Work Efficiency

The reason that the steady-state $\dot{V}O_2$ measurement and cycle ergometer work rate are commonly used interchangeably when describing the level of exercise being performed is because work efficiency (caloric equivalent of the measured work ÷ caloric equivalent of the oxygen consumption for the measured work) varies little from one individual to another.[49] Trained and untrained individuals, whether old or young, male or female, all have similar work efficiencies reflecting the basic biochemical energy yielding reactions to achieve muscle contraction. However, care must be taken not to confuse changes in skill or motor efficiency with practice in the assessment of work efficiency. To evaluate work efficiency, relatively simple tasks must be employed which do not depend on technique, e.g., cycling.

To calculate work efficiency, the caloric equivalent of the *steady-state* $\dot{V}O_2$ (4.86 Cal/L $\dot{V}O_2$ at RQ = 0.85, see Fig. 2-3) and the external work (.014 Cal/min/watt) for at least two *measured* work rates must be known. The work efficiency is the increase in the caloric equivalent of the external work divided by the caloric equivalent of the O_2 used, expressed as a percentage. This is best measured during cycle exercise since the amount of external work can be accurately estimated with this form of ergometry. Normal subjects have an efficiency of approximately 30% for lower extremity cycle work.[28,50]

Dietary Substrate and the Physiological Responses to Exercise

O_2 Consumption

Slightly more high-energy phosphate compounds are generated per molecule of O_2 utilized, when carbohydrate is the substrate instead of fat (~$P:O_2$ = 6.0 and 5.65, respectively). Consequently, steady-state $\dot{V}O_2$ should be slightly less for a given work rate when carbohydrate is the predominant substrate. The $\dot{V}O_2$ required to perform cycle ergometer work after being on a high carbohydrate diet for three days as compared to a high fat diet for a similar duration is shown in Figure 2-22. The $\dot{V}O_2$ is demonstrated to be less when the work task is performed with carbohydrate as the dominant substrate as compared to fat.

Heart Rate

As previously described, cardiac output increases linearly with $\dot{V}O_2$. Since $\dot{V}O_2$ is less when carbohydrate is the dominant substrate, cardiac output might also be less. This is indeed reflected consistently in a slightly lower heart rate when carbohydrate is the predominant substrate as compared to fat (see Fig. 2-22).

Carbon Dioxide Production

While $\dot{V}O_2$ and heart rate are less at a given work rate with carbohydrate as the predominant substrate, $\dot{V}CO_2$ is less with fat as the predominant substrate.[51,52] This may be predicted on the basis of the lower RQ for fat than for carbohydrate.

Minute Ventilation

$\dot{V}E$ has been shown to be less for a given work rate task with a predominant fat substrate, consistent with the hypothesis that the ventilatory control mechanisms appear to cause $\dot{V}E$ to change in proportion to CO_2 flow.[53] When $\dot{V}E$ is plotted against $\dot{V}CO_2$, the relationship is the same whether carbohydrate or fat is the predominant substrate. Thus, when $\dot{V}E$ is plotted against $\dot{V}CO_2$ for a normal population, the individual responses are very consistent (Fig. 2-23). However, when $\dot{V}E$ is plotted against $\dot{V}O_2$ for the same subjects, there is less consistency in the responses. The greater dispersion with $\dot{V}O_2$ as the independent variable is caused by RQ differences amongst the subjects with the high RQ subjects having the steeper $\dot{V}E$-$\dot{V}O_2$ slope.

Interactive Effects of Altered Substrate Utilization

While the O_2 and cardiovascular costs at a given work rate are somewhat less with carbohydrate (more efficient) than with fat as the dominant component of the utilized substrate mixture (see Fig. 2-22), carbohydrate is much less "efficient" with respect to CO_2 production, as shown in Table 2-2. There is a considerable increase in CO_2 generated per high energy phosphate ($\sim$P). Consequently, as ventilation is coupled to CO_2 exchange during exercise

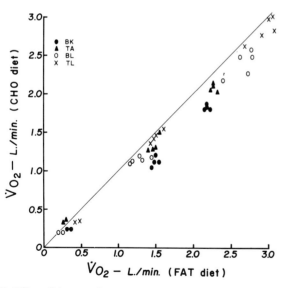

EFFECT OF DIET ON O_2 CONSUMPTION DURING EXERCISE

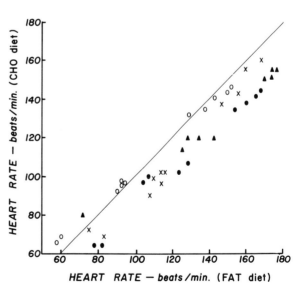

EFFECT OF DIET ON HEART RATE DURING EXERCISE

FIG. 2-22. Effect of dietary substrate on oxygen consumption and heart rate during exercise. Studies were done on four subjects at rest and two levels of work after three days on high carbohydrate diet (RQ at rest = .97) and three days on high fat diet (RQ at rest = .75). It can be seen that the oxygen consumption is higher on the high fat diet than on the high carbohydrate diet during the performance of a given work rate. This is consistent with the biochemical evidence that the high energy phosphate yield from carbohydrate is greater than that from fat for a given O_2 cost. Heart rate during exercise is also shown to be higher on the high fat diet as compared to the high carbohydrate diet reflecting the link between oxygen consumption and cardiac output.

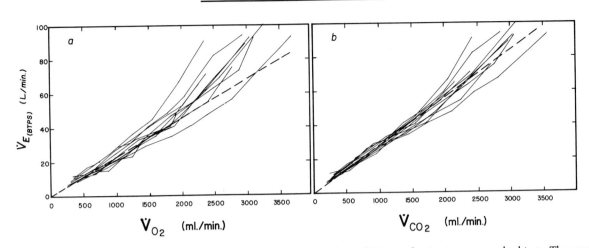

Fig. 2-23. Relationship between steady state minute ventilation and oxygen uptake, and CO_2 production in ten normal subjects. The curvilinear increase in ventilation at high metabolic rates reflects respiratory compensation for the metabolic acidosis. The reduced dispersion noted in the correlation between $\dot{V}_E$ and $\dot{V}_{CO_2}$, as compared to $\dot{V}_E$ and $\dot{V}_{O_2}$, reflects the functional dependence of ventilation on CO_2 flow to the lungs and the effect of differences in RQ amongst the subjects. (From Wasserman, K., VanKessel, A.L., and Burton, G.G.: Interaction of physiological mechanisms during exercise. J. Appl. Physiol., *22*:71–85, 1967.)

and not O_2 uptake, carbohydrate use results in an appreciably greater $\dot{V}_E$ as compared to fat ($\simeq 30\%$ at the extremes of RQ) for a given work rate.

Thus, the substrate mix for energy generation can have important implications for work tolerance. While the O_2 cost and cardiovascular stress are slightly less when the RQ is high, the CO_2 load and ventilatory stress are increased. These substrate considerations are likely to be of importance in patients with limited cardiovascular or ventilatory function, the former benefiting from a high carbohydrate and the latter benefiting from a high fat diet.

Summary

Gas exchange during exercise should be considered from the standpoint of cellular respiration and how cardiovascular and ventilatory mechanisms are coupled to it. Not only does the magnitude of cellular respiration affect external respiration but, importantly, the work rate above the subject's *AT* has a major influence on $\dot{V}_E$. Work above the *AT* causes increased CO_2 and $[H^+]$ production, both having powerful effects on the ventilatory response to exercise. Also, the gas exchange kinetics are altered and exercise endurance is reduced above the *AT*.

The physiological responses to exercise are summarized in Figure 1-1. Approximately 30% of the calories generated during work are transformed into useful external work, while the remaining 70% are lost primarily as heat. The oxidative energy obtained from oxygen creditors (hemoglobin, myoglobin, creatine-PO_4, and pyruvate conversion to lactate) varies with the work rate. At moderate work rates, however, the pyruvate-to-lactate mechanism contributes a very small fraction of the credit, while for very heavy work rates, the pyruvate-lactate mechanism accounts for upwards of 80% of the total O_2 deficit.[20]

The peripheral blood flow distribution appears to depend on work rate and local humoral factors while the cardiac output and heart rate response are dependent upon oxygen consumption. The regional dispersion of ventilation-perfusion ratios in the lungs tends toward being optimized by local control and mechanical factors, while ventilation is determined by the rate of CO_2 production, the physiological

TABLE 2-2. *Effect of different substrates on energetics and carbon dioxide production.*

Substrate	~P:O_2	O_2: ~ P	%Δ*	RQ	CO_2: ~ P	%Δ*
Glucose	6.0	0.167	−5	1.0	0.167	+35
F.F.A.	5.65	0.177		0.71	0.124	

*With respect to free fatty acid (F.F.A.)

dead space ventilation, and the level at which arterial P_{CO_2} is regulated.

Breath-by-breath gas exchange measurements demonstrate that $\dot{V}_{O_2}$, $\dot{V}_{CO_2}$, and $\dot{V}_E$ abruptly increase at the start of exercise (Phase I); this increase appears to respond in relatively precise proportion to the change in cardiac output and may actually result from this change (cardiodynamic). During Phase II, $\dot{V}_{O_2}$, $\dot{V}_{CO_2}$, and $\dot{V}_E$ rise exponentially to a steady-state or an asymptote. Their kinetics are influenced by cellular metabolism and the O_2 and CO_2 storage capacities in tissues. During Phase II and III, $\dot{V}_E$ follows closely the changing rate of CO_2 delivery to the lungs rather than the actual CO_2 produced or the O_2 consumed. Of the various possible control mechanisms for the hyperpnea of muscular exercise, signals dependent on CO_2 flux to the lungs and arterial $[H^+]$ appear to dominate.

References

1. Saltin, B., and Gollnick, P.D.: Skeletal muscle adaptability: significance for metabolism and performance. *In* Handbook of Physiology, Section 10, Skeletal Muscle. Edited by L.D. Peachey. Bethesda, American Physiological Society, 1983, p. 555.
2. Gibbs, C.L., and Gibson, W.R.: Energy production of rat soleus muscle. Am. J. Physiol., *223*:874–881, 1972.
3. Henricksson, J., and Reitman, J.S.: Quantitative measures of enzyme activities in type I and type II muscle fibres of man after training. Acta Physiol. Scand., *97*:392–397, 1976.
4. Buller, A., Eccles, J., and Eccles, R.: Differentiation of fast and slow muscles in the cat hind limb. J. Physiol., *150*:399–416, 1960.
5. Karlsson, J.: Introduction: Basics in human skeletal muscles metabolism. Int. J. Sports Med., *2*:1–5, 1982.
6. Essen, B.: Intramuscular substrate utilization. Ann. NY Acad. Sci., *301*:30–44, 1977.
7. Lehninger, A.L.: Biochemistry. New York, Worth Publishers, 1971, p. 407.
8. Wasserman, K.: The anaerobic threshold measurement to evaluate exercise performance. Am. Rev. Respir. Dis. (Suppl.), *129*:S35–S40, 1984.
9. Lundin, G., and Strom, G.: The concentration of blood lactic acid in man during muscular work in relation to the partial pressure of oxygen of the inspired air. Acta Physiol. Scand., *13*:253–266, 1947.
10. Rosell, S., and Saltin, B.: Energy need, delivery, and utilization in muscular exercise. *In* The Structure and Function of Muscle. Vol.3. Edited by G.H. Bourne. New York, Academic Press, 1973.
11. Simonsen, E.: Depletion of energy yielding substances. *In* Physiology of Work Capacity and Fatigue. Edited by E. Simonsen. Springfield, Charles C. Thomas, 1971.
12. Ahlborg, B., Bergstrom, J., Ekelund, L.G., and Hultman, E.: Muscle glycogen and muscle electrolytes during pro-

longed physical exercise. Acta Physiol. Scand., *70*:129–142, 1967.
13. Bergstrom, J., Hermansen, L., Hultman, E., and Saltin, B., Diet, muscle glycogen and physical performance. Acta Physiol. Scand., *71*:140–150, 1967.
14. Jones, N.L.: Exercise testing in pulmonary evaluation: rationale, methods, and the normal respiratory response to exercise. N. Engl. J. Med., *293*:541–544, 1975.
15. Wasserman, D.H., Lickley, L.A., and Vranic, M.: Interactions between glucagon and other counter-regulatory hormones during normoglycemic and hypoglycemic exercise in dogs. J. Clin. Invest., *74*:1404–1413, 1984.
16. Pozefsky, T., Felig, P., and Tobin, J.D.: Amino acid balance across tissues of the forearm in postabsorptive man. Effects of insulin at two dose levels. J. Clin. Invest., *48*:2273–2282, 1969.
17. Wahren, J.: Substrate utilization by exercising muscle in man. *In* Progress in Cardiology. Vol. 2. Edited by P.N. Yu and J.F. Goodwin. Philadelphia, Lea & Febiger, pp. 255–280, 1973.
18. Wahren, J., Felig, P., Havel, R.J., Jorfeldt, L., Pernow, B., Saltin, B.: Amino acid metabolism in McArdle's syndrome. N. Engl. J. Med., *288*:774–777, 1973.
19. Arsan, R., Rosselin, G., and Dolais, J.: Effects sur la glucagonomie des perfusians et ingestions d'acides animes. J. Ann. Diabet. Hotel Dieu, *7*:25–31, 1967.
20. Wasserman, K., VanKessel, A.L., and Burton, G.G.: Interaction of physiological mechanisms during exercise. J. Appl. Physiol., *22*:71–85, 1967.
21. Wasserman, K., Whipp, B.J., Koyal, S.N., and Beaver, W.L. Anaerobic threshold and respiratory gas exchange during exercise. J. Appl. Physiol., *35*:236–243, 1973.
22. Wasserman, K., Whipp, B.J., Koyal, S.N., and Cleary, M.G.: Effect of carotid body resection on ventilatory and acid-base control during exercise. J. Appl. Physiol., *39*:354–358, 1975.
23. Wells, J.G., Balke, B., and Van Fossan, B.D.: Lactic acid accumulation during work. A suggested standardization of work classification. J. Appl. Physiol., *10*:51–55, 1957.
24. Chance, B., Mauriello, G., and Aubert, X.M.: ADP arrival at muscle mitochondria following a twitch. *In* Muscle as a Tissue. Edited by K. Rodahl and S.M. Horvath. New York, McGraw-Hill, 1962.
25. Guyton, A.C., Jones, C.E., and Coleman, T.G.: Cardiac output in muscular exercise. *In* Circulatory Physiology: Cardiac Output and its Regulation, Ch. 25. Philadelphia, W.B. Saunders Co., 1973.
26. Whipp, B.J., and Mahler, M.: Dynamics of pulmonary gas exchange during exercise. *In* Pulmonary Gas Exchange. Vol. 2. Edited by J.B. West. New York, Academic Press, 1980, pp. 33–96.
27. Whipp, B.J., and Wasserman, K.: Oxygen uptake kinetics for various intensities of constant load work. J. Appl. Physiol., *33*:351–356, 1972.
28. Wasserman, K., and Whipp, B.J.: Exercise physiology in health and disease. Am. Rev. Respir. Dis., *112*:219–249, 1975.
29. Whipp, B.J.: The control of exercise hyperpnea. *In* The Regulation of Breathing. Edited by T. Hornbein. New York, Marcel Dekker, Inc., 1981.
30. Wasserman, K., Whipp, B.J., and Casaburi, R.: Respiratory control during exercise. *In* Handbook of Physiology,

Vol. 2. Edited by N.S. Cherniack and J.G. Widdicombe. Bethesda, American Physiological Society, 1986, pp. 595–619.

31. Krogh, A., and Lindhard, J.: The regulation of respiration and circulation during the initial stages of muscular work. J. Physiol. (Lond.), *47*:112–136, 1913.

32. Eldridge, F.L., Millhorn, D.E., and Waldrop, T.G.: Exercise hyperpnea and locomotion: parallel activation from the hypothalamus. Science, 211:844–846, 1981.

33. DiMarco, A.F., Romaniuk, J.R., von Euler, C., and Yamamoto, Y.: Immediate changes in ventilation and respiratory pattern associated with onset and cessation of locomotion in the cat. J. Appl. Physiol. *343*:1–16, 1983.

34. Weiler-Ravell, D., Cooper, D. M., Whipp, B. J., and Wasserman, K.: Control of breathing at the start of exercise as influenced by posture. J. Appl. Physiol., *55*: 1460–1466, 1983.

35. Wasserman, K., Whipp, B.J., and Castagna, J.: Cardiodynamic hyperpnea: hyperpnea secondary to cardiac output increase. J. Appl. Physiol., *36*:457–464, 1974.

36. Wasserman, K., and Whipp, B.J.: The carotid bodies and respiratory control in man. *In* Morphology and Mechanisms of Chemoreceptors. Edited by A.S. Paintal. Delhi, Vallabhbhai Patel Chest Institute, 1976.

37. Lugliani, R., Whipp, B.J., Seard, C., and Wasserman, K.: Effects of bilateral carotid body resection on ventilatory control at rest and during exercise in man. N. Engl. J. Med., *285*:1105–1111, 1971.

38. Whipp, B.J., and Wasserman, K.: Carotid bodies and ventilatory control dynamics in man. Fed. Proc., *39*:1628–1673, 1980.

39. Oren, A., Whipp, B.J., and Wasserman, K.: Effect of acid-base status on the kinetics of the ventilatory response to moderate exercise. J. Appl. Physiol. *52*:1013–1017, 1982.

40. Phillipson, E.A., Hickey, R.F., Bainton, C.R., and Nadel, J.A.: Effect of vagal blockade on regulation of breathing in conscious dogs. J. Appl. Physiol., *29*:475–479, 1970.

41. Dejours, P.: Control of respiration in muscular exercise. *In* Handbook of Physiology. Section 3, Vol. 1 Edited by W.O. Fenn and H. Rahn. Washington, D.C., American Physiological Society, 1964, pp. 631–638.

42. Kao, F.F.: An experimental study of the pathways involved in exercise hyperpnea employing cross-circulation techniques. *In* The Regulation of Human Respiration. Edited by D.J.C. Cunningham and B.B. Lloyd. Oxford, Blackwell Scientific Publications, 1961.

43. Hornbein, T.F., Sorenson, S.C., Parks, C.R.: Role of muscle spindles in lower extremities in breathing during bicycle exercise. J. Appl. Physiol., *27*:476–479, 1969.

44. Hodgson, H.J.F., and Mathews, P.B.C.: The ineffectiveness of excitation of the primary endings of the muscle spindle by vibration as a respiratory stimulant in the decerebrate cat. J. Physiol. (Lond.), *194*:555–563, 1968.

45. McCloskey, D.I., and Mitchell, J.H.: Reflex cardiovascular and respiratory responses originating in exercising muscle. J. Physiol. (Lond.), *224*:173–186, 1972.

46. Jones, P. W., Huszczuk, A., and Wasserman, K.: Cardiac output as a controller of ventilation through changes in right ventricular load. J. Appl. Physiol., *53*:218–224, 1982.

47. Schneider, E.G., Robinson, S., and Newton, J.L.: Oxygen debt in aerobic work. J. Appl. Physiol., *25*:58–62, 1968.

48. Whipp, B.J., Seard, C., and Wasserman, K.: Oxygen deficit-oxygen debt relationships and efficiency of anaerobic work. J. Appl. Physiol., *28*:452–456, 1970.

49. Astrand, P.O., and Rodahl, K.: Textbook of Work Physiology. 2nd Ed. New York, McGraw-Hill, 1977, pp. 393–411.

50. Whipp, B.J., and Wasserman, K.: Efficiency of muscular work. J. Appl. Physiol., *26*:644–648, 1969.

51. Christensen, E.H., and Hansen, O.: Arbeitsfahigkeit und Ernahrung. Scand. Arch. Physiol., *81*:152–159, 1939.

52. Simonsen, E.: Depletion of energy yielding substances. *In* Physiology of Work Capacity and Fatigue. Edited by E. Simonsen. Springfield, Charles C. Thomas, 1971.

53. Brown, S.E. Wiener, S., Brown, R.A., Maratelli, P.A., and Light, R.W.: Exercise performance following a carbohydrate load in chronic airflow obstruction. J. Appl. Physiol., *58*:1340–1346, 1985.

Measurement of the Physiological Response to Exercise

CHAPTER 3

E XERCISE TESTING enables the simultaneous evaluation of the cardiovascular and respiratory systems' ability to perform their major function, i.e., gas exchange. This chapter describes relatively simple measurements that can be used in the exercise laboratory to assess the physiological responses to exercise. These measurements and the functions that they assess are summarized in Table 3-1. Fortunately, most are noninvasive and can be readily obtained with equipment generally available in most cardiorespiratory laboratories. Detailed descriptions of how these measurements are made can be found in the Appendix if they are not provided here.

Exercise Testing — Incremental

Measurements during incremental exercise testing are useful because they enable the examiner to: 1) titrate the level of the subject's exercise limitation, 2) titrate the adequacy of the performance of various components in the external-internal gas exchange coupling, and 3) determine the organ system limiting exercise performance. All of these are best achieved during short nonsteady-state rather than prolonged steady-state exercise tests.

THE ELECTROCARDIOGRAM (ECG)

The ECG is a valuable measure of the balance between myocardial O_2 availability and O_2 requirement for cardiac work. When the heart muscle contracts without adequate oxygen (ischemia), the muscle cells alter their ionic permeability and the rate of reestablishing the normal ion gradients across the myocardial cell membrane after cardiac systole slows.[1] Consequently, reestablishing the electrical membrane potential during repolarization is slowed

TABLE 3-1. *Assessing Function With Physiological Measurements*

MEASUREMENT	FUNCTION
Electrocardiogram	Myocardial O_2 availability $-$ O_2 requirement balance
$\dot{V}O_2$	Cardiac output $\times$ (arterial-mixed venous O_2 content)
Maximum $\dot{V}O_2$	Highest $\dot{V}O_2$ achieved during presumed maximal effort for an incremental exercise test (specific for type of work)—may or may not equal $\dot{V}O_2$ max.
$\dot{V}O_2$ max	Highest $\dot{V}O_2$ achievable as evidenced by failure of $\dot{V}O_2$ to increase despite increasing work rate (specific for type of work)
$(\Delta\dot{V}O_2/\Delta WR)$ during incremental exercise	Aerobic contribution to exercise (low value suggests high anaerobic contribution)
$\dot{V}O_2$ difference = Expected $\dot{V}O_2$ for maximum WR $-$ maximum $\dot{V}O_2$	O_2 utilization below expected (inability to utilize O_2 normally) or above expected (exceptionally fit for the work task) at the maximum work rate performed by the subject
Cardiac output	Useful when related to vascular pressure or metabolic rate
Anaerobic Threshold (AT)	Highest $\dot{V}O_2$ that can be sustained without developing a metabolic acidosis; important determinant of potential for endurance work (specific for form of work)
O_2 pulse $(\dot{V}O_2/HR) = SV \times C(a - \bar{v}) O_2$	Product of SV and arterial-mixed venous O_2 content difference; under conditions when SV is constant, then O_2 pulse is proportional to $C(a - \bar{v})O_2$
HRR = predicted maximum HR $-$ maximum exercise HR	Heart rate reserve at maximum exercise
Arterial pressure	Detecting systemic hypertension, ventricular outflow obstruction, or myocardial failure (pulsus alternans or decreasing pressure with increasing WR)
$\dot{V}E = \dot{V}A + \dot{V}D$	$\dot{V}D$ is increased at specific work rate due to mismatching of $\dot{V}A$ and $\dot{Q}$. $\dot{V}A$ is increased inversely with decrease in Pa_{CO_2} whether caused by a low CO_2 setpoint, metabolic acidosis, or hypoxemia.
BR = MVV $-$ $\dot{V}E$ at maximum exercise or (MVV $-$ $\dot{V}E$ at maximum exercise)/MVV	Breathing reserve; theoretical additional $\dot{V}E$ available at cessation of exercise
Exercise VD/VT	Measure of mismatching of ventilation and perfusion
$P(a - ET)CO_2$	Detects high $\dot{V}A/\dot{Q}$ components of lung with mismatching of $\dot{V}A/\dot{Q}$
$P(A-a)O_2$	Detects low $\dot{V}A/\dot{Q}$ components of lung with mismatching of $\dot{V}A/\dot{Q}$, diffusion defect, or right to left shunt
Expired flow pattern	Useful for indicating presence of significant airflow obstruction
VT/IC	High with restricted lung expansion
$\dot{V}O_2$ (Phase I) at constant WR	Ability to increase pulmonary blood flow at start of exercise
$\Delta\dot{V}O_2(6 - 3)$	Relationship of steady-state WR to AT
Abrupt change in $\dot{V}E$ and f during hyperoxic (100% O_2) switch	Contribution of the carotid body to ventilatory drive

Abbreviations:

WR = work rate
HR = heart rate
SV = Stroke volume
$C(a - \bar{v}) O_2$ = arterial-mixed venous O_2 content difference
HRR = heart rate reserve
$\dot{V}D$ = physiological dead space ventilation per minute
$\dot{V}A$ = alveolar ventilation per minute

$\dot{V}E$ = minute ventilation
VD = physiological dead space
BR = breathing reserve
MVV = maximal voluntary ventilation
VT = tidal volume
IC = inspiratory capacity
$\Delta\dot{V}O_2(6 - 3)$ = difference between $\dot{V}O_2$ at 6 min and 3 min during constant work rate exercise

in the ischemic areas. This causes the T wave and ST segments to change acutely when the O_2 requirement for the increased cardiac work of exercise exceeds its availability (Table 3-2). An increased frequency of ectopic beats as the work rate increases should also be considered pathologic and suggestive of myocardial ischemia. Some patients, however, manifest occasional premature ventricular or atrial contractions at rest which disappear or become less frequent during exercise. We regard these ectopic

TABLE 3-2. *Electrocardiographic Evidence of Myocardial Ische-mia During Exercise (12 lead)*

ST segment depression
T wave changes
PVC's that appear during exercise

beats as benign and unrelated to a disturbance in the myocardial O_2 availability-requirement balance, as they are overridden by the sinus tachycardia of exercise.

Because exercise causes the heart rate to increase and the diastolic period to decrease, the time for coronary perfusion is decreased. Thus, coronary artery disease is more likely to be detected while exercising rather than during the resting state. However, there are many instances of false positive and borderline changes in the ECG when relying solely on changes in the T wave and ST segments. But when these ECG changes are accompanied by chest pain, a decline in arterial pressure, or a flattening of the $\dot{V}O_2$-work rate relationship, the diagnosis of ischemic heart disease is more certain.

MAXIMAL OXYGEN UPTAKE ($\dot{V}O_2$ MAX) AND MAXIMUM OXYGEN UPTAKE

The body clearly has an upper limit for O_2 utilization at a particular state of fitness or training. This is determined both by the pumping limit of the heart and the potential for O_2 extraction by the exercising tissue, or by having reached the ventilatory limit. Maximal aerobic power (i.e., maximal $\dot{V}O_2$ or $\dot{V}O_2$ max) was originally defined as the $\dot{V}O_2$ at which perform-ance of increasing levels of supramaximal work failed to further increase $\dot{V}O_2$,[2] as illustrated in Figure 3-1*A* and shown experimentally in Figure 2-12. This upper limit in $\dot{V}O_2$ may also be determined by incremental testing, which demonstrates a plateau of $\dot{V}O_2$ despite further increases in the work rate. Thus the maximal $\dot{V}O_2$ represents the highest $\dot{V}O_2$ attainable for a given form of exercise as evidenced by a failure for $\dot{V}O_2$ to increase normally as the work rate is increased. This is contrasted with the maximum $\dot{V}O_2$, which is simply the highest $\dot{V}O_2$ achieved in a given, presumed maximal effort, exercise test. The distinction is diagrammed in Figure 3-1*B*.

Thus the maximum $\dot{V}O_2$ may not equal $\dot{V}O_2$ max. In most normal subjects, however, incremental testing with the legs produces a maximum $\dot{V}O_2$ that closely approximates the predicted $\dot{V}O_2$ max,[3] even when a plateau is not evident. However, if during an incremental test a subject stops exercising because of leg or chest pain, shortness of breath, mechanical limitation to breathing, or lack of motivation, a plateau in $\dot{V}O_2$ may not occur, and the maximum $\dot{V}O_2$ will be less than the $\dot{V}O_2$ max. A plateau of $\dot{V}O_2$ in an incremental exercise test provides the evidence necessary for the judgement that a maximal $\dot{V}O_2$ has, in fact, been attained. Therefore, such tests provide important information regarding a subject's potential for increased metabolic rate and cardiovascular and respiratory performance.

Conditions in which O_2 flow to or O_2 utilization by the tissues is impaired (e.g., cardiovascular diseases, lung diseases, and anemias) cause reductions in the $\dot{V}O_2$ max and maximum $\dot{V}O_2$. Note that at high exercise intensities, the $\dot{V}O_2$ does not describe all of

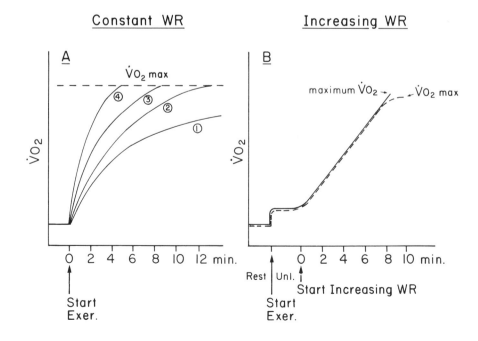

FIG. 3-1. (*A*) Determining the maximal $\dot{V}O_2$ ($\dot{V}O_2$max) from supramaximal work rates tests. 1, 2, 3, and 4 are $\dot{V}O_2$ measurements as related to time for progressively higher work rates. $\dot{V}O_2$ for work rate 1 asymptotes below $\dot{V}O_2$max. Work rate 2 reaches a $\dot{V}O_2$ which is the same as the $\dot{V}O_2$ reached by work rates 3 and 4. Since the maximum $\dot{V}O_2$ for work rates 2, 3, and 4 are same despite increasing work rate, this is regarded as the $\dot{V}O_2$max for the form of work being studied. (*B*) Distinguishing between $\dot{V}O_2$max and maximum $\dot{V}O_2$ from a maximal effort incremental exercise test. When the subject's maximum tolerable work rate results in a flattening of the $\dot{V}O_2$-work rate slope, this is the subject's maximal $\dot{V}O_2$ or $\dot{V}O_2$max. When the $\dot{V}O_2$ does not slow its rate of rise with increasing work rate, but the subject has reached his maximum tolerable work rate, this is the highest or maximum $\dot{V}O_2$ during the test.

the energy expended by the subject because it does not account for the anaerobic (lactic acid generating) contribution to energy production, an important energy source at high work rates.[4]

An incremental exercise test, as in Figure 3-1B, has a number of advantages: 1) the test starts out at relatively low work rates, so it does not require the application of great muscle force or a sudden, large cardiorespiratory stress; 2) the $\dot{V}O_2$ max or maximum $\dot{V}O_2$ can be determined from a test lasting approximately 10 minutes in which the subject is stressed at relatively high work rates for only a few minutes; and 3) the $\dot{V}O_2$-work rate relationship can be determined (cycle ergometry) or estimated (treadmill ergometry). It should be emphasized that in order to obtain the best data for interpreting the measured responses to an incremental exercise test, the work rate increments should be uniform in magnitude and duration. This means that the ergometer must be linear and accurately calibrated.

The maximum $\dot{V}O_2$ is the first measurement to be examined because it establishes whether the patient's physiological responses allow normal maximal aerobic function. Other measurements are needed to differentiate the cause of any exercise limitation whether or not the subject reaches his predicted maximum $\dot{V}O_2$.

OXYGEN UPTAKE AND WORK RATE

Although $\dot{V}O_2$ measurements are made at the mouth, they reflect the O_2 utilization by the cells including the muscle cells performing the work of exercise. The $\dot{V}O_2$-work rate relationship describes how much O_2 is utilized by the exercising subject in relation to the quantity of external work performed. Thus it gives important information concerning the coupling of external to internal respiration. We find it valuable to graph $\dot{V}O_2$ as a function of the work rate. Factors and mechanisms affecting $\dot{V}O_2$ as a function of the work rate during exercise are described below (Fig. 3-2).

Position Displacement of $\dot{V}O_2$ as a Function of the Work Rate

The position of the $\dot{V}O_2$ work rate relationship is dependent on body weight (Fig. 3-2A). Obese subjects require increased $\dot{V}O_2$ to do a given amount of external work (see Chapter 2, Oxygen cost of work). The increase in exercise $\dot{V}O_2$ caused by obesity is considerably greater than the increase in resting $\dot{V}O_2$ because the latter does not include the additional cost of moving the limbs in the case of cycle ergometry and the entire body mass with treadmill exercise. From two separate studies of cycle ergometer exercise on adults, the $\dot{V}O_2$ during unloaded cycling at 60 rpm was displaced upward by an average of 5.8 ml min^{-1} for each kg of body weight;[5,6] thus obesity causes a parallel upward displacement to the normal weight $\dot{V}O_2$-work rate relationship during cycle ergometry. For treadmill exercise a predictable adjustment for body weight may not be possible because of

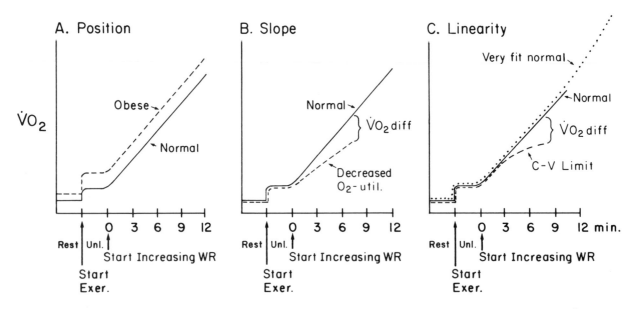

FIG. 3-2. Position displacement (A), slope (B), and linearity (C) of the $\dot{V}O_2$-work rate relationship. Obesity displaces the $\dot{V}O_2$-work rate relationship upward but the slope is unchanged. A decreased slope of the $\dot{V}O_2$-work rate relationship (B) reflects inadequate O_2 availability to the exercising muscles such as when peripheral blood flow is impaired. The linearity of the $\dot{V}O_2$-work rate relationship (C) can be altered in patients with cardiovascular diseases (slope becomes more shallow) because of impaired O_2 flow to the exercising muscles or very fit people (slope becomes more steep—see text). The difference between the expected $\dot{V}O_2$ for the work rate performed and the actual $\dot{V}O_2$ at the maximum work rate of the subject is referred to as the $\dot{V}O_2$ difference.

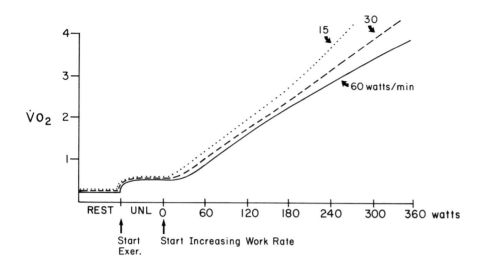

FIG. 3-3. Effect of work rate increment on the slope of the plot of $\dot{V}_{O_2}$ vs. work rate in a normal subject. A work rate increment for which the time from the start of the incrementing period to the maximum $\dot{V}_{O_2}$ is between 6 and 12 minutes generally results in a linear $\dot{V}_{O_2}$-work rate relationship to the subjects' maximum. For work rate increments that are relatively large, causing the subject to fatigue in less than 6 minutes, $\dot{V}_{O_2}$ tends to slow its rate of rise relative to work rate before the maximum $\dot{V}_{O_2}$ is reached. In contrast, for relatively small work rate increments in which it takes 15 minutes or more before the subject fatigues, $\dot{V}_{O_2}$ generally increases more steeply at high work rates.

complex mechanical factors such as the subject's varying center of gravity as the angle of the treadmill is changed and the variable length of the stride as the speed and/or grade are altered. These variables make it difficult to estimate the subject's actual power output.

Slope of $\dot{V}_{O_2}$ as a Function of the Work Rate

The slope of the $\dot{V}_{O_2}$ graphed against the work rate below the anaerobic threshold (*AT*) is important because it measures the aerobic work efficiency. The slope for one-minute incremental cycle ergometer work has been found to be 10.2 ± 1.0 ml O_2/min/watt for normal subjects by Hansen et al.[5] This is similar to the 10.1 ml O_2/min/watt value previously obtained from steady-state measurements below the *AT*.[6] The slope of the $\dot{V}_{O_2}$-work rate plot indicates the increased quantity of O_2 taken up by the exercising subject, and hence by the working muscles, as the work rate is increased. If the muscle is unable to obtain oxygen due to inadequate oxygen delivery, then the slope would be shallower than normal (Fig. 3-2*B*) and the predicted $\dot{V}_{O_2}$ max would not be reached. Although theoretically there may be several reasons why this slope can be reduced, including inadequate O_2 transport and limitation in O_2 diffusion from capillary to mitochondria, a reduction is most likely to be evident in conditions of impaired O_2 flow to the exercising extremities, such as heart disease or stenosis of the conducting vessels to the exercising muscles.

Linearity of $\dot{V}_{O_2}$ as a Function of the Work Rate and the Rate of Work Rate Increment

Because O_2 uptake kinetics becomes more complex than a simple exponential rise above the anaerobic threshold,[7-9] the slope of the $\dot{V}_{O_2}$-work rate relationship is not necessarily constant above the *AT*. If the size of the work rate increment is large relative to the subject's degree of fitness, then a relatively large proportion of energy generated would be anaerobic and the slope would be expected to become more shallow (Fig. 3-3, 60 watt/min). In contrast, when the work rate increments are small, at least three factors can cause an augmented O_2 uptake and thereby cause the $\dot{V}_{O_2}$-work rate slope to be steeper above the *AT*: (1) subjects often use additional muscle groups when performing heavy exercise, e.g., pulling on cycle handlebars to brace one's trunk on the ergometer as the pedals get harder to turn leads to additional and unmeasured arm work; (2) breathing work is increased, nonlinearly, as high levels of ventilation are reached, causing increased O_2 consumption by the breathing muscles; (3) significant lactate conversion to glycogen (Cori cycle) by tissues actively involved in gluconeogenesis (liver and possibly inactive skeletal muscles) requires oxygen consumption to increase in those organs in which this reaction is occurring.

In view of the above considerations, the finding of a deviation in the $\dot{V}_{O_2}$-work rate slope above the anaerobic threshold, such as illustrated in Figure 3-3, is understandable. If the size of the work rate increment was relatively small for a fit subject, then the anaerobic contribution to energy generation (rate of lactate increase) at a given $\dot{V}_{O_2}$ would be relatively small, and the three factors just noted would cause $\dot{V}_{O_2}$ to rise more rapidly relative to the work rate[10-12] than that observed below the *AT*. In contrast, large work rate increments result in a sizable fraction of work done anaerobically above the *AT* (high rate of lactate increase) and $\dot{V}_{O_2}$ would rise more slowly relative to work rate. Thus in the same subject the $\dot{V}_{O_2}$-work rate function above the *AT* can be more steep (small work rate increments) or less steep (large work rate increments) than that observed below the anaerobic threshold (see Fig. 3-3). But regardless of the increment used, the maximum $\dot{V}O_2$ is not markedly affected. In general, work rate increments of 15 to 25 watts per minute in normal adult males and 10 to 20 watts in normal adult females give a similar rate of rise in $\dot{V}O_2$ both above and below the anaerobic threshold. A method of selecting the work rate increment for exercise testing of normals and patients is described in Chapter 5.

With disorders of the cardiovascular system, the linearity of the $\dot{V}O_2$-work rate relationship may be affected regardless of the rate of increment (Fig. 3-2*C*). The $\dot{V}O_2$ may increase normally as the work rate is increased over low levels, but slow its rate of increase as the maximum $\dot{V}O_2$ is approached. This nonlinearity or decrease in slope of the $\dot{V}O_2$-work rate relationship is usually accompanied by a persistently steep $\dot{V}CO_2$-work rate slope, reflecting the simultaneous buffering of lactic acid generated by anaerobiosis. In this situation the subject's $\dot{V}O_2$ max is clearly reduced.

Predicting $\dot{V}O_2$ or Mets from the Work Rate

A unit called a "met." was derived from the resting $\dot{V}O_2$ for a 70 kg, 40-year-old male and its value is 3.5 ml/min per kilogram of body weight. Many laboratories do not measure $\dot{V}O_2$ but, by assuming a certain relationship between the work rate and $\dot{V}O_2$, report an estimate of $\dot{V}O_2$ in ml/min. After obtaining this derived $\dot{V}O_2$ and expressing it per kilogram of body weight, the quotient is divided by 3.5 to obtain the number of mets performed by the subject.

Estimating $\dot{V}O_2$ from the work rate or mets may lead to misinterpretation of the data because, under certain conditions, $\dot{V}O_2$ cannot be accurately predicted for the reasons summarized in Table 3-3. For instance, if the ergometer is not accurately calibrated, the $\dot{V}O_2$ estimated could be in serious error. In addition, if $\dot{V}O_2$ is not in a steady-state, the $\dot{V}O_2$ may be less or more than that extrapolated from the work rate (see Fig. 3-3). Also, the $\dot{V}O_2$ commonly does not increase linearly in patients with cardiovascular diseases as the work rate is increased (see Fig. 3-2 and the cases numbered 15–18, 20, 23, 29, 35, and 36 in

TABLE 3-3. *When Work Rate May Fail to Predict $\dot{V}O_2$*

Faulty ergometer calibration
Steady-state not reached
Obesity
Valvular heart disease
Coronary artery disease
Cardiomyopathy
Peripheral vascular disease
Pulmonary vascular disease

Chapter 8). This will lead to an overestimate of $\dot{V}O_2$ or mets in these patients. Finally, the correct body weight factor must be taken into account to estimate the $\dot{V}O_2$. This factor is often ignored or incorrect estimates of the effect of body weight on cycle ergometer $\dot{V}O_2$ are used. Thus the conversion of work rate to mets without actually measuring $\dot{V}O_2$ is inaccurate, particularly in patients, and should be discouraged.

Analysis of the $\dot{V}O_2$-work rate relationship is of value only if the ergometer is accurately calibrated. Unfortunately, many cycle ergometers are not accurately calibrated, particularly over the low range. We calibrate our cycle ergometer at regular intervals and have added a motor to the flywheel to obviate the initial work of overcoming the flywheel inertia. The inertial work makes initiation of cycling difficult for some elderly patients.

$\dot{V}O_2$ DIFFERENCE

This term refers to the difference between the expected and measured $\dot{V}O_2$ at the subject's maximum work rate (see Fig. 3-2). It is used to describe the obligatory anaerobic component at the maximum work rate during a standardized incremental exercise test. It assumes that $\dot{V}O_2$ increases relatively linearly with the work rate and that, at the subject's maximum work rate, there should be no difference between the expected $\dot{V}O_2$ for that work rate and the measured $\dot{V}O_2$, i.e., a $\dot{V}O_2$ difference of zero. The expected $\dot{V}O_2$ in ml/min for cycle ergometry in which the work rate is increased at one-minute intervals is estimated from the equation:

$$\text{expected } \dot{V}O_2 = \dot{V}O_2 \text{ unloaded} + 10.2 \times (T - 0.75) \times I,$$

where $\dot{V}O_2$ unloaded is $\dot{V}O_2$ measured after 3 min of unloaded pedalling, T is the total time in minutes of incremental work until maximum $\dot{V}O_2$ is reached, 0.75 is the time displacement between the start of the linear increase in work rate and the linear increase in $\dot{V}O_2$ (estimated from normal subjects), and I is the work rate increment in watts per minute. The $\dot{V}O_2$ difference, in percent, is:

$\%\dot{V}O_2$ difference

$$= \frac{\text{expected } \dot{V}O_2 - \text{measured } \dot{V}O_2}{\text{expected } \dot{V}O_2} \times 100$$

If a subject has an O_2 flow problem, a relatively larger fraction of his energy will come from anaerobic mechanisms and, therefore, $\dot{V}O_2$ at the subject's highest work rate will be reduced, i.e., the subject will have a positive $\dot{V}O_2$ difference. Likewise, for a very fit subject, $\dot{V}O_2$ difference may be negative because all three factors described above (Cori cycle, breathing work, and added work of arm muscles) cause total O_2 consumption to increase more steeply than work rate.

CARDIAC OUTPUT

Cardiac output can be estimated by the indirect Fick method during exercise from the measurements of $\dot{V}CO_2$, arterial PCO_2, and mixed venous PCO_2 using the rebreathing method (see Appendix). However, estimation of arterial blood PCO_2 from alveolar or end-tidal measurements has many potential errors, especially in patients.[13]

If a catheter of the Swan-Ganz type is introduced through the heart into the pulmonary artery, the cardiac output can be determined by the direct Fick method. If a thermistor-tip catheter is used, a thermodilution curve can be obtained from the thermistor in the pulmonary artery, following the injection of iced saline into the lumen of the catheter opening into the right atrium. From this curve and the volume of iced saline injected, blood flow through the right atrium can be calculated.[14] However, right heart catheterization is a significantly invasive measurement.

Cardiac output measurements tend not to be very useful during exercise except when accompanied by simultaneous pressure measurements for determining pulmonary vascular resistance or the degree of valvular stenosis. The reason is that the normal range of cardiac output is great, and the measurement, by itself, gives limited information. The major concern of exercise testing should be to determine if the heart is capable of providing the exercise-stressed muscles with enough oxygen. The availability of a cardiac output measurement, even if accurate, does not reveal whether the cardiac output is adequate for the work rate performed. To answer this important question, we have found the measurement of the anaerobic threshold to be of greater theoretical and practical use because it can be measured noninvasively and, therefore, is easily repeated.

ANAEROBIC THRESHOLD *(AT)*

The anaerobic threshold is defined as the level of exercise $\dot{V}O_2$ above which aerobic energy production is supplemented by anaerobic mechanisms, and is reflected by an increase in lactate and lactate/pyruvate ratio in muscle or arterial blood. (see Fig. 2-1 and 2-8). The biochemical and physiological basis of the anaerobic threshold hypothesis is described in Chapter 2. Like the $\dot{V}O_2$ max, the *AT* measurement is influenced by the size of the muscle groups involved in the activity.

Information Derived from the Anaerobic Threshold (AT) Measurement

BLOOD LACTATE. The *AT* is the $\dot{V}O_2$ of the subject above which there is a sustained increase in blood lactate and lactate/pyruvate ratio.

$\dot{V}O_2$ ABOVE WHICH METABOLIC ACIDOSIS OCCURS. Plasma bicarbonate decreases in a close reciprocal relationship to lactate increase (Fig. 3-4).

$\dot{V}O_2$ ABOVE WHICH THERE IS A DELAY IN REACHING A $\dot{V}O_2$ STEADY-STATE. The *AT* demarcates the work rate above which $\dot{V}O_2$ kinetics change. The steady-state in $\dot{V}O_2$, found to occur by 3 minutes when exercising at a constant work rate below the *AT*, is delayed above the *AT*. Thus an increase in $\dot{V}O_2$ between the third and sixth minute of constant work rate exercise can be used as a marker that the work is above the *AT*. This $\Delta\dot{V}O_2$ (6-3) significantly correlates with the lactate increase (see Fig. 2-13).

WORK RATE ABOVE WHICH $\dot{V}E$ INCREASES WITH TIME. Ventilatory drive is stimulated by the metabolic aci-

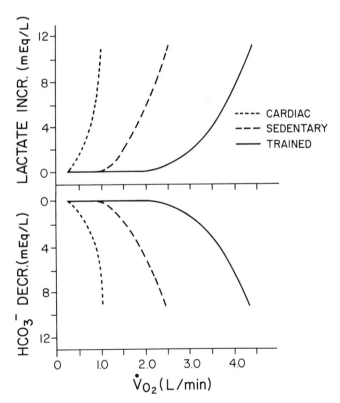

FIG. 3-4. Lactate increase and bicarbonate decrease during incremental exercise in trained and sedentary normal subjects and patients with primary cardiac disease of class II severity as defined by New York Heart Association Classification (37). (From Wasserman, K.: Physiologic basis of exercise testing. *In* Pulmonary Diseases and Disorders. Edited by A.P. Fishman. New York, McGraw-Hill. 1980, pp. 337–347.)

dosis resulting from lactate accumulation. $\dot{V}E$, primarily by increasing breathing frequency, increases as work rates above the AT are sustained (see Fig. 2-21). The rate of increase depends on the degree to which the AT is exceeded.

SUSTAINABLE WORK RATE.   To sustain at a work rate for more than an hour, the work rate must be at or below the AT. The greater the increase in arterial lactate, the less the endurance. In an endurance cycling study on motivated young men, none could sustain pedalling for 50 minutes with an increase in lactate above 2.5 mM/L (see Fig. 2-11).

Methods of Measurement

Because the increase in muscle lactate and $[H^+]$ is associated with an obligatory increase in CO_2 production, it is possible to detect the cellular acidosis by measuring the rate of increase in $\dot{V}CO_2$ relative to that of $\dot{V}O_2$ for an incremental exercise test. A relatively short, progressive work rate test can rapidly determine the $\dot{V}O_2$ at the AT when gas exchange is measured breath-by-breath or as the average of several breaths. A flow diagram describing the sequence of gas exchange and ventilation changes for a one-minute incremental exercise test is illustrated in Figure 3-5. The record of an actual study is shown in Figures 3-6 and 2-10 for illustration (see also Chapter 8). These studies show that as the work rate is increased, the linear pattern of increase in $\dot{V}CO_2$ and $\dot{V}E$ seen at low work rates changes at high work rates. Above the AT lactic acid production results in an acceleration of the rate of increase in $\dot{V}CO_2$ relative to $\dot{V}O_2$. Because, generally, $\dot{V}E$ and $\dot{V}CO_2$ initially accelerate in a proportional manner above the AT, there is a short period in which $\dot{V}E/\dot{V}CO_2$ and PET_{CO_2} do not change while $\dot{V}E/\dot{V}O_2$ and PET_{O_2} increase. Thus there is hyperventilation with respect to O_2 but not CO_2 as the AT is exceeded. The period during which $\dot{V}E/\dot{V}CO_2$ and PET_{CO_2} do not change despite hyperventilation with respect to O_2 normally lasts about 2 minutes. It is referred to as the isocapnic buffering period because of the lack of hyperventilation with respect to CO_2 despite the development of metabolic acidosis.[15] The increase in $\dot{V}E/\dot{V}O_2$ without an increase in $\dot{V}E/\dot{V}CO_2$ is typical of acid buffering rather than other factors (hypoxemia, pain, or psychogenic) affecting ventilation. When observed it is a specific gas exchange demonstration that the AT has been surpassed. As the work rate is increased further, the carotid bodies generally respond to the decreasing pH and cause ventilation to increase faster than CO_2 production. This causes Pa_{CO_2} to decrease and

the reduction in pH to be constrained. This respiratory compensation for the nonrespiratory lactic acidosis is reflected in an increase in $\dot{V}E/\dot{V}CO_2$ and decrease in PET_{CO_2}, as well as by further increases in $\dot{V}E/\dot{V}O_2$ and PET_{O_2} (see Fig. 3-6). The gas exchange ratio, R, which ordinarily slowly increases as the work rate is increased, increases more rapidly above the AT. When the AT is measured as a metabolic stress, i.e., in units of O_2 consumption, it is unaffected by the rate with which the work rate is incremented.[10,16]

The reason for keeping the work rate intervals relatively short during testing is to take advantage of the fact that the CO_2 contribution from buffering is observed only during the buffering process (a period of *decreasing* bicarbonate) and not after the lactate has been buffered. An unchanging although elevated lac-

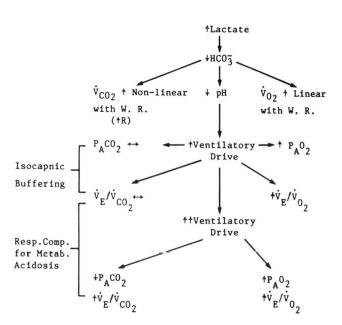

FIG. 3-5. Effect of lactate increase on gas exchange during a one-minute incremental test. Lactate increase causes an approximately equimolar decrease in bicarbonate. This causes $\dot{V}CO_2$ and R to increase more steeply as work rate is increased, while $\dot{V}O_2$ continues to increase in an essentially linear pattern. At the start of metabolic acidosis, ventilation usually increases approximately parallel to the increase in $\dot{V}CO_2$, resulting in no change in end-tidal or arterial P_{CO_2} (isocapnic buffering), while alveolar oxygen tension is increased secondary to the disproportionate increase in ventilation relative to the increase in $\dot{V}O_2$. The increase in ventilation is reflected in an increase in the ventilatory equivalent for oxygen ($\dot{V}E/\dot{V}O_2$) while the ventilatory equivalent for CO_2 ($\dot{V}E/\dot{V}CO_2$) does not change. After several minutes, ventilatory drive increases further and $\dot{V}E$ increases disproportionately to the increase in $\dot{V}CO_2$, resulting in hyperventilation with respect to both O_2 and CO_2. The latter achieves some degree of respiratory compensation for the metabolic acidosis. (From Wasserman, K., Whipp, B.J., and Davis, J.A.: Respiratory physiology of exercise: Metabolism, gas exchange, and ventilatory control. *In* Int. Rev. Physiol. III, Vol. 23. Edited by J.G. Widdicombe. Baltimore, University Park Press. 1981, pp. 149–211.)

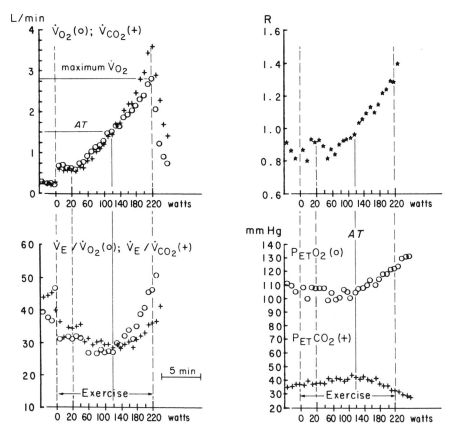

Fig. 3-6. Gas exchange for a normal subject during a one-minute incremental exercise test. In each panel, the far-left dashed line indicates the start of unloaded cycling. The vertical dashed line second from the left indicates the start of the incremental period of exercise and the right vertical dashed line indicates the end of exercise. The maximum $\dot{V}O_2$ is indicated. The anaerobic threshold (AT) is located where the $\dot{V}E/\dot{V}O_2$ curve inflects upward (vertical solid line). The nadir of the $\dot{V}E/\dot{V}CO_2$ curve does not occur until a higher work rate is reached and reflects the start of respiratory compensation for the metabolic acidosis. At the AT, $P_{ET}O_2$ increases reflecting the hyperventilation with respect to $\dot{V}O_2$, while $P_{ET}CO_2$ does not start to systematically decrease until approximately 2 minutes later. At the AT, R increases more steeply, reflecting the increase in $\dot{V}CO_2$ relative to $\dot{V}O_2$.

tate does not generate additional CO_2 since it is already buffered.

Measurement Difficulties and How to Improve Anaerobic Threshold (AT) Estimation

Occasionally, the AT cannot be reliably detected by an examiner because of atypical records caused by irregular breathing, an inappropriate rate of increase in work rate, suboptimal plotting scales, or a poor ventilatory response to the metabolic acidosis on the part of the patient. To obviate these problems, one can measure blood lactate or standard bicarbonate directly. Beaver et al.[17] found that the lactate threshold during exercise can be most reliably selected by plotting log lactate against log $\dot{V}O_2$. Similarly, the start of the [HCO_3^-] fall indicating the start of developing metabolic acidosis can be most reliably de-

tected from a plot of log standard [HCO_3^-] against log $\dot{V}O_2$.[18] There is a slight difference in the time of these thresholds but this is not of clinical significance. But, to obviate blood sampling, dependence on a normal ventilatory response to the metabolic acidosis, and the subjectivity of the examiner in selecting the AT, Beaver et al.[19] developed a computerized method for selecting AT that agrees closely with the lactate and [HCO_3^-] thresholds. This technique is referred to as the V-slope method since it relates the alveolar $\dot{V}CO_2$ to the alveolar $\dot{V}O_2$ as shown in Figure 3-7. The break-point in this relationship is selected by a computer program that defines the $\dot{V}O_2$ above which CO_2 is generated from the buffering of lactic acid. However, the break-point can also be selected visually. While this method uses measured gas exchange ($\dot{V}O_2$ and $\dot{V}CO_2$), it is independent of the subject's ventilatory response. Details of the V-slope method for determining AT are described in the primary report[19] and in the Appendix.

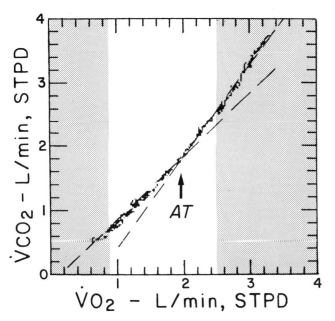

FIG. 3-7. Alveolar CO_2 output plotted against O_2 uptake for anaerobic threshold determination by the V-slope method[19] for a single subject. The data are obtained from breath-by-breath measurements and are smoothed using a 9 second moving average filter. Data in the shaded areas are ignored in the analysis because of nonlinearity in the kinetics at the start of the work rate increment (approximately one minute of data at lower end) and hyperventilation for CO_2 at the upper end. The data in the nonshaded area are analyzed by least squares statistical methods to obtain the best fit to a two component model. The intersecting point that is part of both the lower and upper lines is the anaerobic threshold.

Application of the Anaerobic Threshold Measurement

The *AT* aids in the differential diagnosis of disorders of cardiorespiratory coupling to cellular metabolism. Conditions that limit O_2 flow to the exercising muscles during exercise will most likely cause the *AT* to be low. Combined with other measurements, the pathophysiology of exercise limitation can be subclassified further. The *AT* can also be used for evaluating therapy since it is sensitive to changes in O_2 flow to the tissues and is relatively independent of effort.

HEART RATE-OXYGEN UPTAKE RELATIONSHIP AND HEART RATE RESERVE

Heart rate normally increases linearly with $\dot{V}O_2$ during incremental exercise[20] (Fig. 3-8). In many heart diseases, the heart rate increase is relatively steep for the increase in $\dot{V}O_2$ because the stroke volume is low. In addition, as the patient with heart disease approaches his maximum work rate, $\dot{V}O_2$ commonly slows its rate of increase while the heart rate typically continues to increase. Therefore, the rate of increase

in heart rate relative to $\dot{V}O_2$ becomes even more steep, deviating from the linearity established at lower work rates (see Fig. 3-8). Although this phenomenon is not uniformly seen in patients with heart disease, it is a useful diagnostic observation and suggests a significant cardiac limitation in O_2 transport to the contracting muscles. Pulmonary vascular disease causes the same phenomenon since this disorder limits the rate of venous return to the left side of the heart and, consequently, the left ventricular output.

The estimated heart rate reserve is an expression of the potential heart rate increase that remains at the end of an incremental exercise test. We define this simply as the difference between the predicted maximum heart rate (see the section entitled "maximum heart rate and heart rate reserve" in Chapter 6) and the actual maximum exercise heart rate.

Although the predicted maximum heart rate has considerable variation, as determined from population studies, the heart rate reserve is still a useful concept for differential diagnosis. Table 3-4 lists disorders in which the heart rate reserve may be increased. Normally, the heart rate reserve is relatively small (less than 15 beats). It is also usually normal in patients with primary heart disease and in pa-

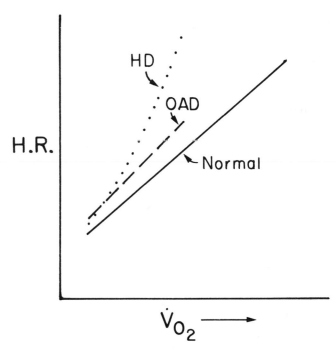

FIG. 3-8. Characteristic changes in heart rate relative to $\dot{V}O_2$ for normal subjects, patients with chronic obstructive airway disease (OAD), and those with heart disease (HD). The higher heart rate-$\dot{V}O_2$ relationship for the obstructive airway disease patient may reflect relative unfitness while the relatively low maximum heart rate reflects respiratory limitation to the maximum level of exercise. The steepening heart rate-$\dot{V}O_2$ relationship in the patient with heart disease reflects the failure of $\dot{V}O_2$ to increase in response to the increasing work rate as illustrated in Figure 3-2C.

TABLE 3-4. *Disorders Associated With Increased Heart Rate Reserve*

Claudication limiting exercise
Angina limiting exercise
"Sick-sinus" syndrome
β-adrenergic blockade
Lung disease
Poor effort

tients with disorders of the pulmonary circulation. In contrast, patients with peripheral vascular disease or coronary artery disease may discontinue exercise because of pain before the maximal heart rate is reached. Patients with disorders of the conducting system of the heart or sinoatrial node disease such as seen with certain cardiomyopathies or consequent to a myocardial infarct may have a low maximum heart rate. Also, patients who take beta-adrenergic blocking drugs or who are limited in exercise because of primary lung disease usually have a large heart rate reserve. Finally, those who make poor effort have an increased heart rate reserve.

OXYGEN PULSE ($\dot{V}O_2$/HR)

The O_2 pulse is calculated by dividing the oxygen uptake by the heart rate. It is the volume of O_2 extracted by the peripheral tissues or the volume of O_2 added to the pulmonary blood per heart beat and can be shown to be equal to the product of stroke volume and the arterial-mixed venous O_2 difference (see Chapter 2, Distribution of Peripheral Blood Flow). As the work rate is increased, the O_2 pulse rises (Fig. 3-9), primarily because of an increasing arterial-mixed venous O_2 difference. If, however, the stroke volume is reduced, the arterial-mixed venous oxygen difference and, therefore, the O_2 pulse reach maximal values at a relatively low work rate, and the O_2 pulse approaches an asymptote at a low value (see Fig. 3-9). The O_2 pulse will also be low with anemia, high levels of carboxyhemoglobin, or severe arterial hypoxemia, all because of a reduced arterial O_2 content.

ARTERIAL PRESSURE

Arterial pressure measurements, particularly direct measurements, are very helpful in certain instances. The normal responses of systolic, diastolic, and pulse pressures are described in Chapter 6, "Brachial Artery Blood Pressure". The systolic pressure increases to a much greater degree than the diastolic resulting in a rise in pulse pressure. This is progressive with work rate. A decrease in the systolic and pulse pressures with an increasing work rate suggests cardiac

dysfunction. The development of a pulsus alternans may also be seen with cardiomyopathies. Finally, the direct arterial pressure tracing recorded at a fast speed may provide evidence for ventricular outflow obstruction, such as seen with aortic stenosis or obstructive hypertrophic cardiomyopathy.

BREATHING RESERVE

The breathing reserve is expressed either as the difference between the maximal voluntary ventilation and the maximum exercise ventilation in absolute terms or the difference as a fraction of the maximal voluntary ventilation (Table 3–1, Fig. 3-10). Except in extremely fit individuals who can attain high levels of $\dot{V}E$, normal males have a breathing reserve of at least 15 liters per minute or 20 to 40% of the maximal voluntary ventilation (Fig. 3-11).[21] A low breathing reserve is characteristic of patients with primary lung disease who are ventilatory limited. The breathing reserve is high in patients with cardiovascular diseases that limit exercise performance.

WASTED VENTILATION AND DEAD SPACE/ TIDAL VOLUME RATIO

Alveolar ventilation is the theoretical ventilation required to eliminate the CO_2 produced by metabolism that would result in the given arterial ("ideal" alveolar) CO_2 tension. The physiological dead space ventilation is the difference between the minute ventilation and the alveolar ventilation. A valuable estimate of the degree of matching of ventilation to perfusion during exercise is the physiological dead

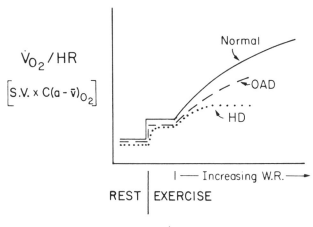

FIG. 3-9. Characteristic changes in $\dot{V}O_2$/heart rate (O_2 pulse) as related to increase in work rate. The $\dot{V}O_2$/HR ratio is equal to stroke volume X C($a - \bar{v}$)$_{O_2}$. Thus patients with low stroke volumes (e.g., heart disease [HD]) will tend to have low $\dot{V}O_2$/HR values at maximal exercise. In contrast, patients with obstructive airway disease (OAD) have a similar pattern as normal subjects, although the values are lower at each work rate reflecting the relatively low stroke volume in these patients.

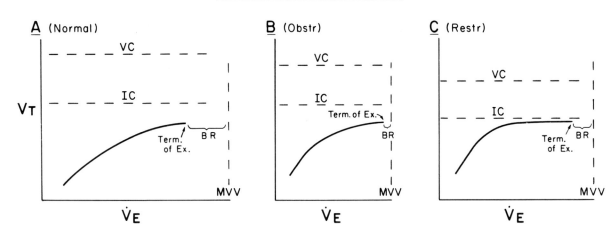

FIG. 3-10. Tidal volume as related to minute ventilation increase during incremental exercise testing in the normal subject (A), and in patients with obstructive (B) and restrictive (C) lung disease. The curve ends at the subjects' maximal exercise performance. The vertical dashed line indicates the subject's MVV and the distance between the highest $\dot{V}E$ and MVV is the subject's breathing reserve (BR). In the case of patients with obstructive lung disease, this is quite small. While the V_T is always less than the vital capacity (VC) and inspiratory capacity (IC), it closely approximates the IC in restrictive lung diseases.

space/tidal volume ratio (V_D/V_T). The V_D/V_T is lowest when alveolar ventilation relative to perfusion is uniform.

At rest the physiological dead space volume is normally about ⅓ of the breath. During exercise it is reduced to about ⅕ of the breath or even less (Fig. 3-12),[22] the major decrement occurring at the lightest work rate. However, in patients with pulmonary disorders in whom ventilation-perfusion relationships are uneven, or in patients with pulmonary vascular disease whose alveoli are poorly or unperfused, the V_D/V_T is increased at rest and fails to decrease normally during exercise.

The V_D/V_T is a valuable measurement because it is typically abnormal in patients with primary pulmonary vascular disease or pulmonary vascular disease secondary to obstructive or restrictive lung disease. It

is sometimes the only gas exchange abnormality evident during exercise testing. Figure 3-12 illustrates the changes in V_D/V_T as the work rate is increased in the normal individual and in patients with lung or pulmonary vascular diseases. The V_D/V_T may be only slightly elevated at rest but remain relatively unchanged, or even increasing rather than decreasing, during exercise. Thus exercise makes the abnormality in ventilation-perfusion mismatching more evident.

When V_D/V_T is increased, $\dot{V}E$ is typically inordinately high for the work rate performed. However, $\dot{V}E$ might also be high in conditions in which the Pa_{CO_2} is relatively low (low CO_2 set-point), e.g., conditions associated with a chronic metabolic acidosis. In this setting, V_D/V_T will be normal if the lungs are normal, despite hyperventilation. Figure 3-13

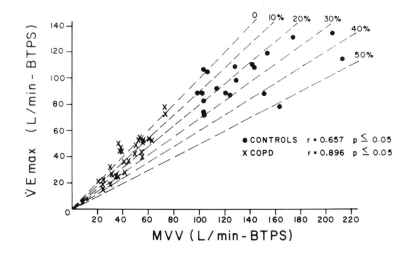

FIG. 3-11. Maximum ventilation ($\dot{V}Emax$) as related to maximum voluntary ventilation (MVV) in patients with chronic obstructive pulmonary disease and normal subjects. The dashed-line isopleths indicate the percent breathing reserve. (Courtesy of Dr. John Andrews.)

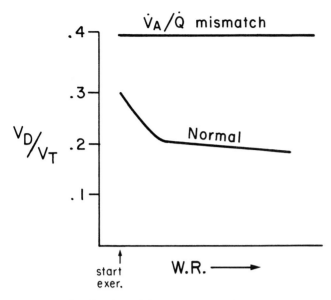

FIG. 3-12. The physiological dead space/tidal volume ratio (V_D/V_T) during rest and increasing work rate for the normal subject and patients with ventilation-perfusion ($\dot{V}_A/\dot{Q}$) mismatching.

shows the minute ventilation required for various metabolic rates ($\dot{V}CO_2$) at designated values of Pa_{CO_2} and V_D/V_T.

ALVEOLAR-ARTERIAL PO_2 DIFFERENCE ($P(A-a)O_2$)

A reduced Pa_{O_2} and increased $P(A-a)_{O_2}$ during incremental exercise typically result from underventilation of regions of lung relative to their perfusion, i.e., mismatching of alveolar ventilation and perfusion ($\dot{V}_A/\dot{Q}$) (Fig. 3-14).[23,24] This is characteristic of patients with airway diseases, particularly during exercise when blood flow increases. Fortunately, the small arteries leading to these poorly ventilated low $\dot{V}_A/\dot{Q}$ areas of the lung constrict under the influence of decreasing alveolar PO_2.[25] This diverts blood flow to areas of relatively good ventilation and generally prevents hypoxemia from becoming progressive and marked as the work rate is increased (Fig. 3-14B). (Exceptions are failure to divert adequately or the presence of a foramen ovale through which venous

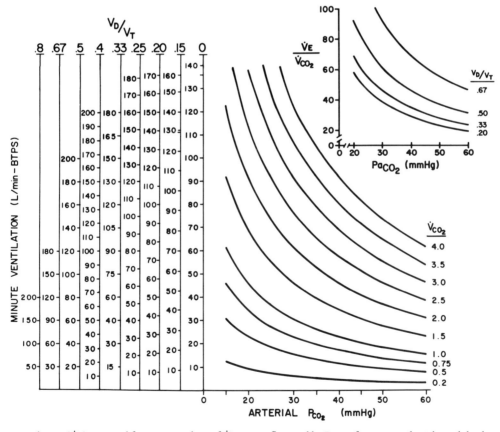

FIG. 3-13. Minute ventilation ($\dot{V}E$) required for various values of $\dot{V}CO_2$ as influenced by Pa_{CO_2} for various physiological dead space/tidal volume (V_D/V_T) fractions. If any three of the above values are known, the fourth might be determined. For instance, if $\dot{V}E$, $\dot{V}CO_2$, and Pa_{CO_2} are measured, V_D/V_T can be determined from the ordinate which agrees with the measured $\dot{V}E$. The insert shows the effect of changing Pa_{CO_2} on the $\dot{V}E/\dot{V}CO_2$ ratio during exercise with a constant V_D/V_T (Modified from Wasserman, K., and Whipp, B.J.: Exercise physiology in health and disease. Am. Rev. Respir. Dis., *112*:219-249, 1975.)

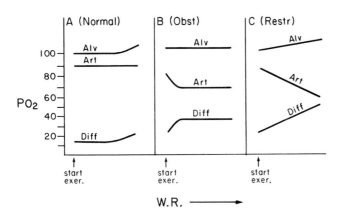

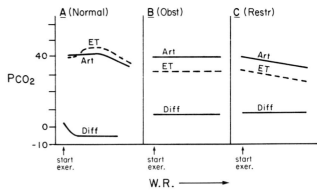

FIG. 3-14. Pattern of arterial and alveolar P_{O_2} and alveolar-arterial P_{O_2} differences in the normal subject (A), and obstructive (B) and restrictive (C) lung disease patients as related to increasing work rate.

FIG. 3-15. Pattern of arterial and end tidal P_{CO_2} values and arterial-end tidal P_{CO_2} difference in the normal subject (A) and obstructive (B) and restrictive (C) lung disease patients as related to increasing work rate, all with normal resting Pa_{CO_2}. In many patients, resting Pa_{CO_2} is increased or decreased but the arterial end-tidal relationship remains abnormal.

blood can shunt from the right to the left atrium during exercise.) In contrast, certain disorders (e.g., pulmonary fibrosis or pulmonary vascular diseases) that have a reduced pulmonary capillary bed have no alternative pathways for the increased blood flow of exercise other than the same capillaries patent at rest. These disorders are characteristically associated with exercise hypoxemia, which becomes systematically more pronounced as the work rate is increased (Fig. 3-14C). This pattern of decreasing Pa_{O_2} and increasing $P(A-a)_{O_2}$ with the work rate probably reflects a loss of capillary volume with a resultant decrease in residence time of red cells in the pulmonary capillaries as the work rate is increased. Thus the time for P_{O_2} in the alveolus to equilibrate with the P_{O_2} in the blood is reduced.

Pa_{O_2} might also decrease as the work rate is increased in conditions in which the alveoli are filled with material in which O_2 is relatively insoluble (e.g., as in pulmonary alveolar proteinosis). As the perfusion rate increases in these lung units, there is failure of O_2 in the gas space to equilibrate with O_2 in the red cell and hypoxemia becomes more marked as the blood flow increases. At rest, however, when the car-

diac output is low, there may be no hypoxemia owing to an adequate capillary residence time.

Calculation of $P(A-a)_{O_2}$, rather than simply relying on the value of Pa_{O_2}, may reveal abnormalities in blood oxygenation masked by hyperventilation. In terms of mechanism, an abnormally elevated $P(A-a)_{O_2}$ is indicative of uneven $\dot{V}A/\dot{Q}$, a diffusion defect, and/or a right-to-left shunt.

ARTERIAL-END TIDAL P_{CO_2} DIFFERENCE ($P(a-ET)_{CO_2}$)

Another valuable measurement that can be used as evidence of uneven $\dot{V}A/\dot{Q}$ or increased alveolar dead space is the $P(a-ET)_{CO_2}$[22] (Fig. 3-15). At rest Pa_{CO_2} is approximately 2 mm Hg greater than $P_{ET_{CO_2}}$. During exercise, however, $P_{ET_{CO_2}}$ increases relative to Pa_{CO_2}. The increase in $P_{ET_{CO_2}}$ comes about because of the increased rate of CO_2 delivery to the lung during exercise, creating an increase in slope of the alveolar phase of the CO_2 expiratory curve (Figure 3-16). Thus the value for $P(a-ET)_{CO_2}$ is slightly posi-

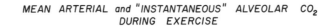

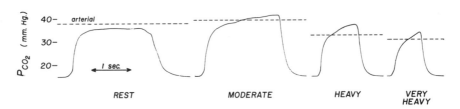

FIG. 3-16. Mean arterial (dashed lines) compared to instantaneous alveolar (solid lines) P_{CO_2} for the resting state and increasing intensities of exercise. The end-tidal P_{CO_2} is normally less than Pa_{CO_2} at rest but greater than Pa_{CO_2} during exercise. (From Wasserman, K., Van Kessel, A., and Burton, G.G.: Interactions of physiological mechanisms during exercise. J. Appl. Physiol. *22*:71–85, 1967.)

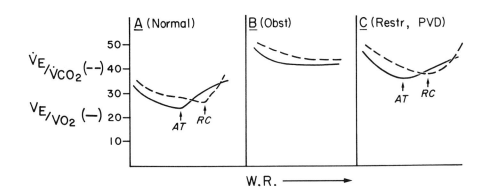

Fig. 3-17. Ventilatory equivalent for CO_2 ($\dot{V}_E/\dot{V}_{CO_2}$) and O_2 ($\dot{V}_E/\dot{V}_{O_2}$) for the normal (*A*) subject, and obstructive (*B*) and restrictive or pulmonary vascular disease (*C*) patients, as related to increasing work rate. The nadir in $\dot{V}_E/\dot{V}_{O_2}$ reflects the anaerobic threshold (*AT*) and the nadir of the $\dot{V}_E/\dot{V}_{CO_2}$ curve reflects the respiratory compensation point (RC).

tive at rest but negative during exercise (normally about −4 mm Hg). The slower the breathing rate the higher the end-tidal P_{CO_2} relative to arterial P_{CO_2}. If the $P(a-ET)_{CO_2}$ remains positive during exercise, this is evidence for decreased perfusion to ventilated alveoli (uneven $\dot{V}_A/\dot{Q}$) (see Fig. 3-15). An extreme situation may be seen when CO_2-rich venous blood is diverted to the left side of the circulation without passing through the lungs during exercise (right to left shunt). In this case, Pa_{CO_2} is higher than $P_{ET_{CO_2}}$ and $P(a-ET)_{CO_2}$ is positive, the magnitude presumably dependent on the size of the shunt.

VENTILATORY EQUIVALENTS AS INDICES OF UNEVEN $\dot{V}_A/\dot{Q}$

Because the measurements of V_D/V_T, $P(A-a)_{O_2}$, and $P(a-ET)_{CO_2}$ require arterial blood sampling, it is helpful to get a clue to an abnormality in $\dot{V}_A/\dot{Q}$ from noninvasive techniques. The nadir of the ventilatory equivalent for CO_2 or O_2 ($\dot{V}_E/\dot{V}_{CO_2}$ and $\dot{V}_E/\dot{V}_{O_2}$, respectively) during incremental exercise can be used as a noninvasive guide to $\dot{V}_A/\dot{Q}$ unevenness. Normally, $\dot{V}_E/\dot{V}_{CO_2}$ and $\dot{V}_E/\dot{V}_{O_2}$ change as illustrated in Figure 3-17*A*. The $\dot{V}_E/\dot{V}_{O_2}$ normally decreases to its nadir at the anaerobic threshold and the $\dot{V}_E/\dot{V}_{CO_2}$ decreases to its nadir when respiratory compensation for metabolic (lactic) acidosis begins. $\dot{V}_E/\dot{V}_{O_2}$ is approximately 25 with a range between 22 and 27 and $\dot{V}_E/\dot{V}_{CO_2}$ is about 28 with a range between 26 and 30. Normal values for these ventilatory equivalents with a $P_{ET_{CO_2}}$ of approximately 40 mm Hg suggest a normal V_D/V_T and uniform matching of $\dot{V}_A$ to $\dot{Q}$ (see Fig. 3-13). Elevated ventilatory equivalents (Figs. 3-17 *B,C*) can reflect either hyperventilation or an increase in V_D/V_T (uneven $\dot{V}_A/\dot{Q}$). Hyperventilation can be distinguished from increased V_D/V_T as a cause of high ventilatory equivalents by measuring Pa_{CO_2} (see Fig. 3-13).

The ventilatory equivalents for O_2 and CO_2 can also be useful in providing evidence for mechanical limitation in ventilation or insensitive chemoreceptors. In a progressive exercise test the $\dot{V}_E/\dot{V}_{O_2}$ normally increases at work rates above the AT, the amount depending on the magnitude of the work rate performed and the sensitivity of the chemoreceptors in response to the metabolic acidosis (see Fig. 3-17). In contrast, patients who have a mechanical limitation to breathe, or those who have insensitive chemoreceptors, have a $\dot{V}_E/\dot{V}_{O_2}$ at the terminal work rate which is hardly different from that at the AT.

EXPIRATORY FLOW PATTERN

The expiratory flow pattern can be useful in detecting airway obstruction during exercise. The normal expiratory flow peaks close to the middle of expiration. The expiratory flow pattern of the patient with obstructive airway disease has a very early peak and appears trapezoidal because the sustained exhalation effort results in an only slightly decreasing flow without an end expiratory pause during expiration (Fig. 3-18). This pattern can normalize in asthmatics, postbronchodilatation (see Fig. 3-18). While the expiratory flow pattern gives only qualitative evidence of airflow obstruction during exercise, it is obtained simply by recording expired airflow with a pneumotachometer. More complex approaches, such as flow-volume analysis, might add further information on disturbances in lung mechanics during exercise.

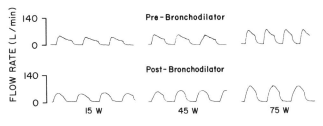

EXPIRATORY FLOW DURING EXERCISE

Fig. 3-18. Expiratory flow pattern in an asthmatic subject at increasing work rates before and after bronchodilator therapy. (From Brown, H.V., Wasserman, K., and Whipp, B.J.: Strategies of exercise testing in chronic lung disease. Bull. Europ. Physiopath. Resp. *13*:409–423, 1977.)

TIDAL VOLUME/INSPIRATORY CAPACITY RATIO (VT/IC)

This ratio is usually abnormal in patients with stiff lung syndromes such as pulmonary fibrosis. Normally, VT increases during exercise but it rarely exceeds 80% of the IC determined from resting pulmonary function tests. However, patients with restrictive lung diseases have a reduced IC and a limited ability to increase their VT in response to exercise (see Fig. 3-10). In these patients, as the work rate is incremented, the VT/IC characteristically exceeds 80% and the VT reaches an asymptote near the IC at a relatively low work rate. This is distinctly abnormal. The limited increase in VT requires a high breathing rate to achieve the $\dot{V}E$ needed for exercise. While we routinely relate VT to both the VC and the IC (see Chapter 8), we have found the VT/IC ratio to be more helpful.

PLASMA BICARBONATE AND ACID-BASE RESPONSE

Subjects making a good effort during an incremental exercise test to their tolerance limit normally develop a significant metabolic acidosis by the terminal work rate, even for relatively short incremental exercise testing protocols (8 to 12 minutes) such as those used routinely in our laboratory (see Fig. 3-19). But the

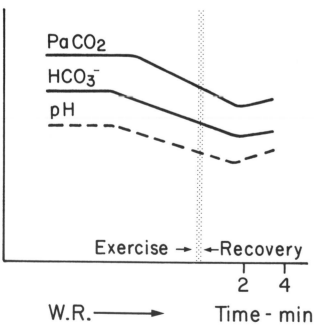

FIG. 3-19. Arterial P_{CO_2}, bicarbonate, and pH as related to increasing work rate and recovery. The stippled vertical bar indicates the point at which exercise stops. Note that the decrease in Pa_{CO_2} is delayed relative to the decrease in [HCO_3^-] and pH (the period of isocapnic buffering). Also note that the P_{CO_2}, [HCO_3^-], and pH continue to decrease in the recovery period with the lowest values at approximately 2 minutes of recovery.

greatest reduction in [HCO_3^-] and pH is noted about 2 minutes after the cessation of the test (see Chapter 6 and Chapter 8). We expect the [HCO_3^-] after 2 minutes of recovery to decrease at least 6 mEq/L from the resting value if the effort is good and the patient is not limited by a respiratory disorder. The further decrease in [HCO_3^-] and pH during the immediate recovery period is probably secondary to the relatively high perfusion of recovering muscles.

Exercise Testing — Constant Work Rate

While the primary gas exchange variables such as $\dot{V}O_2$, $\dot{V}CO_2$, $\dot{V}E$, HR, and blood gas values can be measured during a constant work rate test, much of what we feel are the most important discriminating measurements are easier and quicker to obtain during incremental testing. However, constant work rate tests permit the study of physiological responses reflecting the function of specific organ systems or the investigation of control mechanisms. Figure 2-19 illustrates the physiological determinants of each phase of the gas exchange kinetics in response to constant work rate exercise.

PHASE I OXYGEN UPTAKE KINETICS

Normally, oxygen uptake abruptly increases at the start of exercise (Phase I) because of the immediate increase in blood flow through the lungs, resulting from the increased venous return, cardiac inotropy, and heart rate (see Figs. 2-18 and 2-19). Increased pulmonary blood flow is the predominant mechanism accounting for the increase in $\dot{V}O_2$ during the first 15 sec of exercise. Under conditions in which pulmonary blood flow fails to increase abruptly at the start of exercise, the Phase I increase in oxygen uptake is attenuated (see Fig. 3-20). This reduced Phase I increase in oxygen uptake may be found in disorders that limit the increase in pulmonary blood flow at the start of exercise.[26,27] A reduced ventilatory response in Phase I will not discernibly mask the normal rapid increase in $\dot{V}O_2$.[28]

PHASE II OXYGEN UPTAKE KINETICS

Phase II is the period after the first 15 sec of exercise when blood in the muscles at the time of the start of exercise reaches the lungs and influences gas exchange. Phase II ends when gas exchange reaches a steady state or by 3 minutes. For work below the *AT*, $\dot{V}CO_2$ rises slower than $\dot{V}O_2$ during Phase II because of the relatively high CO_2 solubility in tissues (see Fig. 3-21). Therefore, R transiently decreases.[29] Be-

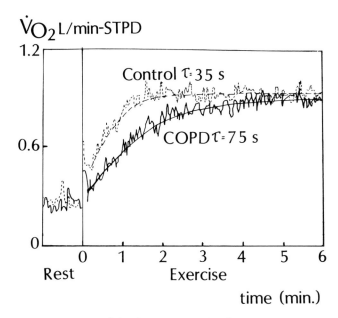

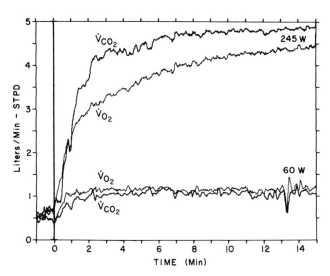

FIG. 3-20. Pattern of alveolar oxygen uptake ($\dot{V}_{O_2}$) in a patient with chronic obstructive pulmonary disease and a matched normal subject during the performance of 40 watts cycle ergometer exercise. Note that $\dot{V}_{O_2}$ during Phase I (the first 15 seconds of exercise) is less in this COPD patient and that the rate of rise of $\dot{V}_{O_2}$ to its asymptote during Phase II is also reduced, as shown by the longer time constant (τ). (Courtesy of Dr. L.E. Nery.)

FIG. 3-21. $\dot{V}_{O_2}$ and $\dot{V}_{CO_2}$ relationships in a normal subject exercising at a work rate below the AT (60W) and above the AT (245W). $\dot{V}_{O_2}$ kinetics are faster than $\dot{V}_{CO_2}$ kinetics below the AT. Above the AT, $\dot{V}_{CO_2}$ rises more rapidly relative to $\dot{V}_{O_2}$ because the latter is slowed due to the mechanisms described in section on metabolic-cardiovascular-ventilatory coupling in Chapter 2, while the former is enhanced by the additional CO_2 produced from $[HCO_3^-]$ as it buffers the $[H^+]$ produced in association with lactate. (Courtesy of Dr. W.L. Roston.)

cause $\dot{V}_E$ increases more closely with $\dot{V}_{CO_2}$ than with $\dot{V}_{O_2}$, this reflects hypoventilation with respect to O_2; therefore, $P_{A_{O_2}}$ decreases causing a transient mild hypoxemia until R reaches its steady-state value.[30] The degree to which gas exchange at the lungs lags behind cell gas exchange depends on the blood flow through the exercising tissues, tissue gas storage characteristics, and the circulation time from the exercising muscles to the lungs (i.e., the physiological components of the transfer between cellular and pulmonary gas exchange). A relatively high blood flow response will limit the decrease in tissue P_{O_2} and increase in tissue P_{CO_2}, thereby resulting in only a small change in tissue gas stores. This should be reflected as a relatively small decrease in R during Phase II. A small increase in tissue blood flow will result in more utilization of tissue and blood (venous) O_2 stores and increased venous P_{CO_2} and tissue CO_2 stores (provided that there is no appreciable lactate production at this time). This should be reflected as a relatively large decrease in R during Phase II. Because bicarbonate buffers lactic acid above the AT, CO_2 coming from $[HCO_3^-]$ breakdown adds to CO_2 from aerobic metabolism and may cause $\dot{V}_{CO_2}$ to rise faster than $\dot{V}_{O_2}$ (see Fig. 3-21).

ANAEROBIC THRESHOLD

When a subject exercises at a constant work rate below his anaerobic threshold, $\dot{V}_{O_2}$ reaches a steady

state or constant value within 3 minutes (see Fig. 3-22). This means that cellular oxidative mechanisms are being satisfied solely by atmospheric O_2, and that Phase II (the component that reflects decreasing mixed venous oxygen content and increasing cardiac output) has been completed. In a steady-state below the AT, there are no anaerobic mechanisms supporting the energetics and the O_2 debt has reached a maximum.[31] However, constant work rate

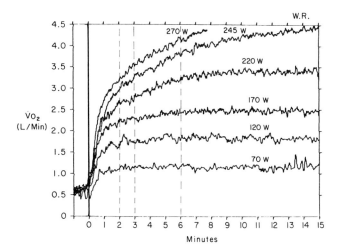

FIG. 3-22. $\dot{V}_{O_2}$ as related to time for various work rates in the same subject. The values to the left of the zero time marks are those for unloaded cycling. For work rates below the AT, the $\dot{V}_{O_2}$ at 6 minutes is the same as that at 3 minutes. For work above the AT, the sixth minute $\dot{V}_{O_2}$ becomes progressively greater than the 3 minute value, the higher the work rate. (Courtesy of Dr. W.L. Roston.)

exercise performed above the anaerobic threshold results in a delay or an inability to reach a constant $\dot{V}O_2$. $\dot{V}O_2$ continues to increase even after 3 minutes, the rate depending on the fractional distance between AT and $\dot{V}O_2$ max (Fig. 3-23). Thus to determine if a specific work rate is above the AT, measurement of $\dot{V}O_2$ at 3 and 6 minutes during a 6-minute constant work rate test is very helpful. If the 6 minute $\dot{V}O_2$ is greater than the 3 minute $\dot{V}O_2$, then the work rate is above the AT. The $\Delta\dot{V}O_2$ (6-3) correlates well with the lactate increase, as shown in Figure 2-13.

CAROTID BODY CONTRIBUTION TO VENTILATION

It is possible to evaluate the role of the carotid bodies in the ventilatory response to exercise by several techniques.[32,33] However, we find a modified Dejours test[34] performed during moderate exercise[5,35,36] to be most informative and particularly applicable to patients with lung diseases. In the steady state of an air breathing exercise test, the surreptitious switch to 100% oxygen results in an almost

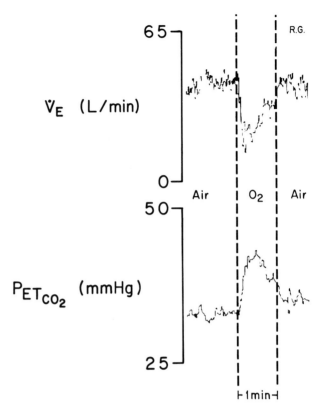

FIG. 3-24. Illustration of a safe test for assessing carotid body contribution to ventilation during exercise. Study is that of a patient with pulmonary alveolar proteinosis with a $Pa_{O_2}=54$ during exercise. A work rate is selected at which the patient can perform without difficulty and for which a steady state in ventilation is reached by 4 to 5 minutes. When $\dot{V}E$ is constant, the inspired gas is switched from air to 100% oxygen for one minute. $\dot{V}E$ decreases to a nadir within several breaths and, as a consequence, PET_{CO_2} rises. After 15 seconds, $\dot{V}E$ spontaneously starts to rebound toward the air-breathing value due to CO_2 stimulation of central chemoreceptors. By 45 seconds, $\dot{V}E$ becomes relatively constant at a reduced value and PET_{CO_2} levels off at an elevated value as compared to the control period. Thus, three phases in ventilation are observed when switching to 100% oxygen breathing: the first 15 seconds when the carotid bodies are attenuated maximally, the period between 15 and 45 seconds which shows a rebound in $\dot{V}E$ caused by the increase in arterial P_{CO_2}, and the period after 45 seconds when $\dot{V}E$ and PET_{CO_2} reach a constant value. The abrupt changes in $\dot{V}E$ in response to the O_2 switch and return to air breathing reflects the very rapid control that the carotid bodies exert in the regulation of ventilation. (From Wasserman, K., Whipp, B.J., and Davis, J.A.: Respiratory physiology of exercise: Metabolism, gas exchange, and ventilatory control. In Int. Rev. Physiol. III, Vol. 23. Edited by J.G. Widdicombe. Baltimore, University Park Press. 1981, pp. 149–211.)

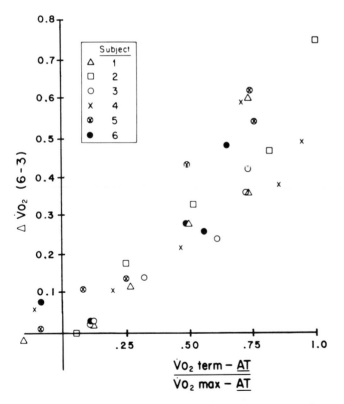

FIG. 3-23. Difference between the 6 minute and the 3 minute $\dot{V}O_2$ for constant work rate exercise [$\Delta\dot{V}O_2(6-3)$], as related to the fraction of the distance between the $\dot{V}O_2$ max and AT of the asymptotic $\dot{V}O_2$ at the termination of exercise ($\dot{V}O_2$ term) and the AT (Modified from Roston, W.L., Whipp, B.J., Davis, J.A., Effros, R.M., and Wasserman, K.: Oxygen uptake kinetics and lactate concentration during exercise in man (to be published).

immediate decrease in ventilation (within one or two breaths) if the carotid bodies actively contribute to the ventilatory drive. By continuously monitoring ventilation, breath-by-breath, the magnitude of the decrement in ventilation can be measured (see Fig. 3-24). This decrement reflects the carotid body contribution to the ventilatory drive. After about 15 to 30 seconds, ventilation will start increasing back toward its control value despite continued breathing of 100% O_2 because the Pa_{CO_2} increases consequent to the transient ventilatory decrease, and this stimulates the central chemoreceptors. This test is rapidly done, lasting only about 1 to 2 minutes of the exercise, and is safe. It could be done at work rates below or above *AT.*

Summary

Changes in O_2 uptake and CO_2 output by the lungs reflect changes in cell respiration induced by exercise. Changes in cardiac output and ventilation also occur in response to changes in cell respiration. Thus measurements that interrelate these variables in response to work rate perturbations can be used to assess the function of the organ systems involved in gas transport. Defects in the coupling of external respiration to internal respiration result in characteristic gas exchange abnormalities which are often unique to the limiting organ system. For example, while diseases of the heart, the lungs, and the peripheral and pulmonary circulations all result in demonstrable abnormalities in gas exchange, each manifests specific and relatively unique abnormalities which are most evident from measurements of function during exercise testing. The effect of various disease states on these measurements is described in Chapter 4.

References

1. Wallace, A.G.: Electrical activity of the heart. *In* The Heart. Edited by J.W. Hurst. New York, McGraw-Hill, 1982.
2. Taylor, H.L., Buskirk, E., and Henschel, A.: Maximal oxygen intake as an objective measure of cardio-respiratory performance. J. Appl. Physiol., *8*:73–80, 1955.
3. Cooper, D.M., Weiler-Ravell, D., Whipp, B.J., and Wasserman, K.: Aerobic parameters of exercise as a function of body size during growth in children. J. Appl. Physiol., *56*:628–635, 1984.
4. DiPrampero, P.E.: Energetics of muscular exercise. Rev. Physiol. Biochem. Pharmacol., *88*:143–222, 1981.
5. Hansen, J.E., Sue, D.Y., and Wasserman, K.: Predicted values for clinical exercise testing. Am. Rev. Respir. Dis., *129*:S49–S55, 1984.
6. Wasserman, K., and Whipp, B.J.: Exercise physiology in health and disease. Am. Rev. Respir. Dis., *112*:219–249, 1975.
7. Linnarsson, D.: Dynamics of pulmonary gas exchange and heart rate changes at start and end of exercise. Acta Physiol. Scand., *415*(Suppl. 1):5–68, 1974.
8. Whipp, B.J., and Wasserman, K.: Oxygen uptake kinetics for various intensities of constant load work. J. Appl. Physiol., *33*:351–356, 1972.
9. Roston, W.L., Whipp, B.J., Davis, J.A., Effros, R.M., and Wasserman, K.: Oxygen uptake kinetics and lactate concentration during exercise in man. (to be published).
10. Whipp, B.J., and Mahler, M.: Dynamics of gas exchange during exercise. *In* Pulmonary Gas Exchange. Vol. II. Edited by J.B. West. New York, Academic Press, 1980.
11. Hesser, C.M., Linnarsson, D., and Bjurstedt, H.: Cardiorespiratory and metabolic responses to positive, negative and minimum-load dynamic leg exercise. Respir. Physiol., *30*:51–67, 1977.
12. Beaver, W.L., and Wasserman, K.: Transients in ventilation at start and end of exercise. J. Appl. Physiol., *25*:390–399, 1968.
13. Jones, N.L., McHardy, C.J.R., and Naimark, A.: Physiological dead space and alveolar-arterial gas pressure differences during exercise. Clin. Sci., *31*:19–29, 1966.
14. Weisel, R.D., Berger, R.L., and Hechtman, H.B.: Measurement of cardiac output by thermodilution. N. Engl. J. Med., *292*:682–684, 1975.
15. Wasserman, K.: Breathing during exercise. N. Engl. J. Med., *298*:780–785, 1978.
16. Buchfuhrer, M.J., Hansen, J.E., Robinson, T.E., Sue, D.Y., Wasserman, K., and Whipp, B.J.: Optimizing the exercise protocol for cardiopulmonary assessment. J. Appl. Physiol.: Respir. Environ. Exercise Physiol., *55*:1558–1564, 1983.
17. Beaver, W.L., Wasserman, K., and Whipp, B.J.: Improved detection of the lactate threshold during exercise using a log-log transformation. J. Appl. Physiol., *59*: 1936–1940, 1985.
18. Beaver, W.L., Wasserman, K., and Whipp, B.J.: Bicarbonate buffering of lactic acid generated during exercise. J. Appl. Physiol, *60*:472–478, 1986.
19. Beaver, W.L., Wasserman, K., and Whipp, B.J.: A new method for detecting the anaerobic threshold by gas exchange. J. Appl. Physiol., (in press), 1986.
20. Donald, K.W., Bishop, J.M., Cumming, C., and Wade, O.L.: The effect of exercise on the cardiac output and central dynamics of normal subjects. Clin. Sci., *14*:37–73, 1955.
21. Sue, D.Y., and Hansen, J.E.: Normal values in adults during exercise testing. *In* Clinics in Chest Medicine. Symposium on Exercise: Physiology and Clinical Applications. Edited by J. Loke., 5:89–97, 1984.
22. Wasserman, K., Van Kessel, A., and Burton, G.G.: Interactions of physiological mechanisms during exercise. J. Appl. Physiol., *22*:71–85, 1967.
23. West, J.B.: Ventilation/Perfusion and Gas Exchange. Oxford, Blackwell Scientific Publications, p. 8, 1965.
24. Farhi, L.E.: Ventilation perfusion relationship and its role in alveolar gas exchange. *In* Advances in Respiratory Physiology. Edited by C. Caro. London, Edward Arnold, Ltd., 1966, p. 177.
25. Fishman, A.P.: Hypoxia on the pulmonary circulation: How and where it acts. Circ. Res., *38*:221–231, 1976.
26. Nery, L.E., Wasserman, K., Andrews, D., Huntsman, D.J., Hansen, J.E., and Whipp, B.J.: Ventilatory and gas exchange kinetics during exercise in chronic obstructive pulmonary disease. J. Appl. Physiol., *53*:1594–1602, 1982.
27. Weiler-Ravell, D., Cooper, D.M., Whipp, B.J., and Wasserman, K.: The control of breathing at the start of exercise as influenced by posture. J. Appl. Physiol., *55*:1460–1466, 1983.
28. Weissman, M.L., Jones, P.W., Oren, A., Lamarra, N., Whipp, B.J., and Wasserman, K.: Cardiac output increase and gas exchange at the start of exercise. J. Appl. Physiol., *52*:236–244, 1982.
29. Wasserman, D.H., and Whipp, B.J.: Coupling of ventila-

tion to pulmonary gas exchange during nonsteady-state work in men. J. Appl. Physiol.: Respirat. Environ. Exercise Physiol., *54*:587–593, 1983.

30. Young, I.H., and Woolcock, A.J.: Changes in arterial blood gas tensions during unsteady-state exercise. J. Appl. Physiol., *44*:93–96, 1978.

31. Schneider, E.G., Robinson, S., and Newton, J.L.: Oxygen debt in aerobic work. J. Appl. Physiol., *25*:58–62, 1968.

32. Rebuck, A.S., and Slutsky, A.S.: Measurement of ventilatory responses to hypercapnia and hypoxia. *In* Regulation of Breathing. Edited by T.F. Hornbein. New York, Marcel Dekker, Inc. 1981, pp. 745–772.

33. Severinghaus, J.W.: Proposed standard determination of ventilatory responses to hypoxia and hypercapnia in man. Chest, *70*(Suppl.):129–131, 1976.

34. Dejours, P.: Control of respiration by arterial chemoreceptors. Ann. NY Acad. Sci., *109*:682–695, 1963.

35. Whipp, B.J., and Wasserman, K.: Carotid bodies and ventilatory control dynamics in man. Fed. Proc., *39*:2668–2673, 1980.

36. Stockley, R.A.: The contribution of the reflex hypoxic drive to the hyperpnea of exercise. Respir. Physiol., *35*:79–87, 1978.

37. Pardee, H.E.B., DeGraff, A.G., Della Chapelle, C.E., Eggleston, C., Kossman, C.E., Maynard, E., Schwedel, J.B., Stewart, H.J., and Wright, I.S.: Functional capacity — Classification of patients. *In* Nomenclature and Criteria for Diagnosis of Diseases of the Heart and Blood Vessels. 5th Ed. New York, New York Heart Association, Inc., 1953, p. 81.

Pathophysiology of Disorders Limiting Exercise

CHAPTER 4

MANY DISORDERS interfere with the normal metabolic-cardiovascular-ventilatory coupling needed for exercise. These include primary disorders of red blood cell production, the peripheral circulation, the heart, the pulmonary circulation, the lungs, the chest wall, respiratory control, and metabolism (see Fig. 4-1). Individually or in combinations, these limit exercise by causing symptoms of dyspnea, fatigue and/or pain. Table 4-1 lists the most common disorders and the pathophysiology causing exercise limitation. Pathophysiological mechanisms contributing to the exercise intolerance of each of these disorders and useful measurements for distinguishing them are described in this chapter.

Obesity (Table 4-2)

While the obese subject has some increase in resting metabolic rate ($\dot{V}_{O_2}$) relative to his lean body mass, the increase is even more marked during dynamic exercise because of the additional energy needed to move his large body. As adipose tissue is added to the body, there is not a commensurate growth of the heart or blood vessels to meet this abnormally elevated metabolic requirement of muscular activity.

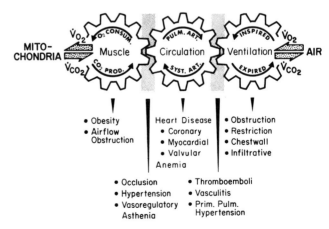

FIG. 4-1. Sites of interference in the metabolic-cardiovascular-ventilatory coupling for various disease states.

TABLE 4-1. *Disorders and Mechanisms Impairing Work Tolerance*

DISORDER	PATHOPHYSIOLOGY	PRIMARY LIMITATION
Obesity	Increased metabolic requirement; cardiorespiratory restriction	Low cardiorespiratory reserve
Peripheral vascular disease	Prevents normal vasodilation	Impaired muscle O_2-supply
Heart disease	Limits cardiac output (stroke volume) increase	Low tissue O_2 delivery
Anemia (or carboxyhemoglobinemia)	Reduced blood O_2-capacity	Impaired tissue O_2 delivery
Pulmonary vascular occlusion	Limited cardiac output increase; decreased efficiency of gas exchange	Impaired tissue O_2 delivery; increased ventilatory requirement
Obstructive lung disease	Increased airway resistance; abnormal $\dot{V}A/\dot{Q}$	Reduced ventilatory capacity; increased ventilatory requirement
Restrictive lung disease	Reduced lung compliance; decreased efficiency of gas exchange; exercise-induced hypoxemia	Reduced ventilatory capacity; increased ventilatory requirement; low tissue O_2 delivery
Chest wall disease	Decreased chest wall compliance; muscle weakness	Reduced ability to breathe
Metabolic acidosis	Reduced buffering capacity; low Pa_{CO_2} set-point	Increased ventilatory requirement
Muscle and Musculo-skeletal abnormalities		
Neuromuscular disease, arthritis	Musculo-skeletal coupling inefficiency; inflammation	Reduced mechanical efficiency; pain
McArdle's Syndrome	Muscle phosphorylase deficiency; lacks the ability to support metabolism with anaerobiosis	Pain
Miscellaneous		
Smoking	CO-Hb, hypertension	Low tissue O_2 delivery
Anxiety reaction	Hyperventilation with respiratory alkalosis; very regular breathing; breath-holding spells	Shortness of breath
Malingering	Very irregular breathing	Secondary gain

Consequently, for the obese individual to do any form of physical work, there must be a greater than normal cardiovascular and respiratory response.

However, constraints are imposed on the maximal performance of the cardiovascular and respiratory

TABLE 4-2. *Discriminating Measurements During Exercise in Obesity.**

high O_2 cost to perform external work

upward displacement of $\dot{V}O_2$-WR relationship

normal O_2 pulse when predicted from height

maximum $\dot{V}O_2$/body weight and *AT*/body weight are low

maximum $\dot{V}O_2$/height and *AT*/height are normal unless patient is extremely obese

high $P(A-a)O_2$ at rest which normalizes during exercise

normal VD/VT

*See Table 3–1 for definition of symbols.

systems by obesity, especially in the extremely obese. Because of the large mass, resting cardiac output per kg lean body weight is already high. During exercise, the further increase in cardiac output is limited.[1] The added mass on the chest wall and the constraining pressure from the abdomen effectively "chest straps"[2-5] the patient and causes the resting end-expiratory lung volume (FRC) to be reduced (in extreme cases, close to the residual volume).[6] This can lead to atelectasis of peripheral lung units and results in hypoxemia at rest. In addition, pulmonary vascular resistance can be increased, primarily as a result of pulmonary insufficiency but also possibly from mechanical kinking of blood vessels at low lung volume. Thus, cor pulmonale may be present.

The increased O_2 cost of performing mechanical work is predictable and well worked out for cycle ergometer work.[7,8] The $\dot{V}O_2$-work rate relationship is displaced upward, depending on the degree of obesity, but without a discernable change in slope (see

Fig. 3-2). The effect of adipose tissue distribution in the body, i.e., legs or trunk, on $\dot{V}O_2$ has not been investigated.

The maximum $\dot{V}O_2$ and AT are low when related to body weight, but are normal when related to height[8] and lean body mass.[9] The hypoxemia commonly present at rest, resulting from atelectasis of peripheral lung units, improves during exercise presumably because the deep breathing re-expands the atelectatic units. It is the only pulmonary condition in which arterial oxygenation improves during exercise. Thus ventilation-perfusion relationships are usually normal during exercise resulting in normal V_D/V_T, $P(A-a)O_2$ and $P(a-ET)CO_2$ values.

Peripheral Vascular Diseases (Table 4-3)

Because of the reduced diameter of, and pathologic changes in, the conducting arteries to the limbs, peripheral vascular diseases impair the normal physiological vasodilation essential for increasing O_2 flow to the working muscles. Thus the O_2 supply to the exercising muscles may not adequately meet the high O_2 requirement and the $\Delta\dot{V}O_2/\Delta$ work rate ratio may be lower than normal. While there is a compensatory increase in mitochondrial number in the ischemic muscle, it is inadequate to make up for the deficiency in O_2 flow.[10] Consequently, the ischemic muscles produce lactic acid and develop a condition inducing pain at relatively low work rates. When the lactic acidosis is evident in the central circulation, breathing is further stimulated.

The maximum $\dot{V}O_2$ and the anaerobic threshold are reduced, although the latter can be so low that it is often not discernible. Since lactate may not enter the central circulation in a detectable quantity because of reduced muscle perfusion, evidence of systemic lactic acidosis may be minimal. Some patients with peripheral vascular disease will have excessively high increases in blood pressure for the low grade of exercise performed. The heart rate at maximum ex-

TABLE 4-3. *Discriminating Measurements During Exercise in Peripheral Vascular Disease.**

low $\Delta\dot{V}O_2/\Delta WR$

leg pain

low maximum $\dot{V}O_2$

low AT

may have abnormal increase in blood pressure

*See Table 3–1 for definition of symbols.

TABLE 4-4. *Discriminating Measurements During Exercise in Heart Diseases.**

may have chest pain

ECG abnormality with coronary artery disease

low maximum $\dot{V}O_2$

low AT

$\Delta\dot{V}O_2/\Delta$ WR more shallow as work rate is increased towards its maximum

low O_2 pulse

heart rate-$\dot{V}O_2$ relationship abnormally steep

high breathing reserve

metabolic acidosis

*See Table 3–1 for definition of symbols.

ercise is usually relatively low because the patient stops exercise from claudication.

Heart Diseases (Table 4-4)

Since gas transport is the major and most immediate role of the cardiovascular system, cardiac dysfunction of all four primary types (i.e., coronary artery, valvular, congenital, and cardiomyopathic) will cause changes in the pattern of $\dot{V}O_2$ and $\dot{V}CO_2$ in response to exercise. Although mild coronary artery disease may only be manifested by ECG changes at high work rates, more significant heart disease will cause the maximum $\dot{V}O_2$ and the AT to be reduced. The $\Delta\dot{V}O_2/\Delta$ work rate ratio is usually normal at low work rates of an incremental exercise test but often decreases as the cardiac patient approaches his or her maximum ability to perform exercise (see Fig. 3-2). This is evidence of a large anaerobic component in the exercise energetics.

Heart diseases limit the increase in stroke volume and cardiac output during exercise. The resultant inadequate O_2 delivery to the skeletal muscles and the associated increased production of lactic acid likely account for the symptom of fatigue. Patients with coronary artery disease may or may not experience chest pain, and ECG changes consistent with ischemia occur when the exercise-induced increase in myocardial oxygen requirement exceeds myocardial oxygen supply. Development of increasingly frequent ectopic beats during exercise as the work rate is increased should also be regarded as evidence of myocardial ischemia. While patients with valvular heart diseases, congenital heart diseases, and cardiomyopathies commonly have distinctive physical, radiological, and echocardiographic findings, the functional measurements during exercise help determine the degree of impairment and guide therapeutic efforts.

During incremental exercise, the increase in HR as a function of $\dot{V}O_2$ is steeper than normal, indicating that the increase in cardiac output is more dependent on the increase in heart rate than normal. While the heart rate-$\dot{V}O_2$ relationship is usually relatively steep in heart disease, there are exceptions in which the heart rate response to exercise is inappropriately low. These include patients taking β-adrenergic blocking drugs and some patients with cardiomyopathies whose sinoatrial node fails to respond appropriately with tachycardia to the low cardiac output state.

Because of the relatively low cardiac output, mixed venous oxygen reaches its lowest value (widest arterial-mixed venous oxygen difference) at a low work rate and stays at this low value as the work rate is increased. Consequently, the O_2 pulse $(C(a-\bar{v})_{O_2} \times SV)$ reaches a plateau at a value that is low and occurs at an unusually low work rate. The $\Delta\dot{V}O_2/\Delta WR$ commonly becomes shallow near the maximum WR (see Fig. 3-2), reflecting the higher proportion of anaerobic metabolism because of limited oxygen delivery.

Patients with heart diseases develop metabolic acidosis at quite low work rates; this may become chronic, being present even at rest, and is accompanied by a low $PaCO_2$.[11] This necessitates a high minute ventilation that becomes more marked the higher the work rate (see Chapter 2, Determinants of the Ventilatory Requirement). In addition, in some patients with congestive heart failure, there is mismatching of ventilation relative to pulmonary perfusion resulting in an increased VD/VT and a further increase in the breathing requirement to maintain blood pH homeostasis.[12] The chronic metabolic acidosis and its acute exacerbation during exercise, and any accompanying increase in VD/VT, are significant contributors to the symptom of dyspnea in patients with chronic heart failure.

Pulmonary Vascular Diseases (Table 4-5)

Diseases of the pulmonary circulation, such as pulmonary emboli and idiopathic pulmonary vascular occlusion, characteristically result in reduced perfusion of some ventilated alveoli. Consequently, unaffected alveoli must accept a greater than normal perfusion and must be ventilated to a proportionately greater degree than normal to remove the metabolic CO_2 and maintain $PaCO_2$ at a normal level; the simultaneous ventilation of the poorly perfused alveoli is wasted (alveolar dead space). Since minute ventila-

TABLE 4-5. *Physiological Findings During Exercise in Diseases of the Pulmonary Circulation.**

high $\dot{V}E$ at submaximal work rates
high VD/VT
high $P(a - ET)_{CO_2}$
Pa_{O_2} decreases as WR is increased
$P(A-a)_{O_2}$ increases with increasing WR
low maximum $\dot{V}O_2$
low AT
$\Delta\dot{V}O_2/\Delta WR$ more shallow toward maximum WR
low O_2 pulse

*See Table 3–1 for definition of symbols.

tion is the sum of the "ideal" or effective alveolar ventilation and the physiological dead space ventilation, minute ventilation is increased in patients with pulmonary vascular diseases at rest and especially during exercise. The increased dead space ventilation results in a high VD/VT and persistently positive $P(a - ET)_{CO_2}$.

Arterial hypoxemia, which becomes progressive as the work rate is increased, is a common occurrence in patients with pulmonary vascular diseases, even when Pa_{O_2} is normal at rest. Several mechanisms may play a role. First, if the time available for diffusion equilibrium of O_2, already shortened by the reduced size of the functional capillary bed, is further shortened by the exercise-induced increase in pulmonary blood flow, equilibration of alveolar and end-capillary PO_2 is less likely to occur. Consequently, Pa_{O_2} decreases as work rate is increased.

Another cause of hypoxemia during exercise in patients with increased pulmonary vascular resistance is that of a right to left shunt secondary to the opening of a potentially patent foramen ovale. Approximately 20% of the population is thought to have an "unsealed" foramen ovale; this is normally closed, however, due to the positive left atrial-right atrial pressure difference. The combination of high pulmonary vascular resistance and increased venous return during exercise may be too much for the right ventricle to tolerate. Consequently, right ventricular end-diastolic pressure and, therefore, right atrial pressure would rise more than normal. If the right atrial pressure exceeds that of the left atrium, some of the right atrial flow passes through the unsealed foramen ovale, creating a right-to-left shunt. The development of a right-to-left shunt can easily be identified by repeating the exercise test while the subject breathes 100% oxygen. If this shunt develops, the arterial PO_2 should decrease well below its normal O_2-breathing value (> 600 mm Hg).

Finally, hypoxemia from low $\dot{V}A/\dot{Q}$ lung units is common in acute pulmonary embolism but is probably a less important cause of arterial hypoxemia in patients with chronic pulmonary vascular occlusive disease. In the latter, high $\dot{V}A/\dot{Q}$ lung units predominate and these do not cause hypoxemia.

Pulmonary vascular occlusions cause a hemodynamic stenosis in the central circulation, making it difficult for the right ventricle to deliver blood to the left atrium at a rate sufficient to meet the increased cardiac output needed for exercise. Because the cardiac output increase in response to exercise is reduced, abnormalities in maximum $\dot{V}O_2$, AT, $\dot{V}O_2$ difference, and O_2 pulse similar to those seen in patients with primary heart disease are also often observed in patients with pulmonary vascular disease. Physiological measurements during exercise are particularly helpful in diagnosing chronic pulmonary vascular occlusive disease. The abnormalities are those associated with a low cardiac output state and disturbances in gas exchange.

Anemia, Hemoglobinopathies, and Carboxyhemoglobinemia (Table 4-6)

Because we have been focusing on defects of the O_2 transport system that might result in exertional dyspnea, it is appropriate to consider changes in the properties of blood that might impair O_2 delivery to the mitochondria. Anemia, of course, results in a reduced O_2 carrying capacity. This compromises O_2 delivery to the mitochondria because the blood PO_2 falls more rapidly than normal as blood travels through the muscle capillaries unloading O_2. Thus the diffusion gradient of O_2 from the blood to the mitochondria might reach critically low levels before the blood exits from the capillaries of the exercising muscle, thereby requiring anaerobic mechanisms at lower than normal work rates to supplement the aerobic generation of ATP.

Similarly, conditions that cause a leftward shift in the O_2 dissociation curve (reduced P_{50}), caused by a decrease in 2,3-DPG, $[H^+]$, PCO_2, or temperature, or increase in carboxyhemoglobin or glycosylated hemoglobin, result in a decrease in capillary blood

PO_2 for a given amount of O_2 unloaded. Thus during exercise the PO_2 difference between the capillary and mitochondrion may not provide adequate O_2 flow to satisfy the mitochondrial needs. Consequently, the mitochondrial membrane proton shuttle (see Fig. 2-1) would not cause reoxidation of $[NADH + H^+]$ rapidly enough to maintain the normal redox state of the cytosol, leading again to anaerobiosis at reduced work rates.[13]

Subjects with anemia commonly experience breathlessness during exercise. Although the O_2 content is low, the arterial PO_2 is not reduced. Because the carotid bodies respond to arterial PO_2 and not O_2 content, the reduced O_2 content, per se, is not the cause of shortness of breath. More likely, the shortness of breath with exercise in the anemic patient is a consequence of the metabolic acidosis that accompanies the low anaerobic threshold. The acidemia results in an increased ventilatory drive (mediated by the carotid bodies) and a high minute ventilation at a relatively low maximum work rate.

The patient with reduced O_2 carrying capacity commonly demonstrates a relatively high cardiac output, with a higher than expected heart rate for a given work rate, i.e., a relative tachycardia. The stroke volume is normal or even increased in contrast to patients with cardiac diseases and disorders of the pulmonary circulation in whom stroke volume is reduced. But, as both the arterial and venous O_2 contents are low at the outset, the potential increase in the arterial-venous O_2 difference in response to exercise is limited and the maximum O_2 pulse is reduced. As in other disorders of O_2 flow, the maximum $\dot{V}O_2$ and AT are reduced. Measurements that reflect ventilation-perfusion mismatching are normal.

Obstructive Lung Diseases (Table 4-7)

Here we consider patients with chronic airflow obstruction, including emphysema, chronic bronchitis,

TABLE 4-6. *Discriminating Measurements During Exercise in Patients With Anemias, CO-Hb, and Conditions Associated With a Low P_{50}.* *

low maximum $\dot{V}O_2$

low *AT*

low O_2 pulse

normal VD/VT, P(a − ET)$_{CO_2}$ and P(A−a)$_{O_2}$

*See Table 3−1 for definition of symbols.

TABLE 4-7. *Discriminating Measurements During Exercise in Patients With Obstructive Lung Diseases.* *

low maximum $\dot{V}O_2$

high VD/VT

high P(a − ET)$_{CO_2}$

high P(A−a)$_{O_2}$

low breathing reserve

failure to develop respiratory compensation for metabolic acidosis

high heart rate reserve

abnormal (trapezoidal) expiratory flow pattern

*See Table 3−1 for definition of symbols.

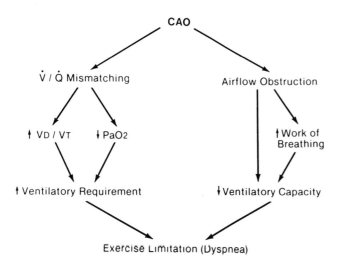

FIG. 4-2. Pathophysiology of exercise limitation in patients with chronic airflow obstruction (CAO)(from reference 31).

bronchial asthma, and mixtures of these three disease entities. The symptom that limits exercise in the obstructive pulmonary patient is almost always dyspnea. This is due to the difficulty in achieving the ventilation needed to eliminate the additional CO_2 generated during exercise at the level of Pa_{CO_2} being regulated by the patient.

Figure 4-2 conceptualizes the pathophysiology leading to dyspnea in patients with chronic airflow obstruction (CAO). The two major contributing factors are the decreased ventilatory capacity and the increased ventilatory requirement. In emphysema the decreased ventilatory capacity is due to increased airflow obstruction combined with reduced lung elastic recoil, while in chronic bronchitis and asthma the decreased ventilatory capacity is due to increased airway resistance. The increased ventilatory requirement is primarily due to inefficient ventilation of the lungs consequent to the mismatching of ventilation to perfusion, i.e., certain regions of the lungs are hypoventilated while others are hyperventilated.

This has the effect of increasing the fraction of the breath that is wasted (V_D/V_T), thereby requiring an increased ventilation to eliminate the CO_2 produced by the patient to maintain the P_{CO_2} at the same value (see Fig. 2-16).

Hypoxemia results from the underventilation of perfused lung units. While this stimulates ventilatory drive through the carotid body chemoreceptors, respiratory alkalosis is virtually never seen in these patients because of ventilatory limitation. In addition, respiratory compensation for the metabolic acidosis, which might develop during heavy exercise, does not occur in those with high grade airway obstruction.

As shown in Figure 4-3, ambulatory patients with stable obstructive lung disease regulate Pa_{CO_2} at a reasonably constant level despite increasing work rates. While regulation of Pa_{O_2} is less precise in these patients (see Fig. 4-4), it usually does not fall to very low levels, even at the patient's maximum work rate. The shape of the oxyhemoglobin dissociation curve generally allows arterial O_2 content to be maintained at satisfactory levels despite a moderate decrease in Pa_{O_2}.

The alveolar-arterial P_{O_2} difference ($P(A-a)_{O_2}$) is usually increased as a consequence of the perfusion of relatively poorly ventilated airspaces. It usually does not increase systematically with increasing work rate as in pulmonary vascular disease or pulmonary fibrosis. The arterial-end tidal P_{CO_2} difference ($P(a-ET)_{CO_2}$) is also high, reflecting mismatching of ventilation to perfusion. In addition, it remains relatively constant and elevated as work rate is increased, rather than decreasing as in normal subjects.

Dyspnea depends on a balance between how much air must be breathed to keep pace with metabolism and how much can be breathed. Patients with chronic airflow obstruction must breathe more to maintain blood gases and pH but cannot breathe as much as a normal subject. The maximal voluntary ventilation (MVV) is probably the best measure of

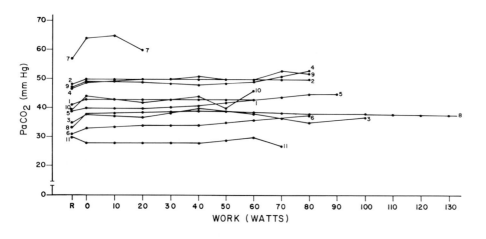

FIG. 4-3. Pa_{CO_2} as related to work rate in 11 patients with stable chronic airflow obstruction (each point is a different work rate). The numbers on each curve identify the patient (courtesy of Dr. John D. Andrews).

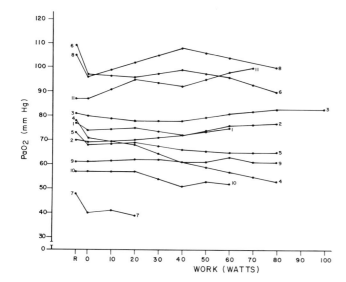

FIG. 4-4. Pa_{O_2} as related to increase in work rate for the same 11 patients shown in Figure 4-3 (each point is a different work rate). The numbers on each curve identify the patient and allow cross correlation with each patient's Pa_{CO_2} shown in Figure 4-3 (courtesy of Dr. John D. Andrews).

the patient's ventilatory capacity. Work tasks requiring ventilation rates in excess of this value obviously cannot be sustained. Thus the breathing reserve is decreased to values close to zero in patients with chronic airflow obstruction (see Fig. 4-5), in contrast to the large reserves found in most normal subjects[14-16] and those with heart disease.

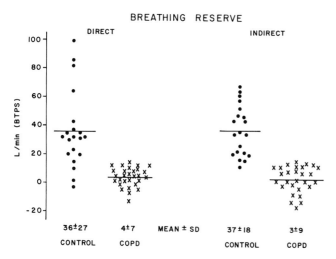

FIG. 4-5. Breathing reserve (MVV—maximum $\dot{V}_E$) for a group of normal subjects and a group of patients with stable chronic obstructive pulmonary disease (COPD). The values under each column show the mean ± standard deviation. Measurements are made using the directly measured MVV and the indirectly measured MVV calculated by multiplying FEV_1 by 40. Note that the breathing reserve in COPD patients is very small and the standard deviation is narrow, reflecting the importance of airflow limitation in determining exercise intolerance (courtesy of Dr. John D. Andrews).

While the maximum $\dot{V}_{O_2}$ is reduced in patients with obstructive lung disease, the $\dot{V}_{O_2}$-work rate relationship usually does not approach a plateau as is commonly seen in patients having circulatory limitation. This is because ambulatory patients with stable obstructive lung disease are usually more limited in their ability to eliminate CO_2 (ventilatory limitation) than in their ability to make O_2 available to the mitochondria. Generally, the AT is in the normal range. However, patients with severe airflow obstruction may not be able to exercise sufficiently to reach an AT.

The heart rate at maximum work rate is generally low (high heart rate reserve)(Fig. 4-6), but can be increased if the patient's maximum work rate can be improved through O_2 breathing or bronchodilatation. In contrast to cardiac disorders, O_2 pulse generally continues to rise normally with increasing work rate, although the absolute values may be reduced.

Examining the expiratory flow pattern can be useful. Typically, as shown in Figure 3-18, it has an early expiratory peak and then a sustained expiratory flow until the point of inhalation giving the recorded pattern a trapezoidal appearance.

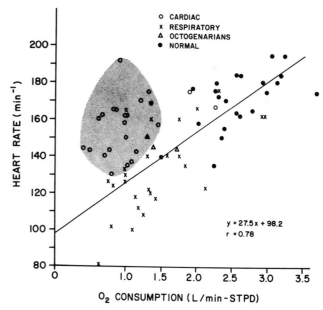

FIG. 4-6. Heart rate at maximal exercise for normal subjects, octogenarians, and patients with chronic respiratory disease or cardiac disease. The normal subjects reach a higher maximum heart rate and $\dot{V}_{O_2}$. Note that the octogenarians fall on the same slope as the younger normal subjects although their maximum heart rate and maximum oxygen uptake are less. Similarly, the patients with respiratory defects have a still lower maximum oxygen uptake and heart rate. The cardiac patients (in stippled area) have a higher maximum heart rate relative to the maximum O_2 uptake than that for the other subjects. (From Wasserman, K., and Whipp, B.J.: Exercise physiology in health and disease (state of the art). Am. Rev. Respir. Dis., *112*:219–249, 1975.)

Restrictive Lung Diseases (Table 4-8)

Pulmonary fibrosis develops from chronic lung inflammation. The severity is usually nonuniform so that some acini, including their blood supply, are completely replaced by scar tissue, whereas neighboring units that are less or uninvolved undergo compensatory hyperinflation. The net effect is a reduction in the total number of acini and, consequently, a relatively noncompliant lung with fewer lung units for gas exchange. While both the total lung capacity and its subcompartments are reduced, the predominant reduction is that of the inspiratory capacity. Thus the extent to which the tidal volume can increase with exercise is limited and the patient must increase breathing frequency to a higher than normal value in order to meet the ventilatory requirement for exercise. Consequently, the VT/IC ratio is high and approaches 1, and the breathing frequency at maximum exercise usually exceeds 50 breaths/min in patients with restrictive lung diseases. Ventilation at the maximum work rate commonly approaches the MVV.

Possibly because of the loss of lung units, the pulmonary vascular bed is reduced and the red cell transit time in the pulmonary capillaries is functionally shortened as the work rate is increased. This effect results in a systematic decrease in Pa_{O_2} as the work rate is increased, similar to that seen in pulmonary vascular disease. (This systematic change in Pa_{O_2} is usually not seen in obstructive lung disease.) In addition, low $\dot{V}A/\dot{Q}$ ratios might also contribute to the hypoxemia in patients with pulmonary fibrosis.[17] The ventilatory response of patients with pulmonary fibrosis is steep because of hyperventilation (reduced Pa_{CO_2} and high VD/VT. Therefore, worsening hypoxemia as the work rate is increased,[17,18] elevated dead space ventilation caused by nonuniform ventilation-perfusion ratios, and a rapid, shallow breathing pattern contribute to the primary symptom of patients with restrictive lung disorders — dyspnea.

TABLE 4-8. *Discriminating Measurements During Exercise in Patients With Restrictive Lung Diseases.**

low maximum $\dot{V}O_2$

high VT/IC

breathing frequency >50 at max WR

low breathing reserve

high VD/VT

high P(a − ET)$_{CO_2}$

Pa_{O_2} decreases and P(A−a)$_{O_2}$ increases as WR is incremented

*See Table 3−1 for definition of symbols.

TABLE 4-9. *Discriminating Measurements During Exercise in Patients With Chest Wall Defects.**

low maximum $\dot{V}O_2$

high VT/IC

high breathing frequency

normal $\Delta\dot{V}O_2/\Delta WR$

low breathing reserve

high heart rate reserve

normal PaO_2

*See table 3− for definition of symbols.

Pulmonary alveolar proteinosis is a good example of exercise hypoxemia that is primarily due to a diffusion defect. This is primarily an alveolar filling disorder with only minimal, or no interstitial pulmonary fibrosis. Commonly, vital capacity and total lung capacity are only slightly reduced and FEV_1 is normal. Because the mean path length from lung gas to capillaries is increased considerably in this disorder, diffusion of O_2 through the insoluble proteinaceous material filling the alveoli may take too long a time to supply sufficient O_2 to saturate hemoglobin. During exercise, when red cell transit time in the capillary bed is further reduced and its residence time shortened, even less time is available for diffusion equilibrium. Thus hypoxemia and increasing P(A−a)$_{O_2}$ result, becoming progressively more abnormal as the work rate is increased. The prominent feature then is a systematic decrease in Pa_{O_2} with increasing metabolic stress.

Chest Wall (Respiratory Pump) Defects (Table 4-9)

Defects of the respiratory pump include muscle weakness, chest deformities, rigidity of the thoracic cage (as in ankylosing spondylitis), and muscle and motor nerve disorders. These patients, like those with restrictive pulmonary disorders, have a limited ability to increase VT. Although their lungs are essentially normal, the maximum intrapleural pressure available to expand the lungs is insufficient to allow VT to increase normally as the work rate is increased. Therefore, to obtain the increase in $\dot{V}E$ required for work, these patients must predominantly increase breathing frequency.

The reduced maximum $\dot{V}O_2$ defines the degree of exercise limitation. The *AT* is generally normal or cannot be determined, and the $\dot{V}O_2$ increases normally with the work rate. Because the lung parenchyma is essentially normal, Pa_{O_2} is usually normal and does not decrease as the work rate is increased.

However, the breathing reserve will be quite low at the termination of exercise, a characteristic of conditions in which the breathing mechanics limit maximum exercise performance. In contrast, heart rate reserve is high because the reduction in maximum work rate results from the breathing limitation.

Metabolic Acidosis (Table 4-10)

Chronic metabolic acidosis can result from poorly controlled diabetes, chronic renal failure, chronic heart failure, or ingestion of certain drugs, such as large amounts of salicylates, which raise the organic acid blood levels and reduce blood $[HCO_3^-]$. This causes the arterial P_{CO_2} to be regulated at a low set point.[19,20] Consequently, for a given work rate, the ventilatory requirement is relatively high (see Fig. 2-15) and leads to an apparent increase in "sensitivity" of the respiratory control mechanisms (i.e., high $\Delta \dot{V}_E/\Delta WR$).

The presence of a chronic metabolic acidosis before exercise begins is evident from the resting arterial blood gases, i.e., a reduced bicarbonate and Pa_{CO_2} with a nearly normal pH. A high resting ventilation for the metabolic rate necessarily accompanies a low Pa_{CO_2}. During exercise, $\dot{V}_E$ will increase proportionally with the increase in CO_2 production. The slope of the $\dot{V}_E$-$\dot{V}_{CO_2}$ relationship, however, becomes more steep the lower the Pa_{CO_2} (see Fig. 2-16). Thus if the Pa_{CO_2} is maintained at 30 mm Hg during exercise, the ventilatory equivalent for CO_2 will be approximately 40 rather than the 30 usually seen in a normal subject maintaining a Pa_{CO_2} of 40 mm Hg (see Fig. 3-13). Without measuring arterial blood gases, a relatively steep slope relationship between $\dot{V}_E$ and $\dot{V}_{CO_2}$ and an elevated ventilatory equivalent for CO_2 during exercise (with R in the normal range) signify either chronic hyperventilation or increased V_D/V_T. Normal values of V_D/V_T, $P(a - ET)_{CO_2}$, and $P(A-a)_{O_2}$ during exercise confirm that there is no abnormality in the distribution of ventilation relative to perfusion as the cause of the increased ventilatory response. Thus the increased $\dot{V}_E$ can be accounted for only by the low Pa_{CO_2}.

Muscle Disorders and Endocrine Abnormalities

Little information is available concerning the metabolic cost of exercise in patients with muscle disorders. Because of a reduced motor efficiency,[21] patients with neuromuscular disorders with accompanying spasticities and motor incoordination presumably have an increased O_2 requirement for per-

TABLE 4-10. *Discriminating Measurements During Exercise in Patients With a Chronic Metabolic Acidosis.**

low $[HCO_3^-]$

steep $\dot{V}_E/\dot{V}_{CO_2}$ relationship

normal $P(A-a)_{O_2}$ and $P(a - ET)_{CO_2}$

normal V_D/V_T

*See Table 3–1 for definition of symbols.

forming physical work. We have not had the opportunity to evaluate these patients in the exercise laboratory.

There are a number of muscle enzyme deficiencies that limit exercise performance. For example, patients with McArdle's syndrome have an absence of muscle glycogen phosphorylase. Consequently, they are unable to exercise to work levels that require anaerobic mechanisms to supplement the energy generated by aerobic mechanisms. They are limited in their maximum work capacity to rates at or below their *AT*, and thus their maximum $\dot{V}_{O_2}$ is of the order of one liter per minute, i.e., the *AT* of a normal sedentary person. These patients experience severe muscle pain when attempting to exercise beyond this level, causing them to quickly stop. The $\dot{V}_{O_2}$-work rate relationship (work efficiency) appears to be normal for work rates below the level that induces pain in these patients.[22]

Diabetes mellitus affects both large arteries by atherosclerosis and small blood vessels by altering the capillary basement membranes. When under poor control, they also have a leftward shift in the oxyhemoglobin dissociation curve. Any one of these abnormalities should reduce the *AT* and $\dot{V}_{O_2}$ max. But, studies suggest that the *AT* and maximum $\dot{V}_{O_2}$ are reduced in diabetic children even when diabetes control is good.[23-25] The effect of exercise on blood glucose for work levels above the *AT*, when glycogen and glucose utilization is increased, has not been studied in these patients.

It has been demonstrated that the ventilatory response to exercise is clearly increased and Pa_{CO_2} is reduced in the female during the progestational phase of the menstrual cycle.[26,27] The effect of this increased ventilatory drive on maximal exercise performance in women is unknown.

Cigarette Smoking, Anxiety, and Malingering

Cigarette smoking can have acute effects on exercise tolerance. It affects primarily the blood, the cardiovascular system, and the lungs. The carboxyhemoglobin level is increased, thereby reducing arterial oxygen content and causing a leftward shift of the oxyhemoglobin dissociation curve. This reduces the maximum V_{O_2} and AT.[28-30] Heart rate, blood pressure, and their double product (heart rate $\times$ systolic blood pressure) are increased when performing exercise immediately after smoking.[30] Ventilation-perfusion relationships become abnormal, as evident from the increased $P(a - ET)_{CO_2}$ during exercise. Unless there is underlying airway disease, the effect of acute smoking on airway resistance is small.

Anxiety reactions occasionally cause dyspnea with exercise. One manifestation of anxiety is intense hyperventilation with development of severe respiratory alkalosis. The hyperventilation pattern is unique in that the breathing frequency is very regular. In addition, the tachypnea starts abruptly, as though "switched on," rather than gradually, as is normally seen during progressive exercise. Hyperventilation might actually start at rest, in anticipation of the exercise.

Another manifestation of an anxiety reaction described as shortness of breath may, in fact, be irregular or hysterical breath-holding. Observing the behavior pattern and the patient's facial expression may be helpful in detecting this problem.

It is important to discern malingering for secondary gain from other disorders. An exercise test in which both heart rate reserve and breathing reserve are high and AT is not reached argues in favor of poor effort. Often, the breathing pattern will be very irregular, with short periods of tachypnea alternating with bradypnea causing wide swings in Pa_{CO_2} and PET_{CO_2} unrelated to the changing work rate.

Summary

The major function of the cardiovascular and respiratory systems is gas exchange between the cells and the atmosphere. Therefore, impairments in cardiovascular and respiratory function will be most apparent during exercise, when cell respiration is stimulated. Since each component of the gas transport system that couples external-to-internal respiration has a different role, the pattern of the gas exchange abnormality might differ according to the pathophysiology. Recognition of these differences is helpful in distinguishing the limiting organ system in the patient experiencing exercise intolerance. Thus, while primary heart disease and primary lung disease both cause a reduction in work capacity, the pattern of the abnormality is different. For instance, in primary heart disease, the V_{O_2} at the maximum work rate performed tends to be low and the slope of the V_{O_2}-work rate relationship commonly decreases. Concurrently, the heart rate-V_{O_2} relationship is steep, the breathing reserve is high, and the heart rate reserve is relatively low. In contrast, in the obstructive lung disease patient, the V_{O_2}-work rate relationship usually increases linearly with a normal V_{O_2}-heart rate relationship, but the breathing reserve is low and heart rate reserve is high. Patients with pulmonary vascular disease and peripheral vascular disease manifest a still different set of abnormalities. By making measurements that address the gas transport function of each site in the external-to-internal respiration coupling, it is possible to deduce the relative physiological status of each component.

References

1. Alexander, J.K., Amad, K.H., and Cole, V.W.: Observations on some clinical features of extreme obesity, with particular reference to circulatory effect. Am. J. Med., *32*:512–524, 1962.
2. Bates, D.V., Macklem, P.T., and Christie, R.V.: Respiratory Function in Disease. 2nd Ed. Philadelphia, W.B. Saunders, 1971, pp. 100–101.
3. Gilbert, R., Sipple, J.H., and Auchincloss, J.H.: Respiratory control and work or breathing in obese subjects. J. Appl. Physiol., *16*:21–26, 1961.
4. Sharp, J.G., Henry, J.P., Sweany, S.K., Meadows, W.R., and Pietras, R.J.: The total work of breathing in normal and obese men. J. Clin. Invest., *43*:728–739, 1964.
5. Cherniack, R.M.: Respiratory effects of obesity. Can. Med. Assoc. J., *80*:613–616, 1959.
6. Ray, C.S., Sue, D.Y., Bray, G., Hansen, J.E., and Wasserman, K.: Effects of obesity on respiratory function. Am. Rev. Respir. Dis., *128*(3):501–506, 1983.
7. Wasserman, K., and Whipp, B.J.: Exercise physiology in health and disease (state of the art). Am. Rev. Respir. Dis., *112*:219–249, 1975.
8. Hansen, J.E., Sue, D.Y., and Wasserman, K.: Predicted values for clinical exercise testing. Am. Rev. Respir. Dis., *129*:S49–S55, 1984.
9. Buskirk, E., and Taylor, H.L.: Maximal oxygen intake and its relation to body composition, with special reference to chronic physical activity and obesity. J. Appl. Physiol., *11*:72–78, 1957.
10. Bylund-Fellenius, A.C., Walker, P.M., Elander, A., and Schersten, T.: Peripheral vascular disease. Am. Rev. Respir. Dis., *129* (Suppl.) S65–S67, 1984.
11. Nery, L.E., et al.: Contrasting cardiovascular and respiratory responses to exercise in severe chronic obstructive pulmonary disease. Chest, *83*:446–453, 1983.
12. Rubin, S.A., and Brown, H.V.: Ventilation and gas exchange during exercise in severe chronic heart failure. Am. Rev. Respir. Dis., *129* (Suppl.): S63–S64, 1984.
13. Butler, W.M., Spratling, L.S., Kark, J.A., and Shoomaker, E.B.: Hemoglobin Osler: report of a new family with exercise studies before and after phlebotomy. Am. J. Hematol., *13*:293–301, 1982.

14. Brown, H.V., Wasserman, K., and Whipp, B.J.: Strategies of exercise testing in chronic lung disease. Bull. Eur. Physiopathol. Respir., *13*:409–423, 1977.
15. Bye, P.T.P., Farkas, G.A., and Roussos, Ch.: Respiratory factors limiting exercise. Am. Rev. Physiol., *45*:439–451, 1983.
16. Pierce, A.K., Luterman, D., Loundermilk, J., Blomquist, G., and Johnson, R.L., Jr.: Exercise ventilatory patterns in normal subjects and patients with airway obstruction. J. Appl. Physiol., *25*:249–254, 1968.
17. Wagner, P.D., Dantzker, D.R., Dueck, R., de Polo, J.R., Wasserman, K., and West, J.B.: Distribution of ventilation-perfusion ratios in patients with interstitial lung disease. Chest, *69*:256–257, 1976.
18. Keogh, B.A., Lakatos, E., Price, D., and Crystal, R.G.: Importance of the lower respiratory tract in oxygen transfer. Am. Rev. Respir. Dis., *129* (Suppl.): S76–S80, 1984.
19. Oren, A., Wasserman, K., Davis, J.A., and Whipp, B.J.: The effect of CO_2 set-point on the ventilatory response to exercise. J. Appl. Physiol., *51*:185–189, 1981.
20. Jones, N.L., Sutton, J.R., Taylor, R., and Toews, J.: Effect of pH on cardio-respiratory and metabolic responses to exercise. J. Appl. Physiol. *43*:959–964, 1977.
21. Whipp, B.J., and Wasserman, K.: Efficiency of muscular work. J. Appl. Physiol., *26*:644–648, 1969.
22. Davis, J.A., Wasserman, K., and Andersen, T.: O_2 consumption as related to work-rate in McArdle's syndrome. (Unpublished observations).
23. Berger, M., Berchtold, P., Cuppers, H.J., Drost, H., Kley, H.K., Muller, W.A., Wiegelmann, W., Zimmerman-Telschow, H., Gries, F.A., Kruskemper, H.L., and Zimmerman, H.: Metabolic and hormonal effects of muscular exercise in juvenile type diabetics. Diabetologia, *13*:355–365, 1977.
24. Rubler, S., and Arvan, S.: Exercise testing in young asymptomatic diabetic patients. Angiology, *27*:539–548, 1976.
25. Storstein, L., and Jervell, J.: Response to bicycle exercise testing in long-standing juvenile diabetes. Acta Med. Scand., *205*:277–280, 1979.
26. Skatrud, J.B., Dempsey, J.A., and Kaiser, D.G.: Ventilatory response to medroxyprogesterone acetate in normal subjects: time course and mechanism. J. Appl. Physiol., *44*:939–944, 1978.
27. Lahiri, S., and Gelfant, R.: Mechanisms of acute ventilatory response. *In* Regulation or Breathing. Part II. Edited by T. Hornbein. New York, Marcel Dekker, Inc., 1981, p. 820.
28. Pirnay, S., Dujardin, J., Deroanne, R., and Petit, J.M.: Muscular exercise during intoxication by carbon monoxide. J. Appl. Physiol., *31*:573–575, 1971.
29. Vogel, J.A., and Gleser, M.A.: Effect of carbon monoxide on oxygen transport during exercise. J. Appl. Physiol., *32*:234–239, 1972.
30. Hirsch, G.L., Sue, D.Y., Wasserman, K., Robinson, T.E., and Hansen, J.E.: Immediate effects of cigarette smoking on the cardiorespiratory responses to exercise. J. Appl. Physiol., *58*:1975–1981, 1985.
31. Brown, H.V., and Wasserman, K.: Exercise performance in chronic obstructive pulmonary diseases. Med. Clin. North Am., *65*:525–547, 1981.

Protocols for Exercise Testing

THE OBJECTIVE of clinical exercise tests should be to learn the maximum about the patient's pathophysiological causes of exercise limitation: 1) with the greatest accuracy, 2) with the least stress to the patient, and 3) in the shortest period of time. The optimal examination will allow the simultaneous evaluation of the adequacy of the muscles, heart, lungs, and peripheral and pulmonary circulations to meet the gas exchange requirements of exercise. The test should enable the investigator to distinguish disorders in these systems from inadequate effort, obesity, anxiety, or unfitness.

For the differential diagnosis of exercise limitation caused by cardiovascular or respiratory disease, relatively complete gas exchange measurements should be made. Exercise with large muscle groups is needed to stimulate internal respiration sufficiently to stress the cardiovascular and pulmonary systems adequately; therefore, either a cycle ergometer or treadmill should be used for testing. Isometric exercise is of limited value since it is largely anaerobic, providing little information about the ability of the cardiovascular and respiratory systems to support the energy requirements of exercise.

The protocol selected for exercise testing depends on the purpose of the test. For instance, if one is certain that the only possible etiology for the patient's symptoms is coronary artery disease, then monitoring the electrocardiogram with 12 leads using the Bruce,[1] Naughton,[2] or Ellestad[3] protocol is satisfactory. The criteria for myocardial ischemia secondary to coronary artery disease are extensively described elsewhere.[3] However, if it is less certain that the exclusive cause of the patient's dysfunction is coronary artery disease, i.e., the patient might have myocardial ischemia or peripheral vascular, pulmonary vascular, lung, muscle, endocrine disease, obesity, or anemia as the underlying pathological disorder causing the patient's symptoms, or is limited by psychogenic factors, then a more comprehensive examination is needed. The protocol that we find most useful in providing a diagnosis of the pathophysiology of exercise limitation is one in which the work rate is increased by a uniform amount each minute (incremental test) as described below.

Description and Use of Incremental Work Rate Tests

With the advent of rapidly responding gas analyzers and computers it has become feasible to obtain a large amount of accurate metabolic, ventilatory, and circulatory data in a brief period of time with minimal stress and maximal safety to the patient. The following is a detailed description of our testing procedures.

PREPARING THE PATIENT

Instructions to Patient

At the time of scheduling, the patient is advised to wear comfortable clothes and low heel or athletic shoes, to adhere to his usual medical regimen, to eat a light meal no less than 2 hours before arrival, and to avoid cigarettes and coffee for at least two hours.

Initial Physician Evaluation

While the exercise system is being calibrated by the technician, the physician takes a history from the patient with particular emphasis on medications, tobacco use, accustomed activity levels, and the presence of angina pectoris or other exercise-induced symptoms. The physician examines the patient with particular attention to the heart, lungs, and peripheral pulses, determines blood pressure from each arm, and obtains an accurate shoeless height and weight.

Informed Consent

The patient is asked to make a maximal effort but is advised that exercise can be stopped at any time. The patient is advised of potential discomforts associated with the procedure and the kinds of information that will be obtained. Finally, the patient is encouraged to ask questions about the testing prior to giving consent.

Resting Respiratory Function

Recent spirometric data are accepted unless the patient has obstructive lung disease or performed erratically when spirometry was last obtained. Under these conditions, the VC, IC, FEV_1, and a direct MVV calculated from a 12 to 15 second maneuver are obtained when arriving at the exercise laboratory for testing. An indirect MVV can be calculated by multiplying the FEV_1 by 40. With poor effort, inspiratory obstruction, and some neuromuscular diseases, the direct MVV will be less than the indirect MVV. However, unless the direct MVV is reduced due to poor effort, it is used as the measure of the patient's maximum breathing capacity.

Equipment Familiarization

If the treadmill is used, time is provided for practice trials so that the patient can get on and off the moving treadmill belt with confidence. If the cycle is used, the seat height is adjusted so that the legs are nearly completely extended when the pedals are at their lowest point. Since during testing a mouthpiece will be in the patient's mouth, the patient is taught to use the signal "thumbs up" if everything is satisfactory and "thumbs down" if he is experiencing any unexpected difficulty. The patient is advised to point to the site of discomfort if chest pain or pressure (symptoms of angina pectoris) or leg pain is experienced. The code of finger signals for intensity is: the index finger if mild, two fingers if moderate, and three fingers if severe. In our laboratory we stop the exercise with a signal of moderate discomfort.

The mouthpiece and noseclip are tried. It is explained to the patient that it is acceptable to swallow with the mouthpiece in place or moisten the inside of the mouth with the tongue. The accumulation of large quantities of saliva in the vicinity of the gas sampling tube orifice can lead to plugging of the tube and erroneous gas concentration measurements. This problem can be minimized by having the gas sampling tube enter the breathing valve-mouthpiece assembly from above with the sampling tube tip free of the inner surface.

Exercise ECG

Silver/silver chloride ECG electrodes with circumferential adhesive provide good electrical contact. For 12 lead tracings the "arm" electrodes are placed at the lateral and superior corners of the scapulae and "leg" electrodes are placed near the right and left inferior rib margins between the midclavicular and anterior axillary lines (Fig. 5-1). (Lower positions increase signal artifact, especially in obese patients). V1 and V2 positions are moved one interspace caudad while V3 through V6 positions are in their usual locations. The three electrodes for the oscilloscope monitor may be positioned as depicted in Figure 5-1.

Arterial Catheter

If the study requires arterial blood sampling, a catheter is inserted into one of the brachial arteries using the Seldinger technique (see Appendix).[4] It is important to check radial and ulnar artery pulsations before

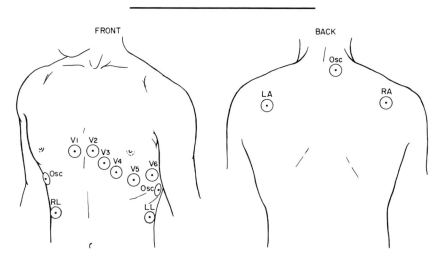

FIG. 5-1. ECG lead placement for upright ergometry. The V1 and V2 electrodes are placed more caudad than usually done for supine tracings while V3, V4, V5, and V6 are in their usual locations. The "arm" electrodes (LA and RA) are placed on the posterior shoulders while the "leg" electrodes (LL and RL) are placed anterolaterally near the lower rib margins. The three oscilloscope (OSC) electrodes are placed separately to minimize electrical interference.

and after catheter insertion. The catheter is attached to a stopcock and a miniature blood pressure transducer via a continuous flush device that provides a slow infusion of a heparinized-saline solution (10 units/ml). The catheter is long enough (20 to 25 cm) so that its hub can be brought around to the lateral aspect of the lower part of the upper arm (Fig. 5-2). The transducer is positioned on the upper arm at a height corresponding to the fourth interspace of the midclavicular line in the exercise position (midatrial level). To avoid spurious dilution of the blood specimen with heparinized saline, about 1/2 ml of blood is discarded before collecting each arterial blood sample. Each sample is collected for an integral number of breaths during an approximate 20 second period so that its gas tensions are representative of the mean arterial value and minimally influenced by ventilatory variations in alveolar gas tensions. Immediately after sampling, the catheter lumen is flushed with heparinized saline. If an arterial catheter is not inserted, arterial O_2 saturation can be monitored with a calibrated ear oximeter as an index of blood oxygenation.

TESTING

Measurements at Rest

An arterial blood gas specimen is obtained with the patient in the sitting position before being moved to the ergometer in order to avoid effects on the breathing pattern induced by the mouthpiece. A noseclip is put on the patient and checked for leaks and the mouthpiece is inserted. In our lab we typically continuously record expiratory and inspiratory airflow,

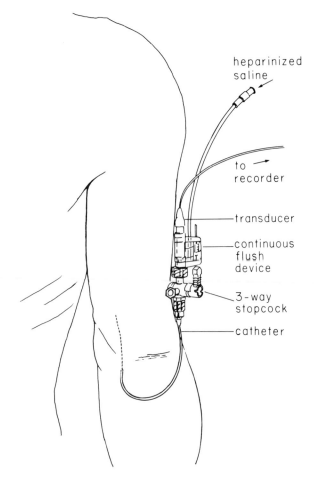

FIG. 5-2. Brachial artery catheter placement. A 25 cm polyvinyl catheter has been placed percutaneously in the left brachial artery. The dressings have been removed to show catheter placement. The hub of the catheter connects to a continuous flush device, three way stopcock, and transducer, the latter located on the lateral arm parallel to the fourth intercostal space in the midclavicular line in the sitting position (at the midatrial level).

continuous O_2 and CO_2 tension at the mouthpiece, and a single lead electrocardiogram on a multichannel recorder. Heart rate (HR), breathing frequency (f), $\dot{V}_E$, $\dot{V}_{O_2}$, $\dot{V}_{CO_2}$, R, PET_{CO_2}, PET_{O_2}, and O_2 pulse ($\dot{V}_{O_2}$/HR) are printed out every 1/2 minute from the breath-by-breath analysis by averaging an integral number of whole breaths, determined during the prior 15 to 20 seconds. These may be plotted out after the test as shown in Chapter 8. If an arterial catheter has been placed, arterial blood pressure is recorded continuously and arterial blood for blood gases and pH (and in some instances for lactate) is sampled at rest and every 2 minutes of exercise. If an arterial catheter is not used, blood pressure is obtained with a pressure cuff and ear oximeter values are recorded. A twelve-lead electrocardiogram is obtained with the subject in the supine position and again while on the ergometer, before exercise.

Unloaded Exercise

In order to overcome the inertia of the cycle flywheel, an accessory motor[5] can be used to rotate the flywheel at a rate of slightly over 60 rpm while the patient's feet are motionless on the pedals. As soon as the patient starts pedalling the accessory motor is turned off. This is particularly helpful for testing patients with limited strength in their legs.

At a verbal signal the patient begins 3 minutes of unloaded pedalling. The patient is advised to look at the rpm meter and to maintain a cycling speed of 60 rpm. A metronome is started at 120 beats per minute, i.e., one leg stroke for each beat of the metronome. A 12 lead ECG, blood pressure, and blood gas sample are obtained near the end of the 3 minutes of unloaded pedalling.

Incremental Exercise

Measurements are continued while the work rate is increased by a uniform amount each minute (Fig. 5-3). A 5, 10, 15, 20, 25, or 30 watt increment is selected, depending on the expected performance of the patient. Twelve lead ECG and arterial samples for blood gas and pH measurement are ordinarily obtained at least every 2 minutes. The technician and physician work cooperatively in observing the patient's facial expression, checking the blood pressure and ECG recordings for inappropriate changes and arrhythmias, looking for leaks at the nose or mouthpiece, observing for signals from the patient, and encouraging the patient to maintain the correct cycle frequency. The resistance of the cycle is removed if the patient evidences distress, if there is a fall in mean

blood pressure greater than 10 mm Hg, if an arrhythmia develops, or if there is ST segment depression of 3 mm or greater. The exercise is also terminated if the patient is unable to maintain cycling frequency above 40 rpm. If practical, an arterial blood sample is obtained during the last half minute of exercise.

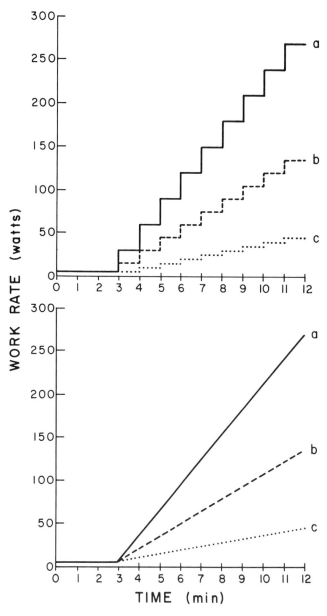

FIG. 5-3. One-minute incremental (upper) and ramp incremental (lower) protocols for cycle ergometry. In both cases the subject initially cycles for 3 minutes of unloaded pedalling. In the example shown, the work rate is incremented 30 (a), 15 (b), or 5 (c) watts per minute depending on the size and health of the subject. The increment is added at the start of each minute for the one-minute test whereas the increment is completed at the end of each minute for the ramp test. Larger or intermediate increments can also be used. The cycle is returned to the unloaded setting when the cycling frequency cannot be maintained over 40 rpm or the physician or subject decides to terminate the incremental exercise.

Recovery

The patient is kept on the mouthpiece during 2 minutes of recovery. In the immediate postexercise period, the patient is advised to continue to pedal at a slow frequency with no load on the ergometer. This prevents the precipitous fall in blood pressure that is occasionally experienced when vigorous exercise is abruptly terminated. A final arterial blood sample is obtained at 2 minutes of recovery.

IMMEDIATE POST-EXERCISE CARE

Immediately after removal of the mouthpiece, the physician questions the patient in a nonleading fashion about his symptoms when stopping exercise. A series of questions may be required in order to assess just what the patient means by his statement of limiting symptoms. It is important to differentiate calf from thigh pain and to determine the exact character of any chest discomfort.

If on review of the data it appears that the test was terminated prematurely because of insufficient effort, a repeat test after a recovery period of 30 to 45 minutes may be indicated. For instance, if the patient made an insufficient effort as suggested by the combination of high breathing and heart rate reserves, a low R, and only a slight fall in bicarbonate, the test bears repeating with greater encouragement from the examiner. The blood gas values are also reviewed before the residual blood in the syringes is discarded to allow remeasurement of any questionable blood values.

If the test is satisfactory and does not need to be repeated, the arterial catheter is removed, keeping direct pressure over the puncture site in the brachial artery for at least 5 minutes. With removal of the pressure, the site is inspected very carefully for evidence of external or internal bleeding. With adequate pressure and observation after removal of the catheter, hematomas can be avoided. With any evidence of bleeding, pressure is continued for at least another 3 minutes. A light dressing covered with an elastic bandage is then applied to the puncture site and the peripheral pulses are checked. The patient is advised not to use his arm for heavy exercise for the next 24 hours. The dressing and elastic bandage can be removed by the patient after several hours have elapsed.

FINAL REPORT

In our laboratory, after the entry of blood gas and blood pressure values, the computer produces graphical and tabular displays of the results of the exercise study such as those shown in Chapter 8. Others may prefer a different format. The physician's final report should include: 1) a short clinical history; 2) a description of the procedure; 3) subjective and objective observation of the patient during testing; 4) tabular and graphical displays (usually one page each) of the detailed data; 5) a summary table with measurements of resting and maximum exercise respiratory and cardiovascular variables; 6) copies of the ECG, expiratory flow, or blood pressure tracings if abnormal; and 7) an interpretation.

CRITIQUE OF ONE MINUTE INCREMENTAL TEST

Cycle or Treadmill (Table 5-1)

The treadmill has been in common use for decades. It allows one to exercise most ambulatory patients except those who are severely dyspneic, uncoordinated,

TABLE 5-1. *Comparison of Treadmill and Cycle Ergometers for Exercise Testing*

FEATURE	TREADMILL	CYCLE
Higher maximum $\dot{V}o_2$ and maximum O_2 pulse	+	
Similar maximum HR and maximum $\dot{V}E$	+	+
Familiarity of exercise	++	+
Quantitation of external work	− −	++
Freedom from artifacts in ECG, gas flow, and pressure tracing	− −	++
Ease of obtaining arterial blood specimens	− −	++
Safe (less musculoskeletal injuries)		+
Useful in supine position		+
Less vertical and horizontal laboratory space		+
Less noise		+
Less expensive		+
Portable	−	+
Greater experience in U.S.	+	
Greater experience in Europe		+

Code: More important advantage (+ +) or disadvantage (− −); Less important advantage (+) or disadvantage (−)

confused, or who have significant lower extremity musculoskeletal disease. The treadmill uses an activity familiar to everyone and allows the investigator the opportunity of varying both speed and grade to change the work rate. However, there are several disadvantages. The treadmill is frightening to some patients and is noisy, bulky, and expensive. Also, the laboratory ceiling height may be too low for use at the higher treadmill grades. With repeated experience on the treadmill there tends to be some increase in the efficiency of walking. Probably the greatest disadvantage of the treadmill is the difficulty in quantifying work. Any connection between the patient and the treadmill, except that between the patient's shoes and the treadmill belt, can decrease the expected energy requirement for body movement at that grade and speed. Railings, arm boards, mouthpieces, blood pressure measuring devices, and steadying hands all have the potential to reduce the patient's actual work rate. Length of stride as speed or grade is changed, shift of center of gravity, and change from walking to jogging all can affect the patient's metabolic requirement.

Even the most athletic patients require several minutes of practice in starting and ending the treadmill exercise before beginning measurement. Although injuries are rarely reported, careful surveillance is necessary. Because patients can lose their balance on the moving belts, it is wise to have additional help immediately available on the sideboard of the treadmill, particularly for elderly patients.

The cycle ergometer allows a more accurate quantitation of external work and can be used in the supine or upright positions. A minor disadvantage is that most individuals have a lower maximum $\dot{V}O_2$ and AT on the cycle than the treadmill, even though their maximum HR, maximum $\dot{V}E$, and maximum lactate are similar on both ergometers. In eight studies of male subjects the mean maximum $\dot{V}O_2$ on the cycle varied from 89 to 95% of treadmill values.[6] The cycle is less expensive, bulky, and noisy than the treadmill. Electrically-braked cycles maintain a given work rate despite minor fluctuations in pedalling frequency. Mechanical cycles are much less expensive but require exact pedalling frequencies for work quantitation. This may be important because some subjects appear unable to cycle at a prescribed rate. None of our patients have been injured using the cycle or treadmill, but we feel that the former is safer for those patients who are less well coordinated. We place the patient's feet in toe clips and sometimes, if necessary, bind their feet to the pedals, so that they do not slip out.

Because of less arm and torso movement on the cycle than the treadmill, there is less artifact in ventilatory and circulatory measurements and greater ease in obtaining blood samples. Because the tubular post supporting our cycle seat once buckled while being used by one very obese patient, we now use a stainless steel rod to support a conventional bicycle seat (covered with sheepskin) or a platform type seat. "Seat pain" can be a problem with prolonged repeated testing but is uncommonly a problem with the clinical protocols described above. In agreement with Astrand[7], we prefer the cycle to the treadmill for clinical testing because we can accurately quantify external work and thereby establish the patient's work rate-$\dot{V}O_2$ relationship, a critical measurement in assessing cardiovascular function.

Duration of Test

Balke and colleagues introduced the use of one-minute incremental treadmill tests for the study of fitness in a large military population.[8,9] Although Balke initially used an increment of 1% in grade per minute with a constant treadmill speed of 3.3 mph, he also used an increment of 2% in grade every minute. Several investigators, including Consolazio,[10] Jones,[11] and Spiro,[12] and their colleagues, used the cycle ergometer with the work increment increased by an equal amount every minute or half minute. Increments of 8, 15, 17, or 25 watts per minute, 10 watts per half minute, or 4 watts every 15 seconds have been reported.[13] We recently introduced the use of a continuously incrementing (ramp pattern) exercise protocol,[14,15] (see Fig. 5-3) and have used it extensively in children.[16] The results and duration of testing are very similar to the one-minute incremental test.

Several investigators[17,18] have stressed the desirability of matching the duration of the test to the patient's cardiorespiratory status. Tests that are too brief, that is with the work rate increased too rapidly, may be terminated too soon and not allow a sufficient quantity of data to be accumulated. Tests that are too long, that is with too small a work rate increase, are likely to be terminated prematurely because of boredom or "seat discomfort." We have found that tests in which the incremental part of the protocol is completed between 6 and 12 minutes duration give the highest maximum $\dot{V}O_2$ in normal subjects, although the differences with durations outside this range are small.[19] We know of no similar study in patients with heart or lung disease; consequently, we can only assume that the findings with patients should be similar. Therefore, we attempt to select a work rate increment that will result in termination of the incremental part of the exercise test in 8 to 10 minutes.

How to Select Increment Size

We select the increment size after considering the patient's history (especially the amount and intensity of his daily activities), physical examination (notably obesity and evidence for cardiac or respiratory disease) and his pulmonary function evaluation (particularly the FEV_1 and MVV).

If we expect the patient to have a near-normal power output, we estimate his $\dot{V}O_2$ at unloaded pedalling from his body weight and his maximum $\dot{V}O_2$ from his age and height. We then calculate the work rate increment necessary to reach the patient's estimated maximum $\dot{V}O_2$ in 10 minutes. The steps that we use to *approximate* the correct increment for the cycle are: 1) $\dot{V}O_2$ unloaded in ml/minute = 150 + (6 × kg); 2) maximum $\dot{V}O_2$ in ml/minute = (Height in cm − age in years) × 20 for sedentary men and ×14 for sedentary women; 3) the work rate (watts) increment/minute = (maximum $\dot{V}O_2$ − $\dot{V}O_2$ unloaded)/100.

For example, given an apparently healthy sedentary man 180 cm in height, 100 kg in weight, and 50 years of age, his anticipated $\dot{V}O_2$ unloaded = 150 + 6 × 100 = 750 ml/minute; his anticipated maximum $\dot{V}O_2$ = (180 − 50) × 20 = 2600 ml/minute. To obtain an incremental test duration of 10 minutes we would calculate an increment size of (2600 − 750)/100 = 18.5 watts/minute. Practically, we would select a 20 watts/minute increment and expect a test duration of slightly less than 10 minutes.

If we know that the patient has a MVV, FEV_1, or DL_{CO} less than 80% of that predicted, we would reduce the expected maximum $\dot{V}O_2$ proportionally; i.e., MVV or DL_{CO} of 50% of that predicted reduces the expected maximum $\dot{V}O_2$ to roughly 1/2 to 2/3 of normal. If the patient has hypertension or resting tachycardia, symptoms suggestive of angina, or evidence of chronic heart failure, we also reduce the expected maximum $\dot{V}O_2$, the amount being judged by our pre-exercise assessment of impairment. In each case we would reduce the size of the work rate increment to keep the total incremental exercise time at about 10 minutes.

Given a choice, we would rather overestimate than underestimate the work rate increment. With too large an increment the test will be brief and the patient will recover quickly, an advantage if retesting is necessary. With too small an increment, the patient may stop for ambiguous reasons and feel too fatigued for retesting.

Validity of Measurements

There has been some concern whether the maximum $\dot{V}O_2$ is as high in continuous incremental protocols as in discontinuous protocols, and whether the highest $\dot{V}O_2$ reached (maximum $\dot{V}O_2$) should be identified as the $\dot{V}O_2$ max. Taylor et al.[20] defined the $\dot{V}O_2$ max from their constant work rate tests as that occurring when an increase in work rate resulted in an increase of $\dot{V}O_2$ of less than 150 ml/min above the $\dot{V}O_2$ from the previous lower work rate. This criterion is appropriate for tests in fit subjects using large work rate increments, such as 2.5% grade change at a treadmill speed of 7 mph. In patients with an imposed increase in work rate of 15 watts, however, the average increase in $\dot{V}O_2$ is normally only 150 ml/min. Therefore, at increments of 15 watts or less, it is invalid to use the criterion of Taylor et al. to determine if the maximum $\dot{V}O_2$ is indeed the $\dot{V}O_2$ max. A single study[21] reported an approximately 10% lower maximum $\dot{V}O_2$ using a continuous rather than a discontinuous graded work rate test; however, the long duration (20 to 30 minutes) of these continuous tests could have accounted for the reduction.[19] In contrast, Maksud,[22] Wyndham,[23] and McArdle,[24] and their associates found no difference in maximum $\dot{V}O_2$ measured in continuous incremental tests compared with discontinuous constant work treadmill tests. Pollack and colleagues[25] found a plateau in $\dot{V}O_2$ in 59 to 69% of the continuous incremental treadmill tests they administered. We found a similar maximum $\dot{V}O_2$ in normal men using a ramp-pattern increase whether the increase was 20, 30, or 50 watts per minute.[15] Thus we believe that the $\dot{V}O_2$ max can be accurately measured with continuous incremental protocols of the proper duration.

Using the ramp-pattern of increasing work rate test, we also found that the *AT*, time constant for $\dot{V}O_2$, work efficiency, maximum $\dot{V}E$, and maximum HR were comparable to values found with constant work rate tests.[14,15]

Because we were concerned that nonsteady state incremental exercise tests might give different values for $\dot{V}E$, $\dot{V}O_2$, $\dot{V}CO_2$, $P(A−a)_{O_2}$, $P(a − ET)_{CO_2}$, and HR as compared to steady state, we studied 23 men (11 normal, 9 with obstructive lung disease and 3 with restrictive lung disease) during steady state constant work rate and one-minute incremental exercise tests (Table 5-2).[26] The steady-state $P(A−a)_{O_2}$ values ranged from 1 to 43 mm Hg and the VD/VT values ranged from 0.12 to 0.44. We found that $\dot{V}CO_2$, $\dot{V}E$, PaO_2, and R were slightly lower during incremental exercise than constant work rate exercise at the same $\dot{V}O_2$. However, the $P(A−a)_{O_2}$, $P(a−ET)_{CO_2}$, $PaCO_2$, $\dot{V}E/\dot{V}CO_2$, and VD/VT values were in close agreement in both protocols for both the normal and patient groups. Thus it is possible to make interpretable measurements of gas exchange and ventilation/perfusion matching equally well during either incremental or steady-state exercise.

TABLE 5-2. *Comparisons of* Pa_{O_2}, $P(A-a)_{O_2}$ *and* V_D/V_T *During One Minute Incremental and Constant Work Rate Cycling at the Same mean* $\dot{V}_{O_2}$ *(0.92 ± 0.03 L/min)*[26]

	N	Pa_{O_2}, mm Hg		$P(A-a)_{O_2}$, mm Hg		V_D/V_T	
		INCR.	CONSTANT	INCR.	CONSTANT	INCR.	CONSTANT
Normal	11	89	94	14	13	0.26	0.25
Restrictive lung disease	3	87	89	18	21	0.21	0.19
Obstructive lung disease	9	79	83	25	22	0.32	0.32
All subjects	23	85*	89	19	17	0.27	0.28

*Indicates significant difference between one minute incremental (Incr.) and constant work rate test at $p < 0.05$ by paired t test; other measurements are not significantly different.

Special Monitoring Requirements for Rapid Incremental Tests

With rapid incremental tests, frequent and accurate measurements are needed. Heart rate and blood pressure are not difficult to measure but accurate measurement of $\dot{V}_E$, $\dot{V}_{CO_2}$, and $\dot{V}_{O_2}$ requires special thought and understanding of the properties of the measuring devices. The reader is referred to the Appendix, Beaver et al.,[27,28] and Sue et al.[29] for descriptions of how to make these measurements and for an analysis of the potential errors.

Description and Use of Constant Work Rate Tests

DETERMINING $\dot{V}_{O_2}$ MAX

Historically, discontinuous constant work rate tests, each with a large increase in work rate with intervening rest periods, were used to measure $\dot{V}_{O_2}$ max.[31] When $\dot{V}_{O_2}$ rose less than 150 ml/minute despite an increase in the work rate, Taylor et al.[20] defined $\dot{V}_{O_2}$ as $\dot{V}_{O_2}$ max.

Advantages of progressively greater constant work rate tests for determining maximum $\dot{V}_{O_2}$ are: 1) the higher intensity work rates selected can be based on the patient's cardiovascular and ventilatory responses to the lower work level tests; 2) timed manual bag collection of mixed expired gas for measurement of $\dot{V}_{CO_2}$ and $\dot{V}_{O_2}$ near the end of each exercise do not require rapidly responding gas analyzers; and 3) there is an obligatory plateau of $\dot{V}_{O_2}$ that provides unequivocal identification of $\dot{V}_{O_2}$ max. Disadvantages are: 1) the repeated tests take considerable patient, physician, and technician time; 2) they are tiring and exhausting and may be more likely to result in injury to the patient; and 3) although such tests are often considered "steady-state" tests, this cannot be true at work rates at or above that necessary to insure a $\dot{V}_{O_2}$ max.

DETERMINING ANAEROBIC THRESHOLD

Constant work rate tests are useful for confirmatory measurement of the *AT* if the *AT* is uncertain after incremental testing. Gas exchange measurements are made for a 6-minute period at a work level expected to require a $\dot{V}_{O_2}$ near the *AT*. If the work rate is significantly above the patient's *AT*, the $\dot{V}_{O_2}$ will not plateau by the end of the 3rd minute but will continue to rise. Alternatively, if the work level is at or below the patient's *AT*, the $\dot{V}_{O_2}$ will typically reach a constant value by the end of 3 minutes and there will be no difference between the 3 and 6 minute $\dot{V}_{O_2}$ values.[32]

MEASURING VENTILATORY AND GAS EXCHANGE KINETICS

Constant work rate tests are used for determining the kinetics of cardiovascular, ventilatory, and gas exchange responses to exercise. Measurement of these variables during the transition from rest to low level exercise or between two levels of exercise using breath-by-breath analysis allows measurement of time constants or half times of the responses.[33] Averaging the data points of repeated breath-by-breath tests may give precise estimates of ventilatory and gas exchange kinetics.[34,35]

DETECTING EXERCISE-INDUCED BRONCHOSPASM

Although exercise induced bronchospasm can often be demonstrated after the usual incremental testing in the afflicted individual, it may be more evident after 6 minutes of near maximal constant load exercise.[36] It is necessary to obtain good baseline measurements of FEV_1 or some other index of airway obstruction immediately before exercise. Most investigators prefer the treadmill to the cycle ergometer for inducing postexercise asthma, although we have used both successfully. To induce postexercise asthma, it is our practice to increase the work rate to approximately 80% of the predicted maximal value for $\dot{V}O_2$ after a one minute warm-up at a lower work level. The patient inspires dry air from a bag filled with compressed air rather than room air since, according to current concepts, dry air aids in the induction of bronchospasm and reduces day-to-day variability if repeated tests are necessary.[37] After cessation of 6 minutes of heavy exercise, spirometric tracings are obtained at 3, 6, 10, 15, and 20 minutes postexercise.

MEASURING CAROTID BODY CONTRIBUTION

The effect of carotid body input to the medullary respiratory centers can be assessed by altering the PO_2 of the blood reaching the carotid bodies.[38] Normally, if the carotid bodies are contributing significantly to ventilatory drive, a rise in carotid artery PO_2 will immediately reduce the carotid body neural outflow and depress ventilation transiently. This can be detected by an immediate fall in $\dot{V}E$, $\dot{V}I$, and f, and a rise in PET_{CO_2} approximately 6 to 10 seconds after an unobtrusive switch of inspiratory gas from room air to 100% O_2 (Fig. 3-24). After one minute of 100% O_2 breathing, a switch back to room air results in a return to baseline $\dot{V}E$ and PET_{CO_2} values. Because ventilation is less variable during exercise than at rest we prefer to perform these measurements during moderate-intensity, constant-rate work. Steady-state levels of $\dot{V}E$ at moderate exercise are usually attained in less than 5 minutes. Thus the effect of the change in FI_{O_2} can be more clearly detected and quantified. Maximal effect is usually seen with an increase in PaO_2 to 250 mm Hg or more. If the patient has a normal arterial O_2 saturation and response, $\dot{V}E$ decreases transiently by about 15%. If a pneumotachograph is used to determine ventilation, an adjustment must be made in calculation to account for the difference in gas viscosity between air and 100% O_2. The calculation adjustment is about 10% if an inspiratory pneumotachograph is used. If an expiratory pneumotachograph is used, the correction will vary between zero and 10% as the expiratory PO_2 rises during the lung O_2 wash-in. On-line recording of ventilatory flow and/or VT and f and gas concentrations is desirable.

EVALUATING THERAPY

Patients with severe heart, lung, or peripheral or pulmonary vascular disease may not be able to tolerate 6 minutes of incremental exercise on either the cycle or treadmill. In such cases, the duration of constant load exercise at low levels (e.g., unloaded cycling or level walking at 1 mph) or changes in gas exchange, ventilation, or cardiovascular responses (heart rate and O_2 pulse) may give critical information regarding the effects of therapy. If the expected effects are subtle, it is desirable to minimize order effects and nonphysiologic effects by adequate patient training on the ergometer prior to definitive testing and by making therapeutic changes single or double blind.

Treadmill Test for Detecting Myocardial Ischemia

METHOD

Bruce[1], Ellestad[3], Naughton[2], and their colleagues and other cardiologists have developed and popularized a number of incremental treadmill protocols for detecting electrocardiographic changes of myocardial ischemia.

The Bruce protocol (Figure 5-4C) begins with 3-minute stages of walking at 1.7 mph at 0, 5, or 10% grade.[1] The 0 and 5% grades are omitted in more fit individuals. Thereafter, the grade is incremented 2% every 3 minutes and the speed incremented 0.8 mph every 3 minutes until the treadmill reaches 18% grade and 5 mph. After this the speed is increased by 0.5 mph every 3 minutes.

Ellestad's protocol (Figure 5-4E) uses seven periods, each of 2 or 3 minutes duration, at speeds of 1.7, 3, 4, 5, 6, 7, and 8 mph, respectively. The grade is 10% for the first four periods with durations of 3, 2, 2, and 3 minutes respectively, and 15% for the last three periods each of 2 minutes duration.[3]

Naughton's protocol (Figure 5-4A) uses 10 exercise periods of 3 minutes duration each separated by rest periods of 3 minutes.[2] The grade and speed of each period are as follows: 0% and 1 mph; 0% and 1.5 mph; 0% and 2 mph; 3.5% and 2 mph; 7% and 2 mph; 5% and 3 mph; 7.5% and 3 mph; 10% and 3 mph; 12.5% and 3 mph; and 15% and 3 mph.

In each of the three treadmill protocols described above, blood pressure is measured and multiple lead ECG's are recorded at each work rate and during recovery. The patient is carefully observed and the test terminated at the physician's discretion (i.e., decline in blood pressure, significant ventricular arrhythmias, progressive ST segment changes, attainment of a given heart rate), or by the patient's symptoms.

CRITIQUE

These treadmill tests have the advantage of having been used extensively for clinical testing. A survey in 1977 concluded that the complication rate for such "exercise stress testing" was 3.6 myocardial infarctions, 4.8 serious arrhythmias, and 0.5 deaths per 10,000 tests.[39] The treadmill was the ergometer used

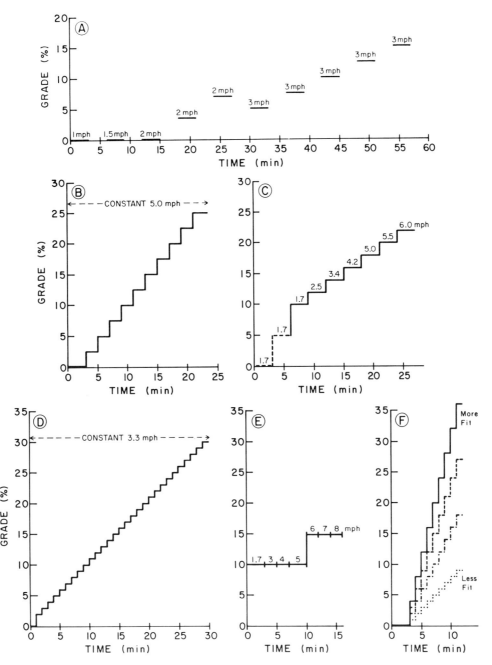

FIG. 5-4. Several treadmill protocols. *A,* Naughton protocol.[2] Three minute exercise periods of increasing work rate alternate with 3 minute rest periods. The exercise periods vary in grade and speed. *B,* Astrand protocol.[31] The speed is constant at 5 mph. After 3 minutes at 0% grade, the grade is increased 2½% every 2 minutes. *C,* Bruce protocol.[1] Grade and/or speed are changed every 3 minutes. The 0% and 5% grades are omitted in healthier subjects. *D,* Balke protocol.[10] After one minute at 0% grade and one minute at 2% grade, the grade is increased 1% per minute, all at a speed of 3.3 mph. *E,* Ellestad protocol.[3] The initial grade is 10% and the later grade is 15% while the speed is increased every 2 or 3 minutes. *F,* Harbor protocol.[19] After 3 minutes of walking at a comfortable speed, the grade is increased at a constant preselected amount each minute: 1%, 2%, 3%, or 4%, so that the subject reaches his maximum $\dot{V}O_2$ in approximately 10 min.

most often (71%) while the favorite protocol (65%) was that of Bruce. The maximum $\dot{V}O_2$ is generally 5 to 11% higher with treadmill as compared to cycle ergometer testing[6] whereas maximum heart rate is similar. As usually performed, $\dot{V}E$, breathing pattern, $\dot{V}O_2$, and gas exchange are not measured during these tests, and so other important cardiovascular and pulmonary system information is not available. Bruce has shown a high correlation of maximum $\dot{V}O_2$ and duration of treadmill exercise in his normal population.[40] Nevertheless, it is invalid to consider the duration of exercise a measure of maximum $\dot{V}O_2$ in patients with cardiovascular disease. The unequal duration of increment and variability in increment size are disadvantages of these tests although interpretation is usually not based on measurements of $\dot{V}O_2$. In addition, heart rate, per se, is a poor measure of exercise intensity in many patients with heart disease. Administration of β-adrenergic blocking drugs also modifies the heart rate-work rate relationship and must be taken into account when interpreting the results of exercise tests.

Rather than using the above protocol for treadmill testing, we[19] and Jones and Campbell[11] prefer using a constant treadmill speed and incrementing the grade by a constant amount each minute for the entire study. After 3 minutes of warm-up at a comfortable walking speed at zero grade (which may range from 1 to 4.5 mph depending on our fitness assessment), we use a constant grade increment of 1, 2, 3, or 4% each minute to the patient's maximum tolerance. We scale speed and grade so that the test will end in approximately 10 minutes after the work rate incrementing begins (Fig. 5-4F). We also make measurements of $\dot{V}E$, $\dot{V}CO_2$, and $\dot{V}O_2$. Following an initial delay of about 1 minute after the incremental period begins, this protocol gives a relatively linear increase in $\dot{V}O_2$ in normal subjects. The additional measures allow us to calculate values such as maximum $\dot{V}O_2$, AT, R, maximum $\dot{V}E$/MVV, $\dot{V}E$/$\dot{V}O_2$, $\dot{V}E$/$\dot{V}CO_2$, and O_2 pulse, thus adding considerable insight into gas exchange, ventilatory, and cardiovascular function.

Tests Suitable for Fitness Evaluation

A variety of tests have been used to evaluate individuals or groups without attempting to ascertain whether a particular system (e.g., cardiovascular, respiratory, or musculoskeletal) or motivation of the performer is limiting exercise. Such tests are likely to be used for children, young adults, military personnel, or laborers exposed to environmental stress (Fig. 5-4B and D). These tests are often considered measures of cardiovascular fitness and may allow division of the population studied into several levels of fitness. Because of their relative simplicity they can be repeated frequently with simple equipment.

HARVARD STEP TEST AND MODIFICATIONS

The original Harvard Step Test consisted of having the subject step up and down at a uniform rate of 30 step-ups per minute on a stool, bench, or platform 20 inches high for a period of 5 minutes, if possible, with measurements of pulse rate for 30 seconds after 1 minute of recovery.[30] Modifications include: 1) the

addition of backpacks, which add approximately 1/3 to the subject's weight, 2) reduction in the duration of the test to 3 minutes, 3) change in the step height to 17 inches for women, 4) measurement of heart rate *during* exercise, 5) change in the time of measurement of recovery pulse, 6) change in test scoring, and 7) use of a gradational step in which the height of the platform could be raised 2 centimeters every minute or 4.5 centimeters every 2 minutes.[30,41,42]

THE 600 YARD RUN-WALK

The 600 yard run-walk requires that the subject cover a 600 yard level distance in the shortest possible time.[43] He may intersperse running with walking but must try to finish as quickly as possible. A properly marked track or football field is suitable. For 87 male university staff and faculty members, time for completion showed a moderately good correlation (r = 0.644) with their maximum $\dot{V}O_2$ measured by an incremental cycle ergometer test (maximum $\dot{V}O_2$ range of 25 to 50 ml/min/kg).[43]

TWELVE MINUTE TEST

In the 12 minute field performance test, the subjects, dressed in running attire cover as much distance as possible by running or walking.[44] The distance covered was shown to correlate fairly well (r = 0.897) with maximum $\dot{V}O_2$ measured during an intermittent incremental treadmill test in 115 military personnel (maximum $\dot{V}O_2$ range of 30 to 60 ml/min/kg).[44]

THREE GRADATIONAL TESTS

The inclined treadmill, cycle ergometer, and step test used in a gradational manner for measurement of cardiorespiratory fitness each have proponents. Shephard reported the results of a study in which experienced users of each technique repeatedly evaluated their methods for 10 successive days on 24 men with maximum $\dot{V}O_2$ of 31 to 69 ml/min/kg.[45] These 24 subjects preferred the treadmill most and the step tests least. When continuous incremental tests were done, without prior information of each subject's previous measures, maximum $\dot{V}O_2$ was highest with the step test and lowest with the cycle test, but the difference was less than 5%. The authors concluded that "central exhaustion" limited treadmill exercise, leg exhaustion limited cycle exercise, and the combination limited stepping. The authors preferred the step test for field experiments on the basis of its cheapness, simplicity, and ease of calibration. They preferred uphill treadmill running for the laboratory tests because the maximum $\dot{V}O_2$ was higher and thigh pain was less than with the cycle.

CRITIQUE

All of the above mentioned tests are designed for studying healthy populations. In the case of the 600 yard run-walk or 12 minute distance tests, it is impractical to measure ventilation, heart rate, gas exchange, or ECG changes during the test; it is also somewhat difficult with the Harvard Step Test. Thus the ability to assess the cause of symptoms or to protect the health of individuals with serious cardiovascular disorders is limited. Although maximum $\dot{V}_{O_2}$, maximum $\dot{V}_E$, maximum HR, and maximum lactate can be measured in the three gradational tests (inclined treadmill, cycle, and increasing step height),[45] the emphasis in all six of these tests is to compare the fitness of communities differing in habitual activities, economic, residential, or nutritional status, or to assess fitness longitudinally. We do not recommend them for the evaluation of patients because of the difficulty in assessing relative contributions of different organ systems to alterations in work capacity and the attendant reduction in patient safety.

Arm Ergometry

METHODS

Arm work-rate protocols are similar to those for lower extremity exercise and are usually done because of dysfunction of the latter. The usual technique is to use a converted cycle ergometer with the axle placed at the level of the shoulders while the subject sits or stands and cycles the pedals so that the arms are alternately fully extended. The most common frequency is 50 rpm. Occasionally, upper extremity exercise is performed using wheel chair wheels coupled to a cycle ergometer, or by rowing, paddling, or swimming in paraplegics, oarsmen, athletes, or normals. To obtain maximal cardiovascular and respiratory stress, arm cycling must be done concurrently with lower extremity exercise.

If the person performing the test is normal and has not undergone specific upper extremity training, the maximum $\dot{V}_{O_2}$ for arm cycling approximates 50 to 70% of that for leg cycling.[46-48] Maximum $\dot{V}_E$ is similarly reduced while the maximum HR was only 2 to 12% less than leg cycle exercise. Thus the maximum O_2 pulse is less with arm compared to leg cycling.

CRITIQUE

Although arm cycling exercise has occasional uses, it does not stress the cardiovascular and respiratory systems as much as leg cycling or treadmill exercise. As such, it is a poor substitute for assessing the cardiovascular and respiratory systems, except when lower extremity exercise is impossible.

Twelve-minute Walking Test

METHOD

The distance covered in 12 minutes of walking (equivalent to the original 12 minute field test described by Cooper) has been used for assessing disability in patients with chronic bronchitis.[49] Each patient is instructed to cover as much distance as he can on foot in 12 minutes, for example, walking over a marked course in a hospital corridor. The patient is told to try to keep going, but not to be concerned if he has to slow down or stop to rest. The aim is for the patient to feel that at the end of the test he could not have covered more ground in the time given. A physician accompanies the patient, acting as timekeeper and giving encouragement as necessary.

Daily repetitions of the 12 minute test in 12 hospital in-patients on three different days showed a significant improvement in distance on day 2 over day 1, but not on day 3 over day 2.[49] In 35 patients with lung disease, the distance correlated significantly with FVC (r = 0.406) but not with FEV_1 (r = 0.283), while it correlated significantly with maximum $\dot{V}_{O_2}$ (r = 0.52) and maximum exercise $\dot{V}_E$ (r = 0.53).[49]

CRITIQUE

This is a relatively simple, practical, and objective measurement of exercise tolerance in patients with respiratory disease. It depends on a variety of factors including motivation, judgement of pace, endurance, cardiovascular fitness, and neuromuscular function. Nevertheless, it may be useful in serially evaluating patients in rehabilitation programs.

Isometric Exercise

METHOD

In this test, the patient's maximal force on a hand dynamometer is recorded. He then sustains 1/4 to 1/3 of this maximal force for 3 to 5 minutes while ECG and blood pressures are recorded.[50] The procedure is sometimes done in the cardiac catheterization laboratory because the patient is immobilized in the supine position by femoral vessel catheterization. Carrying weights in the hands while exercising on the treadmill has also been used as a method of combining dynamic and isometric exercise.

CRITIQUE

Because sustained lifting or forceful handgrip induces angina pectoris in some patients, isometric exercise has been used in the laboratory as a method for detecting ischemic heart disease. Sustained muscle contraction causes compression of the forearm vessels with resulting muscle ischemia, pain, and hypertension. Systolic and mean blood pressure, left ventricular work, and left ventricular end-diastolic pressure rise significantly, but there is a lesser increase in HR or $\dot{V}_{O_2}$.[51] In comparative studies, patients suspected of having coronary artery disease have less angina and less ST segment change, but a higher incidence of ventricular arrhythmia, with isometric than with dynamic exercise.[51,52] Because the muscle groups employed in this test are small, this is not a satisfactory method for inducing cardiorespiratory stress. Even with sustained isometric exercise of a large muscle mass, the increase in $\dot{V}_{O_2}$ is a small fraction of that for maximum dynamic exercise.[53]

Summary

A number of exercise devices, protocols, and physiologic measuring systems are available for the safe and economical evaluation of normal individuals, athletes, or patients suspected of having, or known to have, respiratory, cardiovascular, or neuromuscular disease. The specific exercise performed can be tailored to the diagnostic or therapeutic questions being asked and the facilities and technical and professional expertise available.

Ordinarily, a maximum amount of information can be obtained by making ventilatory, gas exchange, electrocardiographic, blood pressure, and blood gas measurements during a cycle or treadmill test that includes: 1) sitting at rest, 2) unloaded cycling or treadmill walking for 3 minutes, 3) one-minute incremental exercise with an increment size requiring the subject to reach his maximally tolerated work rate in about 10 minutes, and 4) early recovery. At other times, constant work rate tests, exercise tests with supplemental O_2 administration, or arm ergometry may be indicated.

References

1. Bruce, R.A.: Exercise testing of patients with coronary artery disease. Ann. Clin. Res., 3:323–332, 1971.
2. Patterson. J.A., Naughton, J., Pietras, R.J., and Gumar, R.N.: Treadmill exercise in assessment of patients with cardiac disease. Am. J. Cardiol., 30:757–762, 1972.
3. Ellestad, M.H.: Stress Testing, 2nd Ed. Philadelphia, F.A. Davis Co., 1980.
4. Seldinger, S.I.: Catheter replacement of the needle in percutaneous arteriography: a new technique. Acta Radiol., 39:368–376, 1953.
5. Huszczuk, A.: Personal communication, 1985.
6. Hansen, J.E.: Exercise instruments, schemes, and protocols for evaluating the dyspneic patient. Am. Rev. Respir. Dis., 129:(Suppl.) S25–S27, 1984.
7. Astrand, I.: Aerobic work capacity in men and women. Acta Physiol. Scand. 49 (Suppl.169):1–9, 1960.
8. Balke, B.: Correlation of static and physical endurance. I. A test of physical performance based on the cardiovascular and respiratory response to gradually increased work. USAF School of Aviation Medicine Project No. 21-32-004, Report No. 1, April 1952.
9. Balke, J., and Ware, R.W.: An experimental study of "physical fitness" of Air Force personnel. U.S. Armed Forces Med. J., 10:675–688, 1959.
10. Consolazio, C.F., Nelson, R.A., Matoush, L.O., and Hansen, J.E.: Energy metabolism at high altitude (3,475m). J. Appl. Physiol., 21:1732–1740, 1966.
11. Jones, N.L., and Campbell, E.J.M.: Clinical Exercise Testing. 2nd Ed. Philadelphia, W.B. Saunders Co., 1982.
12. Spiro, S.G.: Exercise testing in clinical medicine. Br. J. Dis. Chest, 71:145–172, 1977.
13. Fairshter, R.D., Walters, J., Salvess, K., Fox, M., Minh, V.D., and Wilson, A.F.: Comparison of incremental exercise test during cycle and treadmill ergometry. Am. Rev. Respir. Dis., 125 (Suppl. [abstract]):254, 1982.
14. Whipp, B.J., Davis, J.A., Torres, F., and Wasserman, K.: A test to determine parameters of aerobic function during exercise. J. Appl. Physiol., 50:217–221, 1981.
15. Davis, J.A., Whipp, B.J., Lamarra, N., Huntsman, D.J., Frank, M.H., and Wasserman, K.: Effect of ramp slope on measurement of aerobic parameters from the ramp exercise test. Med. Sci. Sports Exerc., 14:339–343, 1982.
16. Cooper, D.M., and Weiler-Ravell, D.: Gas exchange response to exercise in children. Am. Rev. Respir. Dis., 129 (Suppl.):S47–S48, 1984.
17. Arstilla, M.: Pulse-conducted triangular exercise-ECG test. Acta Med. Scand., 529 (Suppl.):103–109, 1972.
18. Redwood, D.R., Rosing, D.R., Goldstein, A.R., Beiser, G., and Epstein, S.E.: Importance of the design of an exercise protocol in the evaluation of patients with angina pectoris. Circulation, 43:618–628, 1971.
19. Buchfuhrer, M.J., Hansen, J.E., Robinson, T.E., Sue, D.Y., Wasserman, K., and Whipp, B.J.: Optimizing the exercise protocol for cardiopulmonary assessment. J. Appl. Physiol. 55:1558–1564, 1983.
20. Taylor, H.L., Buskirk, E., and Henschel, A.: Maximal oxygen intake as an objective measure of cardio-respiratory performance. J. Appl. Physiol., 8:73–80, 1955.
21. Froelicher, V.F., Brammel, H., Davis, G.D., Noguera, I., Stewart, A., and Lancaster, M.D.: A comparison of three maximal treadmill exercise protocols. J. Appl. Physiol., 36:720–725, 1974.
22. Maksud, M.G., and Coutts, K.D.: Comparison of a continuous and discontinuous graded treadmill test for maximal oxygen uptake. Med. Sci. Sports. Exerc., 3:63–65, 1971.
23. Wyndham, C.H., Strydom, N.B., Leary, W.P., and Williams, C.G.: Studies of the maximum capacity of men for physical effort. Arbeitsphysiol., 22:285–295, 1966.
24. McArdle, W.D., Katch, F.I., and Pechar, G.S.: Compari-

son of continuous and discontinuous treadmill and bicycle tests for max $\dot{V}O_2$. Med. Sci. Sports. Exerc., 5:156–160, 1972.

25. Pollock, M.L., Bohannon, R.L., Cooper, K.H., Ayres, J., Ward, A., White, S.R., and Linnerud, N.D.: A comparative analysis of four protocols for maximal treadmill stress testing. Am. Heart J., 92:39–46, 1976.

26. Furuike, A.N., Sue, D.Y., Hansen, J.E., and Wasserman, K.: Comparison of physiological dead space/tidal volume ratio and alveolar-arterial PO_2 difference during incremental and constant work exercise. Am. Rev. Respir. Dis., 126:579–583, 1982.

27. Beaver, W.L.: Water vapor corrections in oxygen consumption calculations. J. Appl. Physiol., 35:928–931, 1973.

28. Beaver, W.L., Wasserman, K., and Whipp, B.J.: On-line computer analysis and breath-by-breath graphical display of exercise function tests. J. Appl. Physiol., 34:128–132, 1973.

29. Sue, D.Y., Hansen, J.E., Blais, M., and Wasserman, K.: Measurement and analysis of gas exchange during exercise using a programmable calculator. J. Appl. Physiol., 49:456–461, 1980.

30. Consolazio, C.F., Johnson, R.E., and Pecora, L.J.: Physiological Measurements of Metabolic Function in Man. New York, McGraw-Hill, 1963, pp. 368–401.

31. Astrand, P.O., and Rodahl, K.: Textbook of Work Physiology. 2nd Ed. New York, McGraw-Hill, 1977, pp. 333–365.

32. Whipp, B.J., and Wasserman, K.: Oxygen uptake kinetics for various intensities of constant load work. J. Appl. Physiol., 33:351–356, 1972.

33. Nery, L.E., Wasserman, K., Andrews, J.D., Huntsman, D.J., Hansen, J.E., and Whipp, B.J.: Ventilatory and gas exchange kinetics during exercise in chronic airway obstruction. J. Appl. Physiol., 53:1594–1602, 1982.

34. Lamarra, N., Whipp, B.J., Blumenberg, M., and Wasserman, K.: Model-order estimation of cardiorespiratory dynamics during moderate exercise. In Modelling and Control of Breathing. Edited by B.J. Whipp and D.M. Wiberg. New York, Elsevier, Science Publishing Co., Inc. 1983, pp. 338–345.

35. Whipp, B.J., Ward, S.A., Lamarra, N., Davis, J.A., and Wasserman, K.: Parameters of ventilatory and gas exchange dynamics during exercise. J. Appl. Physiol., 52:1506–1513, 1982.

36. Cropp, G.J.A.: The exercise bronchoprovocation test: Standardization of procedures and evaluation of response. J. Allergy Clin. Immunol., 64:627–633, 1979.

37. Deal, E.C., Jr., McFadden, E.R., Jr., Ingram, R.H., Strauss, R.H. and Jaeger, J.J.: Role of respiratory heat exchange in production of exercise-induced asthma. J. Appl. Physiol., 46:467–475, 1979.

38. Wasserman, K.: Testing regulation of ventilation with exercise. Chest, 70:S173–S178, 1976.

39. Stuart, R.J., and Ellestad, M.H.: National survey of exercise stress testing facilities. Chest, 77:94–97, 1980.

40. Bruce, R.A., Kusimi, F., and Hosmer, D.: Maximal oxygen intake and nomographic assessment of functional aerobic impairment in cardiovascular disease. Am. Heart J., 85:546–562, 1973.

41. Nagle, F.J., Balke, B., and Naughton, J.P.: Gradational step tests for assessing work capacity. J. Appl. Physiol., 21:745–748, 1965.

42. Nagle, F.J., Balke, B., Baptista, G., Alleyia, J., and Hawley, E.: Compatability of progressive treadmill, bicycle and step tests based on oxygen uptake responses. Med. Sci. Sports, Exerc., 3:149–154, 1971.

43. Fleishman, E.A.: The Structure and Measurement of Physical Fitness. Englewood Cliffs, Prentice-Hall, Inc., 1964, pp. 171–172.

44. Cooper, K.H.: A means of assessing maximal oxygen intake. J. Am. Med. Assoc., 203:201–204, 1968.

45. Shephard, R.J.: The relative merits of the step test, bicycle ergometer, and treadmill in the assessment of cardiorespiratory fitness. Arbeitphysiol., 23:219–230, 1966.

46. Bar-Or, O., and Zwiren, L.D.: Maximal oxygen consumption test during arm exercise-reliability and validity. J. Appl. Physiol., 38:424–426, 1975.

47. Vokac, Z., Bell, H., Bautz-Holter, E., and Rodahl, K.: Oxygen uptake/heart rate relationship in leg and arm exercise, sitting and standing. J. Appl. Physiol., 39:54–59, 1975.

48. Davis, J.A., Vodak, P., Wilmore, J.H., Vodal, J., and Kurtz, P.: Anaerobic threshold and maximal aerobic power for three modes of exercise. J. Appl. Physiol., 41:544–550, 1976.

49. McGavin, C.R., Gupta, S.P., and McHardy, G.J.R.: Twelve minute walking test for assessing disability in chronic bronchitis. Br. Med. J., 1:822–823, 1976.

50. Helfant, R.H., DeVilla, M.A., and Meister, S.G.: Effect of sustained isometric hand grip exercise on left ventricular performance. Circulation, 44:982–993, 1971.

51. Blomquist, C.G.: Use of exercise testing for diagnostic and functional evaluation of patients with arteriosclerotic heart disease. Circulation, 44:1120–1136, 1971.

52. Haissly, J., Messin, R., Degre, S., Vandermoten, P., Demaret, B., and Denolin, H.: Comparative responses to isometric (static) and dynamic exercise tests in coronary artery disease. Am. J. Cardiol., 33:791–795, 1974.

53. Whipp, B.J., and Phillips, E.E., Jr.: Cardiopulmonary and metabolic responses to sustained isometric exercise. Arch. Phys. Med. Rehabil., 51:398–402, 1970.

Normal Values

INTERPRETATION of the results of exercise tests requires knowing the normal response. In this chapter we have compiled values for important physiological variables that we think represent the best data available for sedentary normal subjects during exercise. In some instances a number of sets of normal values for the same measurement are given. When doing so we have critiqued each set and have put forth our recommendation.

Maximum Oxygen Uptake

Recommended values for maximum $\dot{V}O_2$ are given in Tables 6-1 and 6-2 for sedentary men and women and children of average activity levels performing cycle and, in the case of adults, treadmill exercise. Figure 6-1 gives mean predicted maximum $\dot{V}O_2$ values for leg cycling for adults. Figure 6-2 gives maximum $\dot{V}O_2$ data for leg cycling for children.

At this point, the reader might reconsider the distinction between maximal $\dot{V}O_2$ ($\dot{V}O_2$ max) and maximum $\dot{V}O_2$ described in Chapter 3. In the case of normal values, the predicted maximum $\dot{V}O_2$ is also the predicted $\dot{V}O_2$ max. Maximum $\dot{V}O_2$ in normal subjects during exercise varies with age, sex, body size, level of activity, and type of exercise. Therefore, when comparing the maximum $\dot{V}O_2$ of an individual to the predicted maximum $\dot{V}O_2$, the value must be for a given form of exercise. Also the population from which the data were obtained should have similar characteristics to the subject being tested.

CRITIQUE

Many investigators have reported that maximum $\dot{V}O_2$ declines with age.[1-3] While cross-sectional studies of change in maximum $\dot{V}O_2$ with age are easier to perform, they may be misleading because their maximum $\dot{V}O_2$ values tend to decrease more slowly than longitudinal studies in the same subject.[4] In a longitudinal study, Astrand et al.[5] measured maximum $\dot{V}O_2$ during cycling exercise in 66 well-trained, physically active men and women aged 20 to 33 years and studied them again 21 years later. The mean decrease in maximum $\dot{V}O_2$ was 22% for the 35 women and 20% for the 31 men.

Whether the $\dot{V}O_2$ is expressed as ml/min or ml/kg/min is important when considering changes due to

TABLE 6-1. *Predicted Maximum $\dot{V}O_2$ in Normal Sedentary Adults, ml/min*[6,9,28]

GROUP	ERGOMETER	OVERWEIGHT	MAXIMUM $\dot{V}O_2$, ml/min	LOWER 95% CONFIDENCE LIMIT
Men	Cycle	No*	$W \times (50.72 - 0.372 \times A)$	84% of predicted maximum $\dot{V}O_2$
		Yes*	$(0.79 \times H - 60.7) \times (50.72 - 0.372 \times A)$	
	Treadmill	No*	$W \times (56.36 - 0.413 \times A)$	Predicted maximum $\dot{V}O_2 - 8.2 \times W$
		Yes*	$(0.79 \times H - 60.7) \times (56.36 - 0.413 \times A)$	
Women	Cycle	No†	$(42.8 + W) \times (22.78 - 0.17 \times A)$	
		Yes†	$H \times (14.81 - 0.11 \times A)$	
	Treadmill	No‡	$W \times (44.37 - 0.413 \times A)$	Predicted maximum $\dot{V}O_2 - 8.2 \times W$
		Yes‡	$(0.79 \times H - 68.2) \times (44.37 - 0.413 \times A)$	

Abbreviations: Weight (W) in kg, Height (H) in cm, and Age (A) in years.
*Overweight is $W > (0.79 \times H - 60.7)$.
†Overweight is $W > (0.65 \times H - 42.8)$.
‡Overweight is $W > (0.79 \times H - 68.2)$.

aging. For example, Drinkwater and colleagues[2] found that in *active* women the maximum $\dot{V}O_2$ (ml/min) did not decrease with age from the third to fifth decade, although maximum $\dot{V}O_2$ expressed as ml/kg/min was lower in the older subjects because they were heavier.

Bruce et al.[6] used stepwise multiple regression analysis to identify whether sex, age, physical activity, weight, height, or smoking aided in the prediction of maximum $\dot{V}O_2$ (ml/kg/min) during treadmill exercise in adults. They found that sex and age were the two most important factors. The maximum $\dot{V}O_2$ of women was approximately 77% of maximum $\dot{V}O_2$ of men when adjusted for body weight and activity. Astrand[7] reported 17% lower maximum $\dot{V}O_2$ (ml/kg/min) for 18 women students compared to 17 male students of comparable size.

It is logical to assume that physical size would be a factor in maximal $\dot{V}O_2$ because the mass of the exercising muscles as well as the dimensions of the cardiovascular and pulmonary systems should determine the maximal quantity of O_2 that could be delivered and used. However, the simple measurement of body weight will not suffice. For example, if a woman has a greater proportion of adipose tissue weight than a man, a man will have a higher maximal $\dot{V}O_2$ than a woman of equal body weight, since the capacity to use O_2 in exercise is proportional to the exercising muscle mass, not total weight.

Because obesity adds adipose and not muscle tissue, we believe that maximal $\dot{V}O_2$ should not normally increase with increasing obesity (although the $\dot{V}O_2$ at any submaximal work rate will be increased). This is in agreement with the findings of Buskirk and Taylor[8] who found that maximum $\dot{V}O_2$ correlated better with a measure of fat-free body weight (r = 0.85) than total body weight (r = 0.63) in 43 healthy students and 13 soldiers performing treadmill exercise. But despite the obvious effect of obesity on the predicted maximum $\dot{V}O_2$ given on a per weight basis, many investigators predict maximum $\dot{V}O_2$ from age, sex, and weight, even in obese individuals. We feel that this practice biases the interpretation by giving too high a predicted normal maximum $\dot{V}O_2$.

We found, in a population of 77 middle-aged men (mean age = 54 years, range 34 to 74 years) whom we judged to have normal cardiovascular and respiratory systems and good motivation, that when the subject was overweight,[9,10] there was better agreement with Bruce's data for maximum $\dot{V}O_2$[6] using ideal weight (weight predicted from height) rather than actual weight. This supports the concept that subjects heavier than ideal weight do not have higher values of maximum $\dot{V}O_2$ than individuals of the same

TABLE 6-2. *Predicted Maximum $\dot{V}O_2$ and AT in Normal Children for Cycle Ergometry*[12]

	BOYS≤13	BOYS>13	GIRLS≤11	GIRLS>11
number studied	37	21	24	27
maximum $\dot{V}O_2$, ml/min/kg (mean ± SD)	42 ± 6	50 ± 8	38 ± 7	34 ± 4
lower 95% confidence limit	32	37	26	27
AT, ml/min/kg (mean ± SD)	26 ± 5	27 ± 6	23 ± 4	19 ± 3
lower 95% confidence limit	18	17	16	14

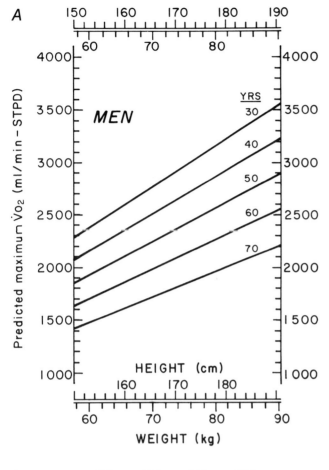

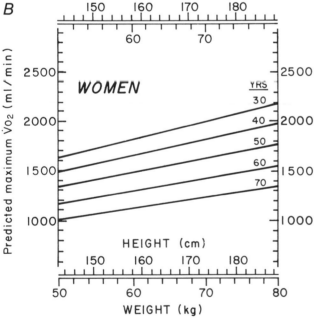

age and sex who are of normal weight. Prediction of maximum $\dot{V}O_2$ in obese subjects from height, age, and sex (see Fig. 6-1) rather than weight has precedent as pulmonary function variables such as vital capacity and airflow are predicted from these same descriptors. Over 60% of the normal working men we studied were over 10% overweight. Since obesity is so prevalent, we predict maximum $\dot{V}O_2$ from height if the patient is above ideal weight and from weight if the patient is at or below ideal weight, using Figure 6-1 or the formulae of Table 6-1.

Although the maximum $\dot{V}O_2$ normalized to height or lean body weight provides the best index of normalcy of cardiovascular and metabolic function in an obese patient, it does not, of course, reflect the patient's ability to perform weight-supported exercise. As such exercise requires the patient to propel the entire weight — and not just the lean fraction — the obese patient may be restricted by the excess weight. The appropriate index of such a patient's ability to perform this kind of task may be the maximum $\dot{V}O_2$ normalized to the total weight, i.e., ml/min/kg.

Cooper and colleagues[11,12] reported maximum $\dot{V}O_2$ for 109 children, aged 6 to 17 years, performing cycle ergometry using a continuously increasing work rate protocol (Fig. 6-2). As the subjects were not obese, maximum $\dot{V}O_2$ correlated similarly with either weight or height. They found, in addition, that their data were quite similar to those of Astrand[7] for the boys, but the girls studied by Astrand had a significantly higher maximum $\dot{V}O_2$ vs. height relationship. They believe that cultural or societal differences might account for this difference.

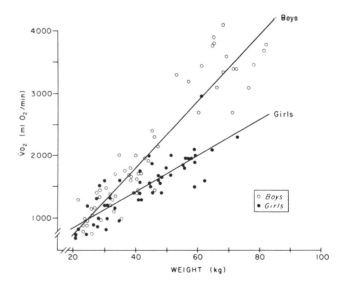

FIG. 6-1. Mean maximum O_2 uptake for sedentary *(A)* men and *(B)* women, using the cycle ergometer.[6,9,28] To use, locate on the horizontal axis both the patient's height and weight. From the more leftward point (which adjusts for obesity) draw a line vertically to the patient's age on the diagonal lines. From this point draw a horizontal line to the vertical axis to read off the predicted maximum $\dot{V}O_2$ in ml/min STPD.

FIG. 6-2. Maximum O_2 uptake of 109 normal North American boys and girls for leg cycling. Regression equations for maximum $\dot{V}O_2$ (ml/min) as function of body weight (kg) were for boys, $\dot{V}O_2 = 52.8 \times$ weight (kg) $- 303.4$, $(r = 0.94)$; for girls, $\dot{V}O_2 = 28.5 \times$ weight (kg) $+ 288.1$, $(r = 0.84)$ (modified from reference 12).

Because the level of physical activity of an individual plays a role in determining maximum $\dot{V}_{O_2}$, it is inappropriate to use "normal values" obtained predominantly from athletes, physical education teachers, servicemen, or participants in organized exercise groups as reference values for sedentary adults. Balke and Ware[13] found the maximum $\dot{V}_{O_2}$ of Air Force personnel to be strongly related to their activity pattern. Also, it has been suggested that the decline in maximum $\dot{V}_{O_2}$ with age is more rapid in habitually inactive men than in active men, even allowing for increasing weight in the inactive group.[4] Finally, it has been found that physical training is capable of acutely increasing maximum $\dot{V}_{O_2}$ by 15 to 20%.[1]

The type of exercise is an important determinant of maximum $\dot{V}_{O_2}$ as already discussed. The maximum $\dot{V}_{O_2}$ during arm cycling ergometer work is about 70% of that of leg cycling exercise[14] because of the smaller mass of muscle and lower work rate being performed. Although Astrand[7] found that young very fit Swedish subjects showed no difference in maximum $\dot{V}_{O_2}$ between cycling and running on a treadmill, six other studies show that maximum $\dot{V}_{O_2}$ during cycling exercise is between 89 and 95% of treadmill values.[15] Thus the form of ergometry and muscle groups involved must be considered when comparing maximum $\dot{V}_{O_2}$.

Maximum Heart Rate and Heart Rate Reserve (HRR)

The mean maximum heart rate for North American children is 187 beats/min.[16] The following are equations for estimating the maximum heart rate (HR) for adults and the heart rate reserve (HRR) for adults and children:

Adult maximum heart rate (beats/min)
$$= 220 - age\ (years).$$

Heart rate reserve (HRR)
= Predicted maximum HR − observed maximum HR
= zero.

CRITIQUE

The maximum heart rate achieved declines with age in all studies. There is no consistent difference between men and women or with the type of exercise used, i.e. leg cycling, stepping, or inclined treadmill, walking or running.

The two most commonly used formulae for predicting maximum HR in adults are: $220 - age$ (years) and $210 - 0.65 \times age$ (years).[17] Data from this laboratory fit the former equation slightly better.

The standard deviation for each formula is 10 beats/min. As reported by Sheffield[18] and Astrand and Rodahl[19] the maximum heart rates derived from fit individuals approximate either formula reasonably well. The study of Cooper et al.[20] shows a lower maximum HR in the less fit than the more fit individual. Similarly, we found that the maximum HR was reduced in obese men, consistent with the suggestion that a sedentary existence may reduce maximum HR even in well-motivated subjects.[9]

Scandinavian children were found to have an average maximum HR of 205 beats/min[19] whereas North American children aged 8 to 18 had an average maximum heart rate of 187 beats/min with a lower 95% confidence limit of 160.[16]

The concept of heart rate reserve can be useful for estimating the relative stress of the cardiovascular system during exercise, but it should be used with caution. The mean predicted maximum HR may not be reached because of normal population variability; poor motivation; medications such as β-adrenergic blockers; or because of heart, peripheral vascular, lung, endocrine, or musculoskeletal diseases.

Maximum Oxygen Pulse

The predicted maximum oxygen pulse is the quotient of predicted maximum $\dot{V}_{O_2}$ and predicted maximum HR as described above. The predicted value is shown graphically in Figure 6-3 for adults and Figure 6-4 for children.

Predicted maximum O_2 pulse (ml/beat)
$$= \frac{\text{Predicted maximum } \dot{V}_{O_2}\ (ml/min)}{\text{Predicted maximum HR (beats/min)}}$$

CRITIQUE

In a given individual there is a close relationship between $\dot{V}_{O_2}$ and HR during exercise (see Fig. 3-7). The quotient of the $\dot{V}_{O_2}$ and HR is the O_2 pulse (see Fig. 3-8). The normal relationship of $\dot{V}_{O_2}$ to HR is linear over a wide range with a positive intercept on the HR axis. Thus the rate of increase of O_2 pulse declines as the O_2 pulse approaches maximum values. The maximum $\dot{V}_{O_2}$ is five to fifteen times resting $\dot{V}_{O_2}$ while the maximum HR is two to three times resting HR. Occasionally just before the end of the incremental exercise test, $\dot{V}_{O_2}$ reaches a maximum before HR, in which case the maximum O_2 pulse (i.e., the highest O_2 pulse *reached*) may be slightly higher than the O_2 pulse at the *end* of exercise.

Either the absolute values of $\dot{V}_{O_2}$, HR, and O_2 pulse or their patterns of increase may be abnormal

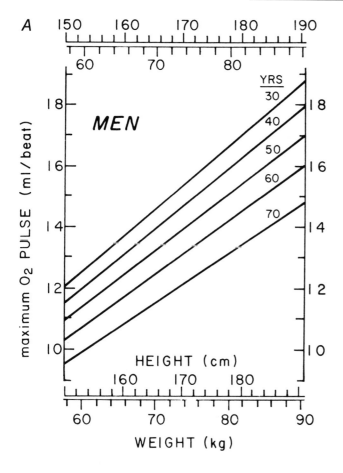

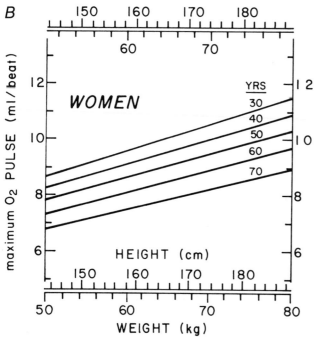

FIG. 6-3. Mean maximum O$_2$ pulse for sedentary *(A)* men and *(B)* women, using the cycle ergometer. To use, locate on the horizontal axis both the patient's height and weight. From the more leftward point (which adjusts for obesity) draw a line vertically to the patient's age on the diagonal lines. From this point draw a horizontal line to the vertical axis to read off the maximum O$_2$ pulse in ml/beat.

in various disease states. The predicted O$_2$ pulse at any given $\dot{V}O_2$, including maximum $\dot{V}O_2$, is strongly dependent on the normal individual's body size, sex, age, degree of fitness, and hemoglobin concentration. This predicted value depends on the predicting equations selected for maximum $\dot{V}O_2$ and HR, described in the Maximum $\dot{V}O_2$ and Maximum Heart Rate sections of this chapter. Normal values for the predicted maximum O$_2$ pulse on the cycle ergometer range from approximately 5 ml/beat in a 7-year-old child to 8 ml/beat in a 145 cm, 70-year-old woman to 17 ml/beat in a 190 cm, 30-year-old man. However, the O$_2$ pulse can be considerably higher than predicted in the cardiovascularly fit person.

Brachial Artery Blood Pressure

The brachial blood pressure values of nonhypertensive men, measured directly (intra-arterial) or by cuff and sphygmomanometer during one-minute incremental exercise, are given in Table 6-3.

CRITIQUE

Blood pressure can be measured by auscultation during exercise by skilled technicians or physicians, but assessing the 4th Korotkoff phase diastolic pressure (muffling of sound) and 5th Korotkoff phase diastolic pressure (disappearance of sound) may be difficult because of the background noise of the ergometer. However, intra-arterial pressures can be accurately and continuously measured by means of a pressure transducer attached to an indwelling catheter whenever arterial blood specimens are not being drawn.

The blood pressure measurements recorded in Table 6-3 are from a predominantly cigarette-smoking and sedentary normal population.[9,21] Values may be somewhat lower in nonsmoking, more active individuals. Noteworthy is the striking rise in systolic (by both cuff and direct intra-arterial recording) and mean pressures, the gradual rise in both intra-arterial and 4th phase cuff diastolic pressures, and the gradual decline in 5th phase cuff diastolic pressures during incremental exercise. Although resting pressures are higher in the older men, the mean maximum exercise systolic and diastolic pressures are similar in both groups.

It is more difficult to obtain accurate intra-arterial blood pressure values during treadmill ergometry because of movement artifacts and baseline shifts. When the subject is using the cycle, the arm and transducer are stabilized by the hand on the handlebar, but tight gripping should be avoided to minimize the hypertensive effect of isometric exercise.

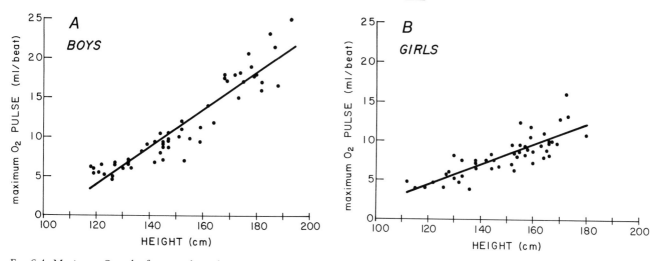

FIG. 6-4. Maximum O_2 pulse for normal North American boys *(A)* and girls *(B)*.[20] For boys the best fit regression line is O_2 pulse (ml/beat) = 0.23 × height (cm) − 24.4. The 95% confidence limit is 3.8 ml/beat below the regression line. For girls the equation is O_2 pulse (ml/beat) = 0.128 × height (cm) − 10.9 with a 95% confidence limit of 3.0 ml/beat below the regression line (Courtesy of Dr. D.M. Cooper).

Anaerobic Threshold (AT)

The mean values for *AT* in normal subjects are given in Figure 6-5 for adults and Table 6-2 and Figure 6-6 for children. The *AT* is expressed in units of oxygen uptake. Many of the same factors that affect maximum $\dot{V}O_2$ affect *AT*, although the latter may vary proportionally more with the degree of training. Any *AT* less than 40% of predicted maximum $\dot{V}O_2$ is below the 95% confidence limits for the *AT* of normal sedentary populations of men, women, and children.

CRITIQUE

The $\dot{V}O_2$ at which blood lactate level begins to be elevated has been used to define the *AT* in normal subjects.[22] However, expired gas measurements per-

mit rapid noninvasive identification of the *AT* if measurements are properly made and interpreted,[23] and values of *AT* in normals using these methods are considered here.

Because we are most often interested in evaluating subjects with exercise limitation, a lower limit of normal for the *AT* is useful for defining an abnormality. Thus while in several series the mean *AT* for men ranged between 49 to 63% of maximum $\dot{V}O_2$,[24–28] the minimum normal value in our study of 77 middle-aged (34 to 74 years) sedentary men was 40% of maximum $\dot{V}O_2$.[9] This lower limit of normal agrees reasonably well with the lowest value for *AT* in normal men suggested by Wasserman et al.[24] at a $\dot{V}O_2$ of 1 l/min, approximately the cost of maintaining a moderate walking pace.

Davis et al.[28] studied 100 nonsmoking, nonobese

TABLE 6-3. *Blood Pressure During One-minute Incremental Cycle Exercise Measured Directly from Catheter in Brachial Artery and in Opposite Arm by Cuff.*[*9,21]

	PRIOR EXAM, AT REST	REST ON CYCLE	EXERCISE NEAR *AT*	EXERCISE NEAR MAXIMUM
SEDENTARY, NONHYPERTENSIVE MEN, AGES 34 TO 74				
Systolic intra-arterial		142 ± 18	182 ± 23	207 ± 27
Systolic cuff	124 ± 11	131	171	200
Diastolic intra-arterial		86 ± 10	92 ± 11	99 ± 12
Diastolic 4th phase	79 ± 7	84	86	88
Diastolic 5th phase		81	80	77
Mean intra-arterial		107	128	142
SEDENTARY, NONHYPERTENSIVE MEN, AGES 19 TO 24				
Systolic intra-arterial		129		203
Diastolic intra-arterial		78		106
Mean intra-arterial		96		141

*Values are mean or mean ± SD in mm Hg.

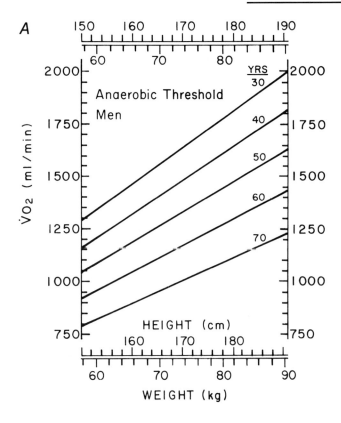

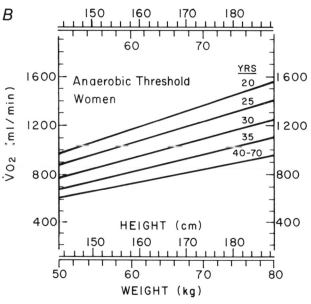

FIG. 6-5. Mean anaerobic threshold *(AT)* for sedentary *(A)* men and *(B)* women, using the cycle ergometer.[9,28] To use, locate on the horizontal axis both the patient's height and weight. From the more leftward point (which adjusts for obesity) draw a line vertically to the patient's age on the diagonal lines. From this point draw a horizontal line to the vertical axis to read off the predicted *AT* in ml/min STPD.

women. Their mean *AT* was about 50% of maximum $\dot{V}O_2$ for those from ages 20 to 59 and 60% of maximum $\dot{V}O_2$ for those 60 to 69 years old. Again, a lower limit of normal of about 40% of maximum $\dot{V}O_2$ was found.

Cooper et al.[12] tested 51 girls and 58 boys between the ages of 6 to 17 years. They were healthy and nonobese, but did not participate in vigorous sports. Mean *AT* was 58% of maximum $\dot{V}O_2$ but, again, the lower limit of normal for this sample of normal children was approximately 40% of maximum $\dot{V}O_2$ (Fig. 6–6). The mode of exercise may affect the value of *AT* in normal subjects. Davis et al.[29] studied 39 healthy college age men. Mean $\dot{V}O_2$ at the *AT* was $46.5 \pm 8.9\%$ of maximum $\dot{V}O_2$ for arm cycling, $63.8 \pm 9.0\%$ of maximum $\dot{V}O_2$ for leg cycling, and $58.6 \pm 5.8\%$ of maximum $\dot{V}O_2$ for treadmill exercise. There was a significant difference between the *AT* during arm cycling and either form of leg exercise, but no difference between the *AT* obtained from cycle and treadmill exercise. Buchfuhrer et al.[30] found similar ratios of *AT*/maximum $\dot{V}O_2$, i.e., $50.3 \pm 9.4\%$ for treadmill and $47.2 \pm 11.0\%$ for the cycle. However, Withers et al.,[31] comparing very well trained cyclists and runners, found a higher *AT* for the total group on the treadmill (mean 75.8% of maximum $\dot{V}O_2$) than on the cycle (mean 63.8% of maximum $\dot{V}O_2$).

Oxygen Uptake-Work Rate (WR) Relationship ($\Delta\dot{V}O_2/\Delta WR$) and O_2 Difference

The overall $\Delta\dot{V}O_2/\Delta WR$ during incremental cycle ergometer exercise of 6 to 12 minutes duration for a population of 54 sedentary adult men was 10.29 ml/min/watt, with a SD of 1.01 ml/min/watt and a lower limit of normal at the 95% confidence level of 8.62 ml/min/watt.[32] The normal O_2 difference at the end of exercise was 0.0% with an SD of 7.0% and an upper limit of normal at the 95% confidence level of 11.6%.

CRITIQUE

A single study[32] compared the relationship between $\dot{V}O_2$ and WR during one-minute incremental exercise, where $\Delta\dot{V}O_2$ is the overall increase in $\dot{V}O_2$ from unloaded pedalling to maximum exercise and ΔWR is the increase in WR when the latter is increased by a constant amount each minute. The formula used for calculation is:

$\Delta\dot{V}O_2/\Delta WR$
$= (\text{maximum } \dot{V}O_2 - \dot{V}O_2 \text{ unloaded})/ [(T - 0.75) \times I]$

where $\dot{V}O_2$ is measured in ml/min, T is the time in minutes of incremental exercise and I is the increment size in watts each minute. The value obtained will be influenced both by the difference in O_2 kinet-

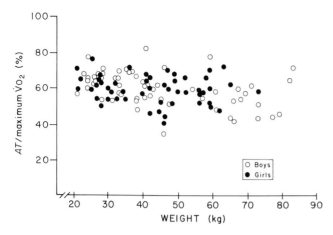

FIG. 6-6. The ratio of anaerobic threshold to maximum O_2 uptake, in percent, for 109 normal North American boys and girls.[12]

ics among individuals and the ratio of anaerobic to aerobic energy generated for the work being performed. Both of these factors may be abnormal in patients with disturbances in O_2 transport and cause $\Delta\dot{V}O_2/\Delta WR$ to decrease. The measured $\Delta\dot{V}O_2/\Delta WR$ may also be slightly decreased in normals if the exercise period selected is too short (the work rate increment is too large) or slightly increased in normals if the exercise period is too long (the work rate increment is too small) (see Chapter 3 and Fig. 3-3).

In a given test, the O_2 difference is positive if the calculated $\Delta\dot{V}O_2/\Delta WR$ is lower than the normal value of 10.29 ml/min/watt. The O_2 difference is negative if the measured $\Delta\dot{V}O_2/\Delta WR$ is higher than 10.29 ml/min/watt.

Ventilation, Tidal Volume, Breathing Frequency and Breathing Reserve

At the subject's maximum work rate, the following values (mean ± SD) have been found for normal adult men, ages 34 to 74, for cycle ergometry using a breathing valve with a dead space of 64 ml.[9,10]

1. Maximum exercise $\dot{V}E/MVV$,% = 72 ± 15%
2. Breathing reserve = MVV − maximum exercise $\dot{V}E$=38 ± 22 L/min; lower limit of normal = 11 L/min.
3. Maximum tidal volume (maximum V_T) < inspiratory capacity (IC) in all subjects
4. Maximum breathing frequency (f) < 50/min in over 95% of all subjects

CRITIQUE

While the $\dot{V}E$ of a given subject is closely linked to the metabolic demand, it is also dependent on the efficiency of ventilation, the degree of respiratory compensation for metabolic acidosis, the appropri-

ateness of the ventilatory control mechanisms, and the mechanical capabilities of the lungs, chest wall, and respiratory muscles.

Maximum Exercise Ventilation

Since the maximal metabolic rate will be lower when smaller muscle groups are used, maximum $\dot{V}E$ for arm cycling is less than that for leg cycling or treadmill walk-running,[29] whereas maximum $\dot{V}E$ is similar for the two latter forms of exercise.[3,30]

Breathing Reserve

The breathing reserve relates the ventilatory response during maximal exercise to the maximal ability to breathe. Because normal untrained subjects are not ordinarily ventilatory limited in their ability to perform work,[33] some ability to increase ventilation further is usually present during maximal exercise. This potential increase in ventilation is generally estimated from the maximal voluntary ventilation (MVV), a test performed at rest. The MVV is highly dependent on the subject's motivation and effort. Normal values for MVV lasting 12 and 15 seconds are available.[34,35] The difference between the measured MVV and the maximum $\dot{V}E$ during exercise is used as a measure of the ventilatory or breathing reserve. A low breathing reserve suggests that a subject's exercise capacity may be limited by his ventilatory capacity. The breathing reserve is markedly reduced in patients with moderate to severe restrictive or obstructive lung disease (see Fig. 4-6).

Many investigators have examined the relationship between MVV and the maximum exercise $\dot{V}E$. In general, maximum exercise $\dot{V}E$ averages 50 to 80% of the 12 or 15 second MVV,[9] indicating a breathing reserve of 20 to 50% of the MVV.

Because the MVV is dependent on subject cooperation, effort, and technique of performance, the MVV is sometimes indirectly estimated from the FEV_1 or $FEV_{0.75}$. Gandevia and Hugh-Jones[36] suggested that the indirect MVV could be estimated as $FEV_1 \times 35$ while Cotes[37] suggested $FEV_{0.75} \times 40$ or $36.8 \times FEV_1 - 2.8$. Miller and colleagues[38] found that $FEV_1 \times 41$ or $FEV_{0.75} \times 46$ estimated MVV. Our data[9] and those of Campbell[39] indicate that $FEV_1 \times 40$ provides a good estimate of the MVV both in normal subjects and in patients with obstructive lung disease; we recommend use of this value if it is necessary to determine MVV indirectly in these two populations. However, the $FEV_1 \times 40$ underestimates the MVV in patients with restrictive lung disease and overestimates the MVV in extreme obesity.

In 77 normal middle-aged subjects during an incremental cycle ergometer exercise test,[9] the mean measured MVV was 131 ± 23.6 L/min (range 81 to 203 L/min) and the mean maximum exercise $\dot{V}E$/MVV, the % was 71.5 ± 14,6; only 13 subjects had a value greater than 80%. When we used $FEV_1 \times 40$ as an indirect estimate of the MVV, the mean maximum exercise $\dot{V}E$/indirect MVV was 71.5 ± 15.3%, i.e., the same percent as for the directly measured MVV. Expressing breathing reserve as MVV − maximum exercise $\dot{V}E$, we obtain an average of 38.1 ± 22.0 L/min using the directly measured MVV and 38.0 ± 21.5 L/min for the indirect MVV.

Tidal Volume and Breathing Frequency During Exercise

The maximum exercise tidal volume (V_T), like VC and other resting pulmonary function measurements, depends on the subject's height, age, and sex. In addition, the dead space or rebreathed volume of the breathing apparatus influences ventilation.[40–42]

Hey et al.[43] recommended that V_T be related to $\dot{V}E$ to analyze the breathing pattern, such as is shown in Figure 3-10. At low work intensity the increase in $\dot{V}E$ is accomplished primarily by an increase in V_T. After the V_T reaches approximately 50 to 60% of the VC, further increases in $\dot{V}E$ are accomplished primarily by increasing breathing frequency (f).[37,44] Using this relationship, f is a curvilinear function of $\dot{V}E$ over this range. Spiro et al.[44] found that the maximum V_T reached in normal subjects was approximately 55% of VC in normal men and 45% in normal women, while Cotes[45] suggested that maximum V_T is about 50% of VC for VC values between 2.0 and 5.0 L in normal men and women of European descent. Astrand[1] found that at maximal exercise the V_T averaged between 1.9 to 2.0 L, or 52 to 58% of the VC, while f at maximal exercise ranged between 34 to 46 breaths/min. There was little difference in V_T/VC between age groups, but f was somewhat lower in the older subjects studied.

Wasserman and Whipp[33] compared exercise V_T to IC. They found that V_T does not usually exceed approximately 70% of the IC during exercise, but increases to a value approaching 100% in patients with restrictive lung disease, suggesting that the IC may limit the increase in V_T (see Figure 4-7). We found in our series of 77 healthy middle-aged men a mean resting V_T of 0.71 ± 0.26 L (mean ± SD) which increased to 1.44 ± 0.43 L at the AT and 2.28 ± 0.43 L at maximum exercise.[9,10] Maximum f was 41.6 ± 9.6 min^{-1}. Maximum V_T averaged 70.0 ± 10.7% of the IC and 55.0 ± 8.7% of the VC. No one had a maximum exercise V_T greater than their resting IC, and only three had a f > 60 min^{-1}.

Partitioning the duration of the ventilatory cycle (T_{TOT}) into the inspiratory (T_I) and expiratory (T_E) components may also prove useful, but to date this measurement is not commonplace in clinical exercise testing.

Ventilatory Equivalents for Carbon Dioxide ($\dot{V}E/\dot{V}CO_2$) and Oxygen ($\dot{V}E/\dot{V}O_2$)

The normal values (mean ± SD) during sea level exercise near the AT for middle-aged normal sedentary men are: 29.1 ± 4.3 for $\dot{V}E/\dot{V}CO_2$ and 26.5 ± 4.4 for $\dot{V}E/\dot{V}O_2$ where the $\dot{V}E$ is expressed at BTPS with apparatus dead space ventilation subtracted, while $\dot{V}CO_2$ and $\dot{V}O_2$ are expressed STPD.

Critique

The ratio $\dot{V}E/\dot{V}CO_2$ gives an index of the dead space ventilation but is, of course, influenced by the Pa_{CO_2} as shown in Figure 3-13. Ratios higher than normal are expected in patients with increased dead space ventilation. Both $\dot{V}E/\dot{V}O_2$ and $\dot{V}E/\dot{V}CO_2$ will necessarily be increased at altitudes at which hyperventilation causes a decrease in Pa_{CO_2}. Wasserman et al.[46] found that $\dot{V}E/\dot{V}CO_2$ declined to approximately 28 during cycle ergometer exercise in 10 healthy young men before $\dot{V}E/\dot{V}CO_2$ increased with the onset of significant metabolic acidosis. In steady-state exercise below the AT, the $\dot{V}E/\dot{V}O_2$ is lower than the $\dot{V}E/\dot{V}CO_2$ because the respiratory quotient is less than 1.[33]

Physiological Dead Space/Tidal Volume Ratio (V_D/V_T)

Figure 6-7 shows the effect of exercise on V_D/V_T at various levels of cycle exercise in young men. We recommend the following predicted values for V_D/V_T at rest and during upright exercise after allowance for valve dead space:

1. For men under age 40: $V_D/V_T \leq 0.40$ at rest, ≤ 0.25 at AT and ≤ 0.21 at maximum exercise.
2. For men over age 40: mean values $V_D/V_T = 0.30 \pm 0.08$ at rest, 0.20 ± 0.07 at AT, and 0.19 ± 0.07 at maximal exercise.
3. Upper 95% confidence limits for men over 40: $V_D/V_T = 0.45$ at rest, 0.33 at AT, and 0.28 at maximal exercise.

Critique

The physiologic dead space (V_D) is dependent on anatomic and physiologic factors while the dead space/tidal volume ratio (V_D/V_T) is also dependent,

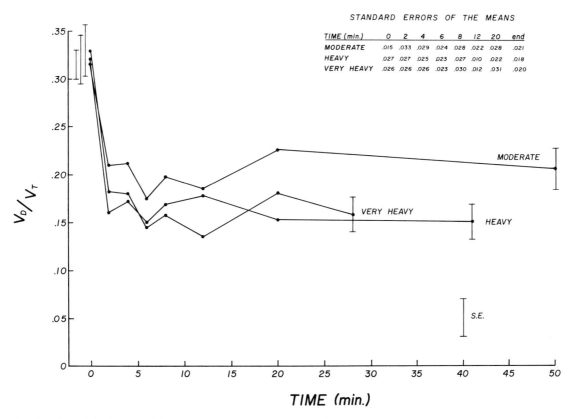

FIG. 6-7. The physiological dead space/tidal volume ratio (V_D/V_T) in 10 normal young men at rest and during 3 intensities of cycle ergometer exercise as related to exercise duration.[46] The SEM are given in the table insert.

even in normals, on the pattern of breathing. At rest the V_D/V_T may be elevated because of the rapid, shallow breathing of anxiety.

Physiologic control mechanisms usually stabilize ventilation at a slower and more efficient breathing pattern soon after the onset of exercise unless anxiety is extreme. Calculation of the V_D and V_D/V_T must be carefully performed, making an adjustment for the apparatus dead space (see Appendix D). In addition, gas exchange measurements must be synchronous with arterial blood sampling for measuring Pa_{CO_2}.

Cotes[48] suggested that V_D (ml) = 140 + 0.07 V_T (ml) with a SD = 90 ml in young men during exercise. Jones et al.[41] found the following relationship during exercise in 17 normal young men: V_D (ml) = 138 + 0.077 V_T (ml), with r = 0.69. Lifshay et al.[42] showed that men aged 50 to 81 had a significantly higher V_D than men and women aged 18 to 37. The prediction equations of Bradley et al.[49] for V_D use sex, age, height, $\dot{V}_{CO_2}$, $\dot{V}_E$, f, and temperature as factors.

All studies have shown a fall in V_D/V_T during exercise in normal subjects. Thus while mean V_D/V_T at rest ranged from 0.28 to 0.35 in several studies of normals, mean V_D/V_T decreased to between 0.20 to

0.25 near the AT and to less than 0.21 at maximum exercise.[9,41,46,50]

Arterial and End-Tidal Carbon Dioxide (Pa_{CO_2}, $P_{ET_{CO_2}}$, and $P(a - {ET})_{CO_2}$

The normal values at sea level during upright exercise in adult men are:

1. Pa_{CO_2}
   a. Resting value = 36 to 42 mm Hg; stable during mild and moderate exercise, declining with heavy exercise.
2. $P_{ET_{CO_2}}$
   a. Resting value = 36 to 42 mm Hg; increases normally by 3 to 8 mm Hg during mild and moderate exercise (depending on breathing pattern), and decreases with heavy exercise.
3. $P(a - {ET})_{CO_2}$ (mean ± SD).
   a. Exercise at the AT = −3 ± 3 mm Hg;
   b. At maximal exercise = −4 ± 3 mm Hg. The $P(a - {ET})_{CO_2}$ becomes negative in more than 95% of normal men at maximal exercise.

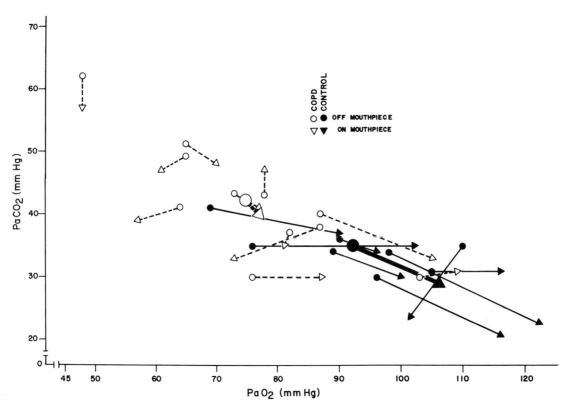

FIG. 6-8. Resting arterial partial pressures of CO_2 (Pa_{CO_2}) and O_2 (Pa_{O_2}) in normal controls and patients with chronic obstructive pulmonary disease (COPD) off and acutely on the mouthpiece while awaiting cycle ergometer exercise. Small arrows show individual values and large arrows show mean values. Note the small mean decline in Pa_{CO_2} and increase in Pa_{O_2} in the COPD patients while breathing on the mouthpiece whereas the controls show a larger decline in Pa_{CO_2} and much larger rise in Pa_{O_2} with the same mouthpiece at rest (Courtesy of Dr. J.D. Andrews).

CRITIQUE

Resting PET_{CO_2} and Pa_{CO_2} values are dependent on the degree of apprehension, anxiety, and training of the subject. Many anxious subjects have a strong tendency to hyperventilate, especially while breathing through a mouthpiece and awaiting the signal to begin exercise (Fig. 6-8). However, once exercise starts, the blood gases and pH are not discernibly different, whether performing the work while breathing through a low resistance breathing valve or breathing normally without a mouthpiece.[51] In more apprehensive individuals, the PCO_2 values rise from rest to moderate exercise as physiologic control mechanisms suppress psychogenic hyperventilation. In the relaxed individual, Pa_{CO_2} values remain stable during rest, mild, and moderate exercise. While Pa_{CO_2} values cannot be predicted accurately from PET_{CO_2} values in an individual person, particularly in a patient with lung disease, measurement of PET_{CO_2} is valuable for following trends in Pa_{CO_2}. Increasing PET_{CO_2} values usually mean that Pa_{CO_2} is rising.

Wasserman et al.[46] found that $P(a - ET)_{CO_2}$ changed from approximately + 2.5 mm Hg at rest to −4 mm Hg during heavy work in 10 normal men (Fig. 6-9). Jones et al.[41] found that, in 17 normal subjects at the highest work rates reached, PET_{CO_2} was

always more than 2 to 3 mm Hg higher than Pa_{CO_2}. In 5 normal men, Whipp and Wasserman[50] found $P(a - ET)_{CO_2}$ was 2.8 ± 1.6 mm Hg at rest and -2.8 ± 0.6 mm Hg at a work rate of 220 watts. All $P(a - ET)_{CO_2}$ values were negative for work rates above 115 watts. In our 77 asbestos-exposed healthy men,[9] mean $P(a - ET)_{CO_2}$ at rest was -0.3 ± 2.9 mm Hg (mean $\pm$ SD) and decreased to -4.1 ± 3.2 mm Hg at maximal exercise. At the peak of exercise it was very rare to find a $P(a - ET)_{CO_2} > 0$.

Arterial, Alveolar, and End-Tidal Oxygen (Pa_{O_2}, Sa_{O_2}, PET_{O_2}, and $P(A-a)_{O_2}$)

The normal blood O_2 level (Pa_{O_2} and Sa_{O_2}) and alveolar-arterial PO_2 difference ($P(A-a)_{O_2}$) at sea level during upright exercise in adult men are:

1. Pa_{O_2}
   a. Rest = 80 mm Hg or greater; usually increasing slightly with heavy exercise.
2. Sa_{O_2}
   a. Rest = 95% or greater; no decrease with exercise.

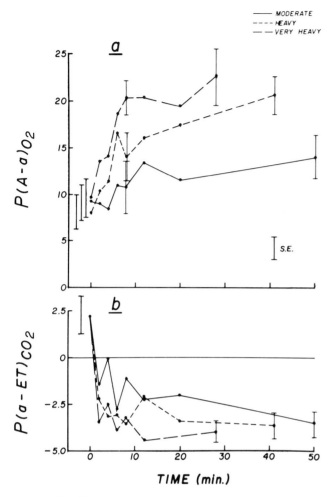

FIG. 6-9. The $P(A-a)_{O_2}$, and $P(a-ET)_{CO_2}$ in 10 normal young men at rest and during 3 intensities of cycle ergometer exercise as related to exercise duration.[46] The mean and SEM are depicted.

3. PET_{O_2}
   a. Rest = 90 mm Hg or greater; increases with heavy exercise.
4. $P(A-a)_{O_2}$
   a. Age 20 to 39: mean $P(A-a)_{O_2}$=8 mm Hg at rest, 11 mm Hg at AT, and 15 mm Hg at maximal exercise.
   b. Age 40 to 69: mean $P(A-a)_{O_2}$=13 ± 7 mm Hg at rest, 17 ± 7 mm Hg at AT, and 19 ± 9 mm Hg at maximal exercise. Upper limit of normal (95% confidence level) = 28 mm Hg at AT and 35 mm Hg at maximal exercise.

CRITIQUE

The normal resting Pa_{O_2} is dependent on age, body position and nutritional status. Values are less with increasing age, obesity, fasting, and in the supine position. Nevertheless, sea-level values less than 80 mm Hg are not seen in normal subjects in the sitting position except in those who are obese. The

PET_{O_2} and PA_{O_2} (the latter calculated from the alveolar air equation; see Appendix) are normally similar, but may differ by 10 or more mm Hg in patients with severe maldistribution of ventilation. The PET_{O_2}, PA_{O_2}, and Pa_{O_2} decrease transiently soon after the start of exercise (since the rise in $\dot{V}E$ is slower than the rise in $\dot{V}_{O_2}$ and R declines) and then rise back to approximately resting values (see Chapter 2, "O_2 uptake kinetics, O_2 deficit, and O_2 debt"). Above the AT, PET_{O_2} increases 10 to 30 mm Hg with maximal exercise due to metabolic acidosis-induced hyperventilation and rising R.

The Sa_{O_2} normally changes less than 2% from rest to maximal exercise. In highly motivated athletes the Sa_{O_2} has been reported to fall below resting values but this is uncommon.

It is commonly reported that the $P(A-a)_{O_2}$ increases during heavy exercise in normal subjects. Both Lilienthal et al.,[52] and Asmussen and Nielsen[53] found a mean $P(A-a)_{O_2}$ of 30 mm Hg at high work rates. Jones et al.[41] found, in 17 normal active men not in physical training, a mean $P(A-a)_{O_2}$ of 12 mm Hg at rest with an increase to approximately 20 mm Hg at work rates with a $\dot{V}_{O_2}$ over 1.5 L/min. Whipp and Wasserman,[50] in 5 healthy young men, found a $P(A-a)_{O_2}$ of 7.4 ± 1.9 mm Hg (mean ± SE) at rest and 10.8 ± 1.6 mm Hg at heavy exercise. Cruz et al.[54] studied four subjects at rest and at work rates approximating 50, 75, and 100% of maximum $\dot{V}_{O_2}$ at sea level and found $P(A-a)_{O_2}$ values (mean ± SEM) of 11.5 ± 2.7, 11.0 ± 2.1, 16.3 ± 1.3, and 20 ± 4.4 mm Hg, respectively. Hansen et al.[55] studied 16 healthy young men, aged 18 to 24, during sea level exercise on a cycle ergometer and found that the mean $P(A-a)_{O_2}$ was 8 mm Hg while sitting at rest, 7 mm Hg during mild, 11 mm Hg during moderate, and 15 mm Hg during maximal exercise. Similar results were obtained by Wasserman et al.[46] in 10 healthy young men and are shown for rest and three work intensities as related to time in Figure 6-9. We found, in our study of 77 normal older men (ages 34 to 74 years) screened by history, chest roentgenograms, resting lung function, and work capacity, $P(A-a)_{O_2}$ values of 12.8 ± 7.4 mm Hg (mean ± SD) at rest and 19.0 ± 8.8 mm Hg at maximum exercise.[9] At maximum exercise, $P(A-a)_{O_2}$ was greater than 35 mm Hg in only 3 of these 77 men.

Acid-Base Balance

Normally, the only acid-base disturbance that develops during exercise is metabolic acidosis. The intensity of the metabolic acidosis can be documented by arterial blood and gas exchange measurements. Normal values for younger[56] and older[9] men for incremental cycle exercise tests are given in Table 6-4.

TABLE 6-4. *Metabolic Acidosis at the End of and During Recovery from Maximum Incremental Cycle Ergometry Exercise in Normal Sedentary Men*[9,56]

TIME AGE, YEARS	AT END OF EXERCISE		TWO MINUTES INTO RECOVERY	
	18–24	34–74	18–24	34–74
Number studied	10	77	10	77
Average exercise duration, min	18	9	18	9
Arterial lactate, mEq/L*	6.6 ± 1.4		7.6 ± 1.8	
Arterial HCO_3^- decline from rest, mEq/L*	6.2 ± 2.3	4.0 ± 2.5	8.7 ± 2.6	8.5 ± 2.9
Arterial pH*	7.31 ± 0.04	7.37 ± 0.04	7.29 ± 0.04	7.33 ± 0.03
Gas exchange ratio (R)*		1.21 ± 0.12		1.59 ± 0.19

*Values are mean ± SD

CRITIQUE

Measurements of the acid-base status and R at the termination of an incremental exercise test are valuable in deciding whether or not the subject made a good effort to perform maximally. Resting venous and arterial lactate values are normally less than 1 mEq/L and typically rise significantly before the termination of maximal exercise. During exercise, venous lactate values can be dependent on the site of lactate production and the sampling site, whereas arterial lactate gives a better indication of the total body lactate burden. As described in Chapter 2, the rise in blood lactate during exercise is accompanied by a nearly equimolar decline in bicarbonate and a decrease in pH. This metabolic acidosis results in hyperventilation, a decline in Pa_{CO_2}, and a further increase in $\dot{V}_{CO_2}$ so that R increases. The lactate and R reach their peak and the pH and bicarbonate reach their nadir at about 2 minutes of recovery after an incremental exercise test. The magnitude of these changes indicates the severity of exercise-induced metabolic acidosis. Small changes signify a mild degree of exercise stress secondary to low motivation or disorders that preclude the performance of exercise at a significant level above the *AT*.

Summary

Normal exercise values for maximum $\dot{V}_{O_2}$, anaerobic threshold, heart rate, heart rate reserve, O_2 pulse, arterial blood pressure, ventilation, ventilatory equivalents, breathing pattern, breathing reserve, arterial blood gases, $P(A-a)_{O_2}$, $P(a-ET)_{CO_2}$, V_D/V_T, and acid base balance are presented in this chapter for use in subject assessment. We also provide a critique of each measurement in which we discuss the recommended and other normal values and their sources.

In the future, new and more versatile sets of normal values will undoubtedly be compiled.

References

1. Astrand, I.: Aerobic work capacity in men and women with special reference to age. Acta Physiol. Scand., *49* (Suppl. 169):1–89, 1960.
2. Drinkwater, B.L., Horvath, S.M., and Wells, C.L.: Aerobic power of females, ages 10 to 68. J. Gerontol., *30*:385–394, 1975.
3. Hermansen, L., and Saltin, B.: Oxygen uptake during maximal treadmill and bicycle exercise. J. Appl. Physiol., *26*:31–37, 1969.
4. Dehn, M.M., and Bruce, R.A.: Longitudinal variations in maximal oxygen intake with age and activity. J. Appl. Physiol., *33*:805–807, 1972.
5. Astrand, I., Astrand, P.O., Hallback, I., and Kilborn, A.: Reduction in maximal oxygen uptake with age. J. Appl. Physiol., *35*:649–654, 1973.
6. Bruce, R.A., Kusumi, F., and Hosmer, D.: Maximal oxygen uptake and nomographic assessment of functional aerobic impairment in cardiovascular disease. Am. Heart J., *85*:546–562, 1973.
7. Astrand, P.O.: Human physical fitness with special reference to sex and age. Physiol. Rev., *36*:307–335, 1956.
8. Buskirk, E., and Taylor, H.L.: Maximal oxygen intake and its relation to body composition, with special reference to chronic physical activity and obesity. J. Appl. Physiol., *11*:72–78, 1957.
9. Hansen, J.E., Sue, D.Y., and Wasserman, K.: Predicted values for clinical exercise testing. Am. Rev. Respir. Dis., *129* (Suppl.):S49–S55, 1984.
10. Sue, D.Y., and Hansen, J.E.: Normal values in adults during exercise testing. Clin. Chest Med., *5*:89–98, 1984.
11. Cooper, D.M., and Weiler-Ravell, D.: Gas exchange response to exercise in children. Am. Rev. Respir. Dis., *129* (Suppl.):S47–S48, 1984.
12. Cooper, D.M., Weiler-Ravell, D., Whipp, B.J., and Wasserman, K.: Aerobic parameters of exercise as a function of body size during growth in children. J. Appl. Physiol., *56*:628–634, 1984.

13. Balke, J., and Ware, R.W.: An experimental study of "physical fitness" of air force personnel. U.S. Armed Forces Med. J., *10*:675–688, 1959.

14. Astrand, P.O., and Saltin, B.: Maximal oxygen uptake and heart rate in various types of muscular activity. J. Appl. Physiol., *16*:977–981, 1961.

15. Hansen, J.E.: Exercise instruments, schemes, and protocols for evaluating the dyspneic patient. Am. Rev. Respir. Dis., *129* (Suppl.):S25–S27, 1984.

16. Cooper, D.M., Weiler-Ravell, D., Whipp, B.J., and Wasserman, K.: Growth-related changes in oxygen uptake and heart rate during progressive exercise in children. Pediatr. Res., *18*:845–851, 1984.

17. Jones, N.L., and Campbell, E.J.M.: Clinical Exercise Testing. 2nd Ed. Philadelphia, W.B. Saunders Co., 1982, p. 119.

18. Sheffield, L.T., Maloof, J.A., Sawyer, J.A., and Roitman, D.: Maximal heart rate and treadmill performance of healthy women in relation to age. Circulation, *57*:79–84, 1978.

19. Astrand, P.O., and Rodahl, K.: Textbook of Work Physiology. 2nd Ed. New York, McGraw-Hill, 1977, p. 190.

20. Cooper, K.H., Purdy, J., White, S., Pollock, M., and Linnerud, A.C.: Age-fitness adjusted maximal heart rates. Med. Sci. Sports, *10*:78–86, 1977.

21. Robinson, T.R., et al.: Intra-arterial and cuff blood pressure responses during incremental cycle ergometry (to be published).

22. Wasserman, K., and McIlroy, M.B.: Detecting the threshold of anaerobic metabolism in cardiac patients during exercise. Am. J. Cardiol., *14*:844–852, 1964.

23. Wasserman, K.: The anaerobic threshold measurement to evaluate exercise performance. Am. Rev. Respir. Dis., *129* (Suppl.):S35–S40, 1984.

24. Wasserman, K., Whipp, B.J., Koyal, S.N., Beaver, W.L.: Anaerobic threshold and respiratory gas exchange during exercise. J. Appl. Physiol., *35*:236–243, 1973.

25. Nery, L.E., Wasserman, K., French, W., Oren, A., and Davis, J.A.: Contrasting cardiovascular and respiratory responses to exercise in mitral valve and chronic obstructive pulmonary diseases. Chest *83*:446–453, 1983.

26. Orr, G.W., Green, H.J., Hughson, R.L., and Bennett, G.W.: A computer linear regression model to determine ventilatory anaerobic threshold. J. Appl. Physiol., *52*:1349–1352, 1982.

27. Davis, J.A., Frank, M.H., Whipp, B.J., and Wasserman, K.: Anaerobic threshold alterations caused by endurance training in middle-aged men. J. Appl. Physiol., *46*:1039–1046, 1979.

28. Davis, et al.: Personal communication, 1985.

29. Davis, J.A., Vodak, P., Wilmore, J.H., Vodak, J., and Kurtz, P.: Anaerobic threshold and maximal aerobic power for three modes of exercise. J. Appl. Physiol., *41*:544–550, 1976.

30. Buchfuhrer, M.J., Hansen, J.E., Robinson, T.E., Sue, D.Y., Wasserman, K., and Whipp, B.J.: Optimizing the exercise protocol for cardiopulmonary assessment. J. Appl. Physiol: *55*:1558–1564, 1983.

31. Withers, R.T., Sherman, W.M., Miller, J.M. and Costillo, D.L.: Specificity of the anaerobic threshold in endurance trained cyclists and runners. Eur. J. Applied Physiol., *47*:93–101, 1981.

32. Hansen, J.E., Sue, D.Y., Oren, A., and Wasserman, K.: Reduced oxygen uptake during incremental work: a marker of cardiovascular dysfunction (to be published).

33. Wasserman, K., and Whipp, B.J.: Exercise physiology in health and disease. Am. Rev. Respir. Dis., *112*:219–249, 1975.

34. Kory, R.C., Callahan, R., Boren, H.G., and Syner, J.C.: The Veterans Administration-Army cooperative study of pulmonary function. I. Clinical spirometry in normal men. Am. J. Med., *30*:243–258, 1961.

35. Lindall, A., Medine, A., and Grismor, J.T.: A re-evaluation of normal pulmonary function measurements in the adult female. Am. Rev. Respir. Dis., *95*:1061–1064, 1967.

36. Gandevia, B., and Hugh-Jones, P.: Terminology for measurements of ventilatory capacity. Thorax, *1*:290–293, 1957.

37. Cotes, J.E.: Lung Function: Assessment and Application in Medicine. 3rd Ed. Oxford, Blackwell Scientific Publications, 1975, p. 104.

38. Miller, W.F., Johnson, R.L., Jr., and Wu, N.: Relationships between maximal breathing capacity and timed expiratory capacities. J. Appl. Physiol., *14*:510–516, 1959.

39. Campbell, S.C.: A comparison of the maximum voluntary ventilation with forced expiratory volume in one second: an assessment of subject cooperation. J. Occup. Med., *24*:531–533, 1982.

40. Bradley, P.W., and Younes, M.: Relation between respiratory valve dead space and tidal volume. J. Appl. Physiol., *49*:528–532, 1980.

41. Jones, N.L., McHardy, G.J.R., Naimark, A., and Campbell, E.J.M.: Physiological dead space and alveolar-arterial gas pressure differences during exercise. Clin. Sci., *31*:19–29, 1966.

42. Lifshay, A., Fast, C.W., and Glazier, J.B.: Effects of changes in respiratory pattern on physiological dead space. J. Appl. Physiol., *31*:478–483, 1971.

43. Hey, E.N., Lloyd, B.B., Cunningham, D.J.C., Jukes, M.G.M., and Bolton, D.P.G.: Effects of various respiratory stimuli on the depth and frequency of breathing in man. Respir. Physiol., *1*:193–205, 1966.

44. Spiro, S.G., Juniper, E., Bowman, P., and Edwards, R.H.T.: An increasing work rate test for assessing the physiological strain of submaximal exercise. Clin. Sci. Molec. Med., *46*:191–206, 1974.

45. Cotes, J.E.: Lung Function: Assessment and Application in Medicine. 3rd Ed. Oxford, Blackwell Scientific Publications, 1975, p. 392.

46. Wasserman, K., VanKessel, A.L., and Burton, G.G.: Interaction of physiological mechanisms during exercise. J. Appl. Physiol., *22*:71–85, 1967.

47. Hansen, J.E.: Exercise testing. *In* Pulmonary Function Testing Guidelines and Controversies. Edited by J.L. Clausen. New York, Academic Press, 1982, p. 272.

48. Cotes, J.E.: Lung Function: Assessment and Application in Medicine. 3rd Ed. Oxford, Blackwell Scientific Publications, 1975, pp. 147, 394.

49. Bradley, C.A., Harris, E.A., Seelye, E.R., and Whitlock, R.M.L.: Gas exchange during exercise in healthy people. I. The physiological dead-space volume. Clin. Sci. Molec. Med., *51*:323–333, 1976.

50. Whipp, B.J., and Wasserman, K.: Alveolar-arterial gas tension differences during graded exercise. J. Appl. Physiol., *27*:361–365, 1969.

51. Ward, S.A., Wasserman, K., Davis, J.A., and Whipp, B.J.: Breathing-valve encumbrance and arterial blood gas and acid-base homeostasis during incremental exercise. Fed. Proc., *43*:634 (Abstract), 1984.

52. Lilienthal, J.L., Riley, R.L., Proemmel, D.D., and Franke, R.E.: An experimental analysis in man of the oxygen pressure gradient from alveolar air to arterial blood during rest and exercise at sea level and at altitude. Am. J. Physiol., *147*:199–216, 1946.

53. Asmussen, E., and Nielsen, M.: Alveolo-arterial gas exchange at rest and during work at different O_2 tensions. Acta Physiol. Scand., *50*:153–166, 1960.

54. Cruz, J.C., Hartley, L.H., and Vogel, J.A.: Effect of altitude relocations upon AaD_{O_2} at rest and during exercise. J. Appl. Physiol., *39*:469–474, 1975.

55. Hansen, J.E., Vogel, J.A., Stelter, G.P., and Consolazio, C.F.: Oxygen uptake in man during exhaustive work at sea level and high altitude. J. Appl. Physiol., *23*:511–522, 1967.

56. Beaver, W.L., Wasserman, K., and Whipp, B.J.: Bicarbonate buffering of lactic acid generated during exercise. J. Appl. Physiol., *60*:472–478, 1986.

Principles of Interpretation

CHAPTER 7

Introduction to Flow Charts

When a subject complains of exercise intolerance, it is usually because he is unable to accomplish a task that he expects to complete with comparative ease and without unusual effort or undue feelings of fatigue or shortness of breath. Identifying the cause of this exercise intolerance is the major objective of clinical exercise testing.

The measurements needed for physiological assessment were discussed in Chapter 3, and their patterns of change in response to the pathophysiology of specific diseases were described in Chapter 4. Having chosen the optimum exercise protocol (Chapter 5) and carefully determining the predicted values for the discriminating physiological variables (Chapter 6), there still remains the task of identifying the probable cause(s) of the exercise intolerance. In this chapter we show how the measurements made during exercise may be used in a systematic fashion to deduce pathophysiology. Although the analytical procedure to be presented is unlikely ideal in all instances, we have found a flow chart strategy, described in Figures 7-1 through 7-5, to be useful.

Analysis begins on flow chart 1 (Fig. 7-1) and then proceeds to specific flow charts depending only on the measured maximum $\dot{V}O_2$ and AT, i.e., to flow chart 2 (Fig. 7-2) if maximum $\dot{V}O_2$ is normal; to flow chart 3 (Fig. 7-3) if maximum $\dot{V}O_2$ is low and AT is normal; to flow chart 4 (Fig. 7-4) if maximum $\dot{V}O_2$ and AT are low; and to flow chart 5 (Fig. 7-5) if maximum $\dot{V}O_2$ is low and AT has not been determined. To facilitate the description of the diagnostic flow, branchpoints are numbered on the flow charts. The symbol $-R$ refers to the right branch of the numbered branchpoint and $-L$ to the left branch of the numbered branchpoint.

Establishing the Pathophysiological Basis of Exercise Intolerance

EXERCISE INTOLERANCE WITH NORMAL MAXIMUM $\dot{V}O_2$ [FLOW CHARTS 1 AND 2]

If maximum $\dot{V}O_2$ is normal, but the patient complains of exercise intolerance, the conditions to the

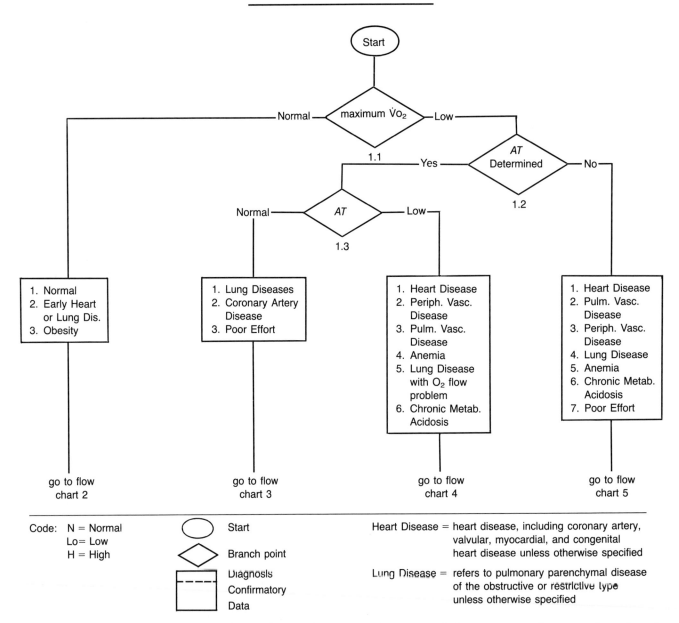

FIG. 7-1. Flow chart for differential diagnosis of cause of exercise limitation. Analysis starts with the measurement of maximum $\dot{V}O_2$. Ellipsoids indicate starting points, diamonds indicate branch points, and boxes indicate diagnoses. Branch points are numbered to correspond to text. Measurements listed under diagnoses are used to confirm them. If the confirmatory information does not fit well, try a closely related branch point leading to a different diagnosis in which the confirmatory measurements fit better. The code shown at the bottom of this figure pertains to all five flow charts.

left of branchpoint 1.1 of Figure 7-1 are considered. The diagnostic possibilities, which are further described in Figure 7-2, are: 1) a normal patient who is anxious about his condition and needs reassurance; 2) a person who had been quite fit but has recently developed a defect in the cardiovascular or respiratory system; or 3) an obese individual who, consequent to the higher-than-normal metabolic cost of work, has increased cardiovascular and respiratory stress during exercise and reduced ability to perform physical work. It should be noted that a normal maximum $\dot{V}O_2$ with a low anaerobic threshold is unusual. However, this might be observed in a cardiac patient.

The measurements that confirm each of the diagnoses associated with a normal maximum $\dot{V}O_2$ are described here and shown in flow chart 2 (see Fig. 7-2):

Normal with anxiety state (2.1-L, 2.2-L)

People with this condition tend to be physically active and try to maintain their general state of health, otherwise they would not be concerned. Therefore, their maximum $\dot{V}O_2$ is generally on the high side of normal, and they are not obese. If the exercise electrocardiogram, O_2 pulse and arterial blood gases are

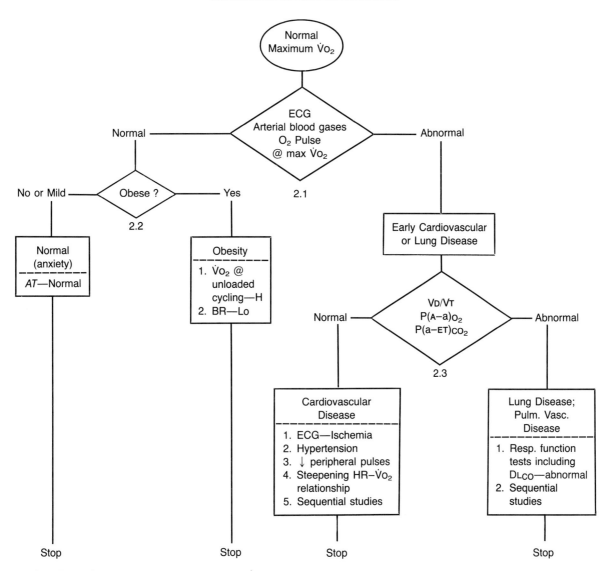

FIG. 7-2. Flow chart 2 for conditions in which maximum $\dot{V}O_2$ is normal but the patient feels exercise limited. If the confirmatory information does not fit well, try a closely related branch point leading to a different diagnosis in which the confirmatory measurements fit better. Symbols and flow chart method are as described in "Introduction to Flow Charts" and Figure 7-1, pp. 87–88.

normal at all work rates, including the maximum, the subject is probably normal. The breathing reserve is normal, but may be on the low side of normal if the subject has a maximum $\dot{V}O_2$ which is considerably better than the predicted normal value, i.e., the subject is in very good physical condition. A confirmatory measurement is an *AT* which is clearly normal. A patient with these findings would benefit from reassurance.

Obesity (2.2-R)

When the obese individual is relatively young, he generally tolerates the increased oxygen cost for work caused by his large body mass quite well. However, when the normal deteriorating effects of aging on the maximum ability to transport O_2 are combined with

the extra O_2 cost of moving the large body, further increases in cardiac and ventilatory responses are constrained and the cardio-respiratory reserve decreases at any given work rate. Thus, since the O_2 cost of work for the obese individual does not decrease with aging but the ability to transport oxygen to the tissues does, the oxygen cost for even ordinary walking might eventually exceed the *AT*. Although the *AT* is normal when adjusted for height or lean body mass, the O_2 cost for walking may be too great to perform without developing a metabolic acidosis. The patient's heart rate reserve is normal at maximum exercise, although his breathing reserve may be reduced because of respiratory restriction. Weight loss would be particularly beneficial when obese individuals start to experience exercise limitation.

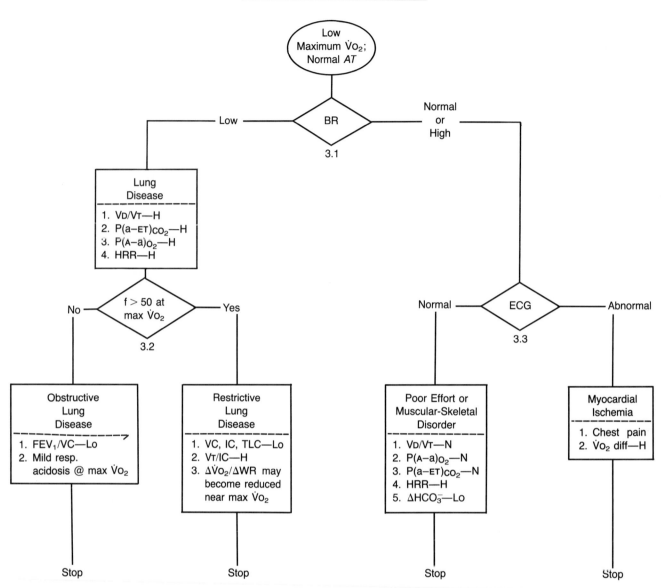

FIG. 7-3.   Flow chart 3 for conditions in which maximum $\dot{V}O_2$ is low but anaerobic threshold *(AT)* is normal. If the confirmatory information does not fit well, try a closely related branch point leading to a different diagnosis in which the confirmatory measurements fit better. Symbols and flow chart method are as described in ''Introduction to Flow Charts'' and Figure 7-1, pp. 87–88.

Early cardiovascular or lung disease (2.1-R, 2.3)

Although a defect may not be severe enough to cause the maximum $\dot{V}O_2$ to be less than that predicted, specific measurements become abnormal depending on the site of the defect in the metabolic-cardiovascular-ventilatory coupling. Thus, a patient may have a maximum $\dot{V}O_2$ value that falls in the normal range and yet still have a mild defect, only recently developed. It is often difficult to document such a developing abnormality except by sequential studies demonstrating deterioration in the maximum $\dot{V}O_2$ and *AT*. Because this patient might have coronary artery disease, the most common problem limiting the

middle-aged adult, examination of the electrocardiogram at various work rates including the patient's maximum $\dot{V}O_2$ is essential. Also, the relationship between heart rate and $\dot{V}O_2$ should be examined to document that linearity is maintained up to the maximum value; a faster rise in HR than $\dot{V}O_2$ toward the end of exercise may be a sign of heart disease. Similarly, flattening of the O_2 pulse at submaximal exercise levels also suggests the presence of heart disease. These changes, associated with evidence of myocardial ischemia on the ECG, make a strong case for the diagnosis of coronary artery disease (2.3-L).

It may also be important to measure arterial blood gases during incremental exercise testing to determine the VD/VT, $P(a–ET)_{CO_2}$, and $P(A–a)_{O_2}$. Normal values rule out mild or developing pulmonary vascular, lung parenchymal, or airway diseases. One or all of these measurements are usually abnormal in these conditions (2.3-R).

LOW MAXIMUM $\dot{V}O_2$ WITH NORMAL AT [FLOW CHART 3]

The measurement that provides a good first branchpoint for the differential diagnosis of the disorders with a low maximum $\dot{V}O_2$ and normal AT is the breathing reserve (3.1). Those patients with a normal or high breathing reserve (3.1-R) include patients making a poor effort, patients limited by muscular and skeletal diseases, or patients with coronary artery disease limited by chest pain at relatively low work rates. Patients with a low breathing reserve (3.1-L) include patients with lung diseases.

Normal or high breathing reserve (3.1-R)

POOR EFFORT OR LOW CARDIORESPIRATORY STRESS (3.3-L). Perhaps for secondary gain, the subject may make a poor effort and thereby have a low maximum $\dot{V}O_2$ during testing. Both the breathing reserve and heart rate reserve are high, indicating that the patient has not used the full potential of either his cardiovascular or his ventilatory systems. The absence of metabolic acidosis at the end of exercise is also evidence of poor effort. Additional confirmatory features include normal exercise V_D/V_T, $P(A-a)O_2$, and $P(a-ET)CO_2$, demonstrating that the distribution of ventilation relative to perfusion is uniform, virtually ruling out primary lung or pulmonary vascular disease.

A low cardiorespiratory stress is also found in conditions associated with musculoskeletal pain or weakness. Optimal cardiovascular and pulmonary evaluation will be impossible when exercise is limited by arthritis or neuromuscular diseases, but this information is, of course, not without value if previously unsuspected.

MYOCARDIAL ISCHEMIA (3.3-R). The 12 lead ECG generally becomes abnormal when the myocardium becomes ischemic as the work rate is increased to the patient's symptom-limited maximum. The ECG abnormality may be evident only at high work rates and the patient may or may not experience chest pain. While coronary artery disease is the most frequent cause of myocardial ischemia, it may also occur in aortic valve disease or marked systemic hypertension, with or without coronary artery disease. The ECG may be normal in patients with posterior myocardial ischemia, but when myocardial ischemia develops, the $\dot{V}O_2$ usually fails to increase normally as the work rate is increased. If the patient exercises

sufficiently, a normal AT without ECG abnormalities makes primary heart disease unlikely.

Low breathing reserve (3.1-L)

A low BR suggests lung disease. The breathing frequency may be a useful next branchpoint to distinguish obstructive from restrictive lung disease. However, the confirmatory data listed under each should also be noted. If the confirmatory data do not support the diagnosis well, the alternate branch should be tried, or a mixed disorder considered.

OBSTRUCTIVE LUNG DISEASES (3.2-L). Although the maximum $\dot{V}O_2$ achieved during incremental exercise testing is low in this disorder, the anaerobic threshold is commonly normal. This suggests that these patients do not have a problem with oxygen flow to the tissues. Characteristically, these patients have abnormal Pa_{O_2}, V_D/V_T, $P(a-ET)CO_2$, and $P(A-a)O_2$ values during exercise consequent to ventilation-perfusion mismatching. Decreases in Pa_{O_2} commonly occur in a single step at low work rates with little further change as the work rate is increased (see Fig. 4-4). This is probably because the increased perfusion goes predominantly to normal and high $\dot{V}A/\dot{Q}$ regions of the lungs. Except in mild obstructive disease, the breathing reserve is decreased due to the ventilatory limitation. However, in contrast to O_2 flow limiting disorders, the $\dot{V}O_2$ continues to increase linearly as the work rate is increased to the patient's maximum $\dot{V}O_2$; i.e., there is no flattening of the $\dot{V}O_2$-work rate relationship. The heart rate reserve is commonly increased because the cardiovascular capacity cannot be fully challenged due to the breathing limitation. Finally, expiratory flow frequently has an obstructive pattern (trapezoidal in appearance, with an early peak as illustrated in Figure 3-18).

In patients with marked airflow obstruction, the AT will usually be indeterminate by gas exchange methods of determination. Thus flow chart 5 becomes a better guide to the differential diagnosis than flow chart 3.

RESTRICTIVE LUNG DISEASES (3.2-R). Functional disturbances in restrictive lung diseases have much in common with those of the obstructive lung diseases but there are very clear differences. The V_D/V_T and $P(a-ET)CO_2$ are increased in both types of lung disorders as reflections of ventilation-perfusion mismatching. However, in contrast to obstructive lung diseases, the $P(A-a)O_2$ usually increases systematically at each work rate during the incremental test. Also, the V_T increases to its maximum at a relatively low work rate and the V_T/IC ratio nears a value of one. Since V_T cannot increase normally, the ventilatory response to the increasing work rate is achieved primarily by increasing the breathing frequency, usually exceeding 50 breaths/min. Patients with restrictive lung diseases often manifest an O_2-flow problem. In this situation, $\dot{V}O_2$ fails to increase normally as the work rate is incremented to the patient's maximum. This may be caused by both the low arterial O_2 content and the increased pulmonary vascular resistance (resulting from destruction of pulmonary blood vessels by the fibrosing process) that limits the cardiac output increase.

LOW MAXIMUM $\dot{V}O_2$ WITH LOW AT [FLOW CHART 4]

Breathing reserve (BR) serves as a good primary branchpoint (4.1) for the differential diagnosis of disorders having a low maximum $\dot{V}O_2$ and low AT. But further branching is needed to distinguish the various conditions in this category. The VD/VT is a good second branchpoint (4.2) for the conditions that have a low BR; while $\dot{V}E/\dot{V}CO_2$ at the AT is a useful second branchpoint (4.3) for the conditions with a normal or high BR.

Normal or high breathing reserve (4.1-R)

NORMAL $\dot{V}E/\dot{V}CO_2$ AT AT (4.3-L). If the breathing reserve is normal or high and the $\dot{V}E/\dot{V}CO_2$ at AT is normal (4.3-L), then we must consider non-lung disease O_2-flow problems such as heart disease, peripheral vascular disease, and anemias or hemoglobinopathies. Hematocrit (4.4) and O_2 pulse ($\dot{V}O_2/HR$) (4.6) are further branchpoints which distinguish these diagnoses.

Heart diseases (4.6-R). Patients with primary heart diseases (coronary artery disease, valvular heart disease, and cardiomyopathies) usually have a low maximum $\dot{V}O_2$ with a low AT. In these disorders, $\dot{V}O_2$ usually slows its rate of rise relative to the work rate as the maximum $\dot{V}O_2$ is approached. The heart rate often continues to increase as the work rate is increased despite $\dot{V}O_2$ increasing more slowly. This results in a steepening of the heart rate-$\dot{V}O_2$ relationship as the work rate is increased and a plateau of the O_2 pulse at subnormal values (see Fig. 3-9). In coronary artery disease, the ECG during exercise usually provides evidence of myocardial ischemia (see Table 3-2).

Patients with heart failure secondary to valvular heart diseases or cardiomyopathies may have a chronic metabolic acidosis, maintaining arterial PCO_2 and bicarbonate at relatively low values with a nor-

mal pH. An acute metabolic acidosis is superimposed during exercise. In rare instances, VD/VT may be elevated because of ventilation/perfusion mismatching. These acid-base changes and the increased VD/VT presumably contribute to the symptom of dyspnea.

Peripheral vascular disease (4.6-L). In contrast to primary heart diseases, the heart rate reserve is generally high in this condition since the patient stops exercising because of claudication before the heart can be maximally stressed. Because of the failure of normal systemic vasodilatation during exercise, hypertension often occurs. Commonly, the increase in oxygen uptake relative to the increase in work rate is diminished, resulting in a relatively shallow slope for the $\dot{V}O_2$-work rate relationship (low $\Delta\dot{V}O_2/\Delta WR$). Finally, in the absence of concomitant lung disease, the measurements of VD/VT, $P(a-ET)CO_2$, and $P(A-a)O_2$, which reflect the distribution of ventilation relative to perfusion, are normal.

Anemia (4.4-R). Because of the reduced O_2 carrying capacity of the blood, lactic acidosis occurs at a relatively low work rate causing the AT to be reduced. The low oxygen content of the arterial blood caused by the anemia means that a high cardiac output is required to meet the tissue O_2 requirement. Consequently, heart rate is increased relative to $\dot{V}O_2$ causing the O_2 pulse to be reduced at the maximum $\dot{V}O_2$. The arterial blood gas tensions and the VD/VT are normal, even at maximal exercise.

HIGH $\dot{V}E/\dot{V}CO_2$ AT AT (4.3-R). If the breathing reserve is normal or high (4.1-R) but the $\dot{V}E/\dot{V}CO_2$ at AT is high (4.3-R), then the most likely primary disorder is an abnormal pulmonary circulation with or without a right-to-left intracardiac shunt. The pattern of change in O_2 saturation (4.5) in response to exercise helps distinguish these conditions.

Pulmonary vascular diseases (4.5-L). In this category, we include those disorders that originate in the pulmonary vascular bed and cause pulmonary vascular resistance to be increased, e.g., pulmonary thromboembolic disease, primary pulmonary hypertension, and diseases that cause a pulmonary vasculitis. These disorders, when chronic, have little effect on pulmonary mechanics, but cause abnormalities in gas exchange as well as limit the cardiac output response to exercise.

If the pulmonary circulation, interposed between the right and left sides of the heart, cannot dilate normally, the increased venous return that accompanies exercise cannot be readily transmitted to the left ventricle. Thus, since the right side of the heart cannot "feed" blood to the left side at a rate commensurate with that required for normal exercise, cardiac

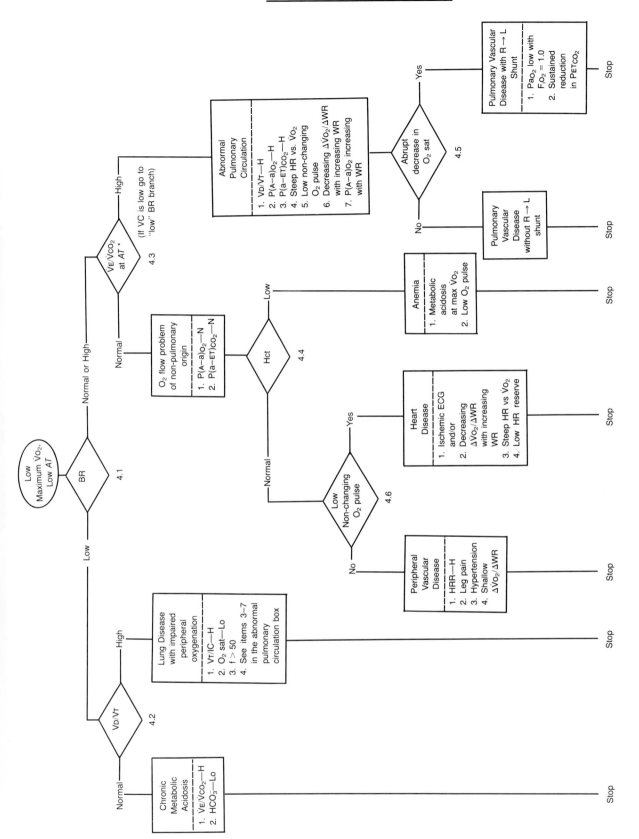

*When the patient is hyperventilating, rely on Vᴅ/Vᴛ, P(A–a)o₂ and P(a–ET)co₂ as indices of ventilation-perfusion mismatching or see insert in Figure 3-13 to correct V̇ᴇ/V̇co₂ for hyperventilation.

Fɪɢ. 7-4. Flow chart 4 for conditions in which maximum V̇o₂ is low and anaerobic threshold (AT) is low. If the confirmatory information does not fit well, try a closely related branch point leading to a different diagnosis in which the confirmatory measurements fit better. Symbols and flow chart method are as described in "Introduction to Flow Charts" and Figure 7-1, pp. 87–88.

output cannot respond appropriately to the exercise stimulus. Because the cardiac output increase is limited, the $\dot{V}O_2$-work rate relationship may flatten at a relatively low work rate during an incremental exercise test, resulting in a low maximum $\dot{V}O_2$. Also, heart rate increases steeply relative to $\dot{V}O_2$ and gets steeper as the maximum $\dot{V}O_2$ is approached. The O_2 pulse is reduced at maximum work and fails to increase as the work rate is increased. These findings are similar to those seen in many patients with primary heart disease.

However, unlike uncomplicated heart disease, high VD/VT and positive $P(a–ET)_{CO_2}$ values provide evidence of poor perfusion of ventilated air spaces. Also, the $P(A–a)_{O_2}$ increases abnormally as the work rate is increased probably due to the shortened pulmonary capillary transit time described in Chapter 4. While these changes are similar to those seen in primary lung diseases, other measurements made during exercise contrast these particular disorders. For instance, the breathing reserve is normal. Also, rather than the mild respiratory acidosis that commonly accompanies obstructive lung diseases, a metabolic acidosis develops with pulmonary vascular diseases in response to exercise.

Primary lung diseases can cause major disturbances in function of the pulmonary circulation and the abnormal pulmonary circulation might become the dominant pathophysiology limiting exercise. In such instances, the abnormalities noted in the "abnormal pulmonary circulation" diagnostic box of flow chart 4 become evident during exercise testing.

Pulmonary vascular disease with a right to left shunt or cyanotic congenital heart disease (4.5-R). During incremental exercise, patients with pulmonary vascular disease who open a potentially patent foramen ovale or have congenital heart disease with a right-to-left shunt may demonstrate markedly decreased arterial O_2 saturation during air and O_2 breathing and flattening of the $\dot{V}O_2$-work rate relationship. The VD/VT, $P(a–ET)_{CO_2}$, and $P(A–a)_{O_2}$ values are very abnormal, depending on the degree of pulmonary hypoperfusion and size of the shunt. These values generally increase as the work rate is increased. These disorders can be distinguished from patients with other pulmonary vascular diseases by the abrupt and sustained decreases in arterial O_2 saturation and PET_{CO_2} (changes that occur as soon as exercise begins). Also, $\dot{V}CO_2$ may exceed $\dot{V}O_2$ during the first few minutes of exercise even at the lowest work rates.

Repeating the exercise test while the patient breathes 100% O_2 is particularly helpful in distinguishing a right-to-left shunt from other causes of hypoxemia. If a right-to-left shunt exists, Pa_{O_2} falls precipitously and the $P(A–a)_{O_2}$ increases markedly as the venous return shunts from right to left.

Low breathing reserve (4.1-L)

In the category of patients with a low maximum $\dot{V}O_2$ and low AT accompanied by a low breathing reserve and high VD/VT (4.2-R), the most likely disorder is a primary lung disease such as pulmonary fibrosis. In contrast, a low breathing reserve with a normal VD/VT in this category is caused by diseases associated with chronic metabolic acidosis (4.2-L). The following discussion describes further physiological measurements that help confirm the diagnosis of each of these disorders.

LUNG DISEASE WITH IMPAIRED PERIPHERAL OXYGENATION (4.2-R).   In certain patients, primarily those with severe interstitial lung disease in which the pulmonary circulation is also markedly impaired, and where there is considerable O_2 desaturation as the subject exercises, the AT as well as the maximum $\dot{V}O_2$ is reduced. Also, the slope of the $\dot{V}O_2$-work rate relationship may be reduced as the work rate is increased. Other abnormalities in gas exchange characteristic of restrictive lung disease will be present as described in the earlier section of this chapter on Restrictive Lung Diseases.

CHRONIC METABOLIC ACIDOSIS (4.2-L).   Patients with chronic heart failure, diabetes mellitus, renal failure, and those taking large doses of aspirin may have a chronic metabolic acidosis. Because Pa_{CO_2} is reduced in these conditions, exercise ventilation is also elevated (low Pa_{CO_2} set-point). Therefore, higher than normal alveolar ventilation is needed to clear the increased metabolic CO_2 generated during exercise (see Fig. 2-15). This reduces the breathing reserve and causes the ventilatory equivalents for CO_2 and O_2 to be increased. Because of the high ventilation requirement, these patients may experience exertional dyspnea before reaching their predicted maximum $\dot{V}O_2$. Their AT is generally reduced because of their underlying disease process. The chronic metabolic acidosis is easily identified from arterial blood gas and pH measurements.

LOW MAXIMUM $\dot{V}O_2$ (1.1-R) WITH AT NOT DETERMINED (1.2-R) [FLOW CHARTS 1 AND 5].

The AT may not be measured during a test or the AT may be too difficult to determine to be reliable. The latter usually results from a very irregular breathing pattern or because the AT occurs at such a low work

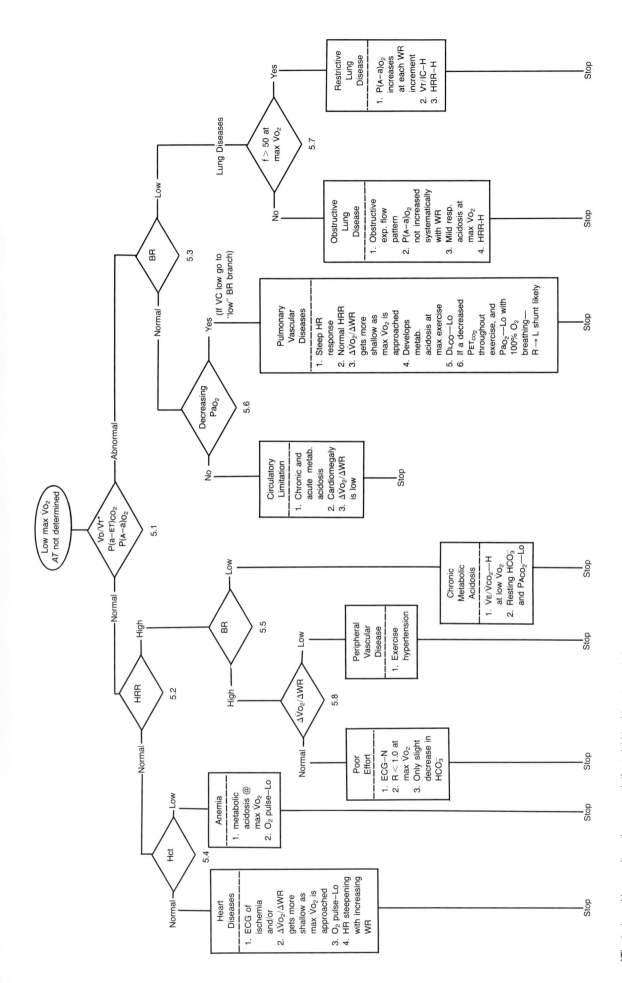

Fig. 7-5. Flow chart 5 for conditions in which maximum $\dot{V}O_2$ is low but anaerobic threshold has not been reliably determined. If the confirmatory information does not fit well, try a closely related branch point leading to a different diagnosis in which the confirmatory measurements fit better. Symbols and flow chart method are as described in "Introduction to Flow Charts" and Figure 7-1, pp. 87–88.

*The text provides an alternative approach if arterial blood is not sampled.

rate that the dynamics of gas exchange at the start of exercise blur the changes in gas exchange that accompany the *AT.* Also, patients with respiratory insufficiency may not manifest the normal ventilatory changes associated with the development of a metabolic acidosis. If it is particularly important to know the patient's *AT,* it can be ascertained by doing several constant work rate tests and measuring the increase in $\dot{V}O_2$ from 3 to 6 minutes (see Fig. 3-23). The highest work rate at which there is no difference between the 6 minute and 3 minute $\dot{V}O_2$ is approximately the *AT* (see the section on "Oxygen Cost of Work," Chapter 2, and the section "Exercise Testing — Constant Work Rate," in Chapter 3). This, however, requires repeated constant work rate tests that are time consuming and, therefore, may be inconvenient.

An alternative to *AT* as the second major branchpoint (1.2) in the decision-making process shown in flow chart 1 is given in flow chart 5 (see Fig. 7-5). After finding a reduced maximum $\dot{V}O_2$, we next consider tests that detect mismatching of ventilation to perfusion. This allows us to distinguish disorders associated with inefficiency of lung gas exchange from disorders with normal lung function but limited ability to increase O_2-flow to the tissues. The decision requires simultaneous arterial blood gas and pulmonary gas exchange information. As shown in flow chart 5, if VD/VT, $P(a-ET)_{CO_2}$, and $P(A-a)_{O_2}$ values are normal (5.1-L), we examine the heart rate reserve (HRR) (5.2); if VD/VT, $P(a-ET)_{CO_2}$, and $P(A-a)_{O_2}$ values are abnormal (5.1-R), we examine the breathing reserve (BR) (5.3) in the decision-making process. The possible diagnoses at each of these branch points separate into two major groups depending on whether the heart rate reserve is normal or high, or the breathing reserve is normal or low. The next level of branching allows specific diagnoses to be made.

While the first step in flow chart 5 (5.1) depends on knowledge of arterial P_{CO_2} and P_{O_2}, we realize that it may not be feasible to collect arterial blood under some circumstances. An alternative is to approximate Pa_{CO_2} from venous blood drawn from a superficial vein of a warmed hand or from capillary blood from a finger or ear lobe, and from these measurements, estimate VD/VT and $P(a-ET)_{CO_2}$.* Normal values would direct the analysis to the left (5.1-L) and abnormal values would direct the analysis to the right (5.1-R).

---

*A less satisfactory alternative is to look at $\dot{V}E/\dot{V}CO_2$ and $\dot{V}E/\dot{V}O_2$ values at moderate work rates. If these values are normal, $\dot{V}A/\dot{Q}$ disturbances are unlikely; but normal values associated with hypoventilation and elevated VD/VT cannot be excluded. If the $\dot{V}E/\dot{V}CO_2$ and $\dot{V}E/\dot{V}O_2$ are elevated, $\dot{V}A/\dot{Q}$ disturbances are likely, but hyperventilation as the cause cannot be excluded.

Normal distribution of ventilation-perfusion (5.1-L)

Heart disease, anemia, poor effort, peripheral vascular disease, and chronic metabolic acidosis are all associated with a low maximum $\dot{V}O_2$ but have normal indices of gas exchange efficiency (uniform $\dot{V}A/\dot{Q}$). The HRR allows this group to be further subdivided into those with a normal HRR (5.2-L) (heart disease and anemia) and a high HRR (5.2-R) (poor effort, peripheral vascular disease, and chronic metabolic acidosis).

The two disorders with a low maximum $\dot{V}O_2$, uniform $\dot{V}A/\dot{Q}$, and normal HRR (5.2-L) are heart diseases (ischemic, valvular, cardiomyopathic or noncyanotic congenital) and anemia. They can be distinguished on the basis of the hematocrit (5.4) and the diagnosis can be confirmed by examining the measurements listed in the diagnostic boxes in flow chart 5.

The causes of a low maximum $\dot{V}O_2$, uniform $\dot{V}A/\dot{Q}$, and high HRR (5.2-R) are poor effort, peripheral vascular disease, or chronic metabolic acidosis. The last is associated with low breathing reserve (5.5-R) and could be confirmed from arterial blood gas and pH measurement.

The patient making a poor effort can be confirmed by other measurements, including his high breathing reserve (5.5-L), failure to develop a significant metabolic acidosis at end-exercise, an R of <1.0 at the maximum $\dot{V}O_2$, and a normal ECG.

The low $\Delta\dot{V}O_2/\Delta WR$ value (5.8-R) also distinguishes peripheral vascular disease from poor effort. The measurements listed in the respective diagnostic boxes in flow chart 5 confirm these diagnoses.

Abnormal distribution of ventilation-perfusion (5.1-R)

Chronic heart failure, pulmonary vascular diseases, and obstructive and restrictive lung diseases are all associated with a low maximum $\dot{V}O_2$ and abnormal indices of gas exchange efficiency (nonuniform $\dot{V}A/\dot{Q}$). The breathing reserve (5.3) allows this group to be further subdivided into those with a normal breathing reserve (heart failure and pulmonary vascular diseases) and a low breathing reserve (obstructive and restrictive lung diseases).

The two disorders with a low maximum $\dot{V}O_2$ and a nonuniform $\dot{V}A/\dot{Q}$ but a normal breathing reserve (5.3-L), can usually be distinguished by the Pa_{O_2} or arterial O_2 saturation (5.6) measurement. The patient with pulmonary vascular disease without a right to left shunt will generally have a mildly reduced Pa_{O_2} or arterial O_2 saturation at rest that decreases progressively as the work rate increases (5.6-R). If the pulmonary vascular disease is accompanied by a right to left shunt, such as in cyanotic congenital heart disease or the opening of an unsealed foramen ovale, then the decrement in O_2 saturation at the start of exercise will be marked. Item 6 in the diagnostic box for pulmonary vascular diseases describes other confirmatory data for a right to left shunt.

The patient with chronic heart failure will have a normal or only a slightly reduced O_2 saturation at rest that remains largely unaffected by exercise (5.6-L). The box identifying this diagnosis lists confirmatory measurements.

The two lung disorders with a low maximum $\dot{V}_{O_2}$ and a nonuniform $\dot{V}_A/\dot{Q}$ but with a low breathing reserve (5.3-R) can generally be distinguished by the breathing frequency. A breathing frequency of >50 at the patient's maximum $\dot{V}_{O_2}$ is commonly associated with restrictive lung disease (5.7-R), whereas a breathing frequency of <50 at the maximum $\dot{V}_{O_2}$ is characteristic of the patient with obstructive lung disease (5.7-L). These diagnoses are supported by the measurements listed in the respective diagnostic boxes of the flow chart.

Interpretation of Constant Work Rate Tests

While the analyses just given use measurements obtained from incremental exercise tests, certain information can best be obtained from constant work rate tests. For example, it is possible to evaluate the role of the carotid bodies in the exercise hyperpnea by surreptitiously switching the inspired gas from air to 100% oxygen during steady-state exercise. (see Fig. 3-24). There will be a decrease in ventilation within two breaths or so as arterial blood with a high P_{O_2} reaches the carotid bodies. The maximum decrement in ventilation can be measured by monitoring ventilation breath-by-breath. The proportional decrease in ventilation is the minimum that the carotid bodies contribute to ventilatory drive since the degree of hyperoxia obtained may not have completely attenuated the carotid bodies. Also, the consequent increase in Pa_{CO_2}, as the ventilation falls, might lead to chemoreceptor stimulation and offset some of the carotid body inhibition.

Exercise of moderately severe intensity can also be used to identify exercise induced bronchospasm (see Chapter 5) by comparing indices of airflow obstruction during the first 20 minutes of recovery with those before exercise. Normally, the FEV_1 is unchanged or increased after exercise, but reductions in FEV_1 of 10% or greater accompany exercise-induced asthma.

Summary

To determine the likely pathophysiological causes of exercise limitation, we have found that a logical approach can be expressed in a series of five flow charts. Physiological measurements relating heart rate, ventilation, and gas exchange to work rate are used in the decision-making process of the patient with exercise intolerance. The first flow chart separates four major categories of patients: 1) those with a normal maximum $\dot{V}_{O_2}$, 2) those with a reduced maximum $\dot{V}_{O_2}$ but with a normal anaerobic threshold, 3) those with a reduced maximum $\dot{V}_{O_2}$ but with a reduced anaerobic threshold, and 4) those with a reduced maximum $\dot{V}_{O_2}$ but with the anaerobic threshold not determined. Flow charts 2 to 5 analyze these four categories further, usually allowing a specific organ-related physiological diagnosis to be made. However, the flow charts are designed only as guides to an orderly decision-making process. The final judgement must be made by the examiner.

Case Presentations

W E SELECTED THE cases presented in this section because they are either representative of specific pathophysiology or they teach a unique lesson. They were not selected because they show data from especially cooperative subjects or are pretty records. In fact, these studies were done on typical patients evaluated in our clinical exercise laboratory and therefore include records that range between the best and the worst with respect to appearance. The primary goal of this chapter is to offer a systematic approach to interpretation of exercise performance. We demonstrate how measurements can be used as decision-making branchpoints for reaching an appropriate diagnosis and apply these measurements to a spectrum of abnormalities.

The data given in these case presentations are restricted to information needed to interpret the exercise test. Generally, two sets of resting blood gas data are included in Table 3 of each report. The first is obtained with the subject sitting on the ergometer but before breathing on the mouthpiece (i.e., *without* accompanying respiratory gas exchange data), and the second is obtained with the subject on the ergometer while breathing on the mouthpiece prior to exercise (i.e., *with* accompanying gas exchange data). Both sets of data are reported for comparison.

The graphical data given in Figures A and B display data points every 30 seconds, calculated as the average of whole breath-by-breath measurements over the preceding 15 to 20 second period. On graphs 1, 2, 3, 6, 8, and 9 of these figures, after a period of rest and unloaded pedalling (0 watts), the work rate is increased in equal increments each minute; various variables are plotted on the vertical axes. The increments begin at the left vertical dashed line, and the termination of exercise or return to unloaded cycling is indicated by the right vertical dashed line. Two minutes of recovery data are also plotted. On graph 3, the predicted change in $\dot{V}_{O_2}$, as work rate is increased, is shown by the stippled diagonal bar. Interrelated ventilatory and cardiovascular variables are plotted on graphs 4, 5, and 7 during rest and exercise, but not recovery. On graph 5 the mean predicted maximum $\dot{V}_{O_2}$ and maximum HR for a sedentary person of the same sex, age, and body size are marked with a small circle. The summary data shown in Table 2 are taken from Table 3 (and Table 4, if given) and Figure A (and Figure B, if given).

The predicted values given for each case are the mean values taken from Chapter 6. As with any predicted values there are normal ranges. To the best of our knowledge, our interpretations take the range of normal values into account.

Fifty-two cases are presented for interpretation. Practical considerations limited our ability to provide more examples, and of course, there are many disorders of exercise performance that we have not studied directly. But because each category of disease can have perturbations that are instructive to review, we find it desirable sometimes to present more than one case of each type of disorder. Also, patients frequently have more than one abnormality. Thus, we thought it important to present some of these complex cases and to provide our rationale for our conclusions regarding the dominant pathophysiology.

Of the *52 cases,* the first *12* are of men and women whom we concluded were normal. They were selected to show the effect of age, gender, form of ergometry used for testing, effect of O_2 breathing, effect of beta-adrenergic blockade, and effect of cigarette smoking on the test results.

Cases *13* and *14* are examples of poor effort during exercise testing.

Cases *15-20* are examples of valvular heart disease, coronary artery disease, and cardiomyopathies. Other examples of heart diseases are provided in the "complex" case category described below.

Cases *21-23* are examples of peripheral vascular diseases. Again, some examples are included in the "complex" case category since these disorders are commonly associated with primary heart disease.

Cases *24-29* include several types and severity of diseases primarily associated with airflow obstruction. Other examples of obstructive airway disease can be found in the "complex" category.

Cases *30-34* are examples of various types of pulmonary fibrosis or respiratory restriction. Two cases show results before and after treatment.

Cases *35-39* are examples of chronic pulmonary vascular diseases of several types. One of the major roles of exercise testing is diagnosis and evaluation of the effect of therapy in these disorders. Other examples of pulmonary vascular diseases are presented in cases *40-43*; these represent a group of patients with complex kinds of lung disease and pathophysiology.

Examples of disorders of the respiratory "pump" are presented in cases *44-46*. These disorders can be found in many forms, and the three cases presented are representative.

The last and perhaps the most challenging and interesting group of patients, cases *47-52*, are those with multiple abnormalities (complex cases). We have analyzed these cases with the intent of diagnosing the limiting disorder or disorders.

In a few instances, the conclusions we reached in the case analysis will not be easily obtained from the logical sequence suggested by the flow charts. Nevertheless, we started each analysis by using the flow charts in all cases. The supporting data listed under each diagnosis should always be considered to confirm the diagnosis derived from the flow chart analysis.

We recommend, therefore, that students of these cases ought not be too rigid in the use of the flow charts. For instance, we point out that a measurement (branchpoint) that distinguishes obstructive from restrictive lung disease is the breathing frequency at the maximum work rate performed. Generally this value is greater than 50 per minute in patients with restrictive lung disease and less than 50 per minute in patients with obstructive lung disease. Although this distinction usually exists, exceptions will almost inevitably occur.

Finally, although certain disorders are not specifically presented here, we hope that the principles taught in this and the preparatory chapters will provide the reader with the necessary physiological background to interpret the many pathophysiological conditions not described.

CASE 1 *Normal man*

CLINICAL FINDINGS

This 55-year-old executive was referred for exercise testing because of his complaint of decreased exercise tolerance. He complained of weakness, fatigue, and some dyspnea after jogging one block, but he could walk 3 miles on the level without difficulty. He became symptomatic following recovery from an ankle injury two years earlier and felt unable to satisfactorily improve his exercise tolerance. He denied chest pain, syncope, palpitations, coughing, or wheezing. He smoked one half pack of cigarettes per day for 10 years but had reduced his smoking to 3 to 4 cigarettes per week. He took no medications. Physical examination, chest roentgenograms, and resting ECG were normal.

EXERCISE FINDINGS

The patient performed exercise on a cycle ergometer. He pedalled at 60 rpm without added load for 3 minutes. The work rate was then increased 20 watts per minute to his symptom limited maximum. Blood was sampled every second minute and intra-arterial blood pressure was recorded from a percutaneously placed brachial artery catheter. The patient stopped exercise because of thigh fatigue. Twelve-lead ECG recordings remained normal during exercise.

TABLE 1-1. *Selected Respiratory Function Data*

MEASUREMENT	PREDICTED	MEASURED
Age, yr		55
Sex		Male
Height, cm		182
Weight, kg	83	80
Hematocrit, %		41
VC, L	4.75	6.06
IC, L	3.17	4.16
TLC, L	7.08	8.24
FEV_1, L	3.76	4.52
FEV_1/VC, %	79	75
MVV, L/min	151	200
DL_{CO}, ml/mm Hg/min	28.8	28.3

TABLE 1-2. *Selected Exercise Data*

MEASUREMENT	PREDICTED	MEASURED
Maximum $\dot{V}O_2$, L/min	2.42	2.53
Maximum HR, beats/min	165	176
Maximum O_2 pulse, ml/beat	14.7	14.5
$\Delta\dot{V}O_2/\Delta WR$, ml/min/watt	10.3	9.8
$\dot{V}O_2$ difference, %	0.0	3.7
AT, L/min	>0.97	1.1
Blood pressure, mm Hg (rest, max)		144/81,225/87
Maximum $\dot{V}E$, L/min		107
Exercise breathing reserve, L/min	>15	93
Pa_{O_2}, mm Hg (rest, max ex)		98,110
$P(A-a)_{O_2}$, mm Hg (rest, max ex)		5,15
$P(a-ET)_{CO_2}$, mm Hg (rest, max ex)		0,−5
VD/VT (rest, heavy ex)		0.26,0.15
HCO_3^-, mEq/L (rest, 2 min recov)		25,12

TABLE 1-3.

TIME min	WORK RATE W	BP mmHg	HR min⁻¹	f	VE BTPS —L/min—	VCO₂ STPD	VO₂ —L/min	O₂ pulse ml/beat	R	pH	HCO₃⁻ mEq/L	PO₂ ET	PO₂ a —mmHg—	PO₂ A-a	PCO₂ ET	PCO₂ a —mmHg—	PCO₂ a-ET	VE VCO₂	VE VO₂	VD VT
Rest	153/ 87									7.42	25	97			39					
Rest		144/ 81	78	13	9.8	0.25	0.31	4.0	0.81			105			38			35	28	
Rest			80	11	9.2	0.26	0.34	4.3	0.76	7.42	24	103	98	5	38	38	0	32	24	0.26
Rest			76	10	13.2	0.38	0.43	5.7	0.88			106			37			32	29	
Unloaded			91	12	17.1	0.58	0.69	7.6	0.84			104			38			28	23	
Unloaded			83	19	14.5	0.42	0.53	6.4	0.79			103			39			31	24	
Unloaded		171/ 87	85	25	16.4	0.50	0.62	7.3	0.81	7.41	25	101	100	2	40	40	0	28	23	0.21
1.0	20		86	28	18.1	0.58	0.67	7.8	0.87			104			40			27	23	
2.0	40	183/ 84	93	18	19.9	0.69	0.82	8.8	0.84	7.40	25	101	99	5	42	40	−2	27	22	0.17
3.0	60		104	17	26.0	0.91	1.03	9.9	0.88			102			42			27	24	
4.0	80	195/ 81	110	16	28.4	1.07	1.16	10.5	0.92	7.33	24	103	93	9	43	40	−3	25	23	0.14
5.0	100		123	17	38.1	1.44	1.41	11.5	1.02			107			43			25	26	
6.0	120	207/ 87	135	19	44.5	1.67	1.62	12.0	1.03	7.37	23	107	103	7	43	41	−2	26	26	0.17
7.0	140		146	20	49.4	1.87	1.74	11.9	1.07			109			42			26	27	
8.0	160	213/ 90	155	19	58.3	2.23	1.99	12.8	1.12	7.35	21	110	101	13	42	39	−3	25	28	0.13
9.0	180		163	22	69.5	2.55	2.16	13.3	1.18			112			42			27	31	
10.0	200	225/ 87	170	27	90.7	3.10	2.42	14.2	1.28	7.31	18	115	105	15	40	36	−4	29	37	0.16
11.0	220	216/ 90	176	30	102.9	3.20	2.36	13.4	1.36	7.30	15	118	110	15	37	32	−5	31	43	0.14
Recovery			158	21	71.5	2.10	1.26	8.0	1.67			124			35			33	55	
Recovery		165/ 75	149	19	52.7	1.44	0.91	6.1	1.58	7.22	12	126	124	5	32	30	−2	35	56	0.18

FIGURE 1-A

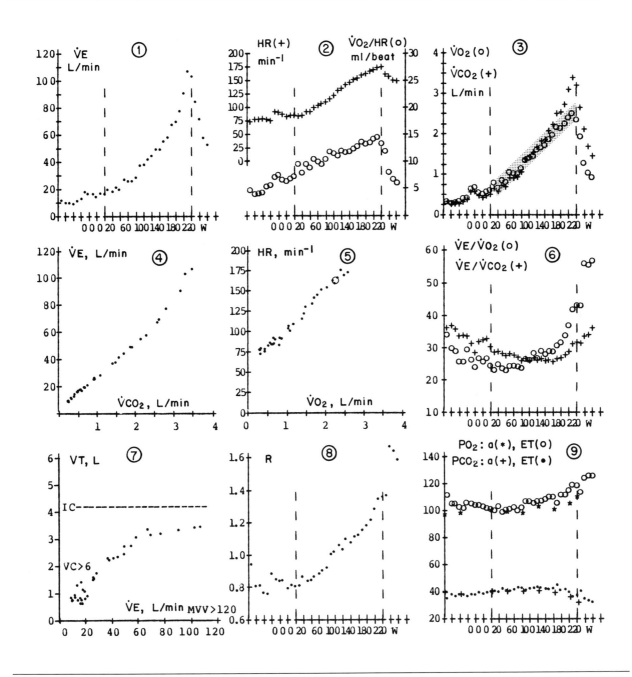

Interpretation

COMMENTS

The results of the respiratory function studies are within normal limits (Table 1-1).

ANALYSIS

Flow Chart 1: The maximum $\dot{V}O_2$ and anaerobic threshold are normal (Table 1-2). See *Flow Chart 2:*

The electrocardiogram and arterial blood gases (Table 1-3) are normal throughout exercise; the O_2-pulse at the maximum work rate is normal.

CONCLUSION

Normal man, with high level of anxiety regarding his physical status.

CASE 2 *Normal athlete*

CLINICAL FINDINGS

This 31-year-old physiologist was a frequent marathon runner. He had no known health problems and trained several times weekly.

EXERCISE FINDINGS

The subject performed exercise on a cycle ergometer. He pedalled without added load at 60 rpm for 2 minutes. The work rate was then increased 30 watts every minute to his symptom limited maximum. There were no arrhythmias and ECG remained normal.

TABLE 2-1. *Selected Respiratory Function Data*

MEASUREMENT	PREDICTED	MEASURED
Age, yr		31
Sex		Male
Height, cm		182
Weight, kg	83	81
Hematocrit, %		43
VC, L	5.48	6.27
IC, L	3.65	3.56
FEV_1, L	4.43	4.51
FEV_1/VC, %	81	72
MVV, L/min	182	185

TABLE 2-2. *Selected Exercise Data*

MEASUREMENT	PREDICTED	MEASURED
Maximum $\dot{V}O_2$, L/min	3.20	4.95
Maximum HR, beats/min	189	175
Maximum O_2 pulse, ml/beat	16.9	28.3
$\Delta\dot{V}O_2/\Delta WR$, ml/min/watt	10.3	11.5
$\dot{V}O_2$ difference, %	0.0	−10.2
AT, L/min	>1.28	2.2
Maximum $\dot{V}E$, L/min		186
Exercise breathing reserve, L/min	>15	−1

TABLE 2-3.

TIME min	WORK RATE W	BP mmHg	HR min⁻¹	f	$\dot{V}E$ BTPS L/min	$\dot{V}CO_2$ STPD L/min	$\dot{V}O_2$ STPD L/min	O_2 pulse ml/beat	R	pH	HCO₃ mEq/L	PO₂ ET mmHg	PO₂ a mmHg	PO₂ A-a mmHg	PCO₂ ET mmHg	PCO₂ a mmHg	PCO₂ a-ET mmHg	$\dot{V}E/\dot{V}CO_2$	$\dot{V}E/\dot{V}O_2$	VD/VT
Rest			74	31	17.0	0.35	0.52	7.0	0.67			94			36			48	33	
Rest			68	10	14.5	0.33	0.41	6.0	0.80			112			30			44	35	
Unloaded			76	25	20.4	0.53	0.82	10.8	0.65			94			37			38	25	
Unloaded			64	26	15.7	0.39	0.60	9.4	0.65			93			39			40	26	
1.0	30		76	24	20.1	0.52	0.77	10.1	0.68			96			38			39	26	
2.0	60		85	27	23.8	0.69	1.01	11.9	0.68			93			40			35	24	
3.0	90		94	24	29.6	0.99	1.37	14.6	0.72			92			42			30	22	
4.0	120		101	22	36.5	1.31	1.65	16.3	0.79			97			42			28	22	
5.0	150		106	25	43.1	1.50	1.85	17.5	0.81			93			44			29	23	
6.0	180		117	25	53.2	2.03	2.39	20.4	0.85			92			46			26	22	
7.0	210		127	30	71.7	2.61	2.79	22.0	0.94			96			46			27	26	
8.0	240		135	31	80.6	2.97	3.05	22.6	0.97			105			41			27	26	
9.0	270		142	32	85.0	3.27	3.38	23.8	0.97			97			47			26	25	
10.0	300		155	37	104.4	3.88	3.80	24.5	1.02			99			46			27	27	
11.0	330		162	48	142.4	4.81	4.31	26.6	1.12			102			46			30	33	
12.0	360		168	53	162.3	5.38	4.64	27.6	1.16			115			38			30	35	
13.0	390		175	63	186.0	6.01	4.95	28.3	1.21			116			38			31	38	
Recovery			134	38	99.1	3.29	2.05	15.3	1.60			119			40			30	48	

FIGURE 2-A

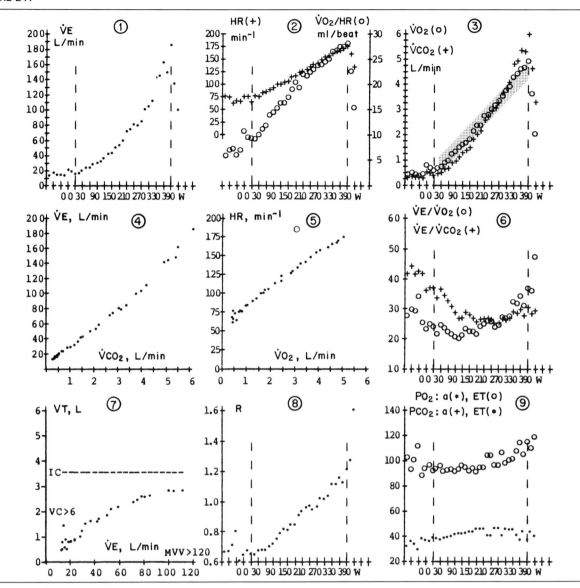

Interpretation

COMMENTS

This case is presented to illustrate results of a normal, athletic subject.

ANALYSIS

Flow Chart 1: The maximum $\dot{V}O_2$ and the anaerobic threshold are considerably above the predicted values (Table 2-2). The predicted values are, of course, those for a sedentary population. The results of this study demonstrate how much better an athlete can perform than the average member of the sedentary group. The exceptionally high O_2 pulse at maximum work rate reflects the very large stroke volume and $C(a-\bar{v})_{O_2}$ that this subject must have. Assuming that the mixed venous O_2 saturation were as low as 20%, the O_2 pulse of 28.3 ml/beat would indicate that the subject's stroke volume must be approximately 175 ml. The normal ventilatory equivalent for O_2 and CO_2 at the anaerobic threshold (Graph 6, Figure 2-A) reflects the normal ventilation/perfusion matching of a normal subject. It should be noted that the maximum exercise ventilation is approximately equal to his MVV. Thus his breathing reserve is approximately zero, a common finding in exceptionally fit people.

CONCLUSION

Exceptionally fit, normal subject.

CASE 3 *Normal man: Air and oxygen breathing*

CLINICAL FINDINGS

The patient was a 59-year-old retired shipyard worker with a history of asbestos exposure and 2 pack year history of cigarette smoking. He stopped working 4 years previously. He was asymptomatic at the time of this examination. Physical and laboratory examinations were normal; chest roentgenograms revealed focal pleural plaques with calcification.

EXERCISE FINDINGS

After we obtained informed consent, the patient participated in a blind-crossover exercise study on a cycle ergometer, receiving one of two humidified gas mixtures, (compressed air or 100% oxygen) just prior to and during each study. He pedalled at 60 rpm without added load for 3 minutes. The work rate was then increased 15 watts per minute to his symptom limited maximum. Blood was sampled every second minute, and intra-arterial blood pressure was recorded from a percutaneously placed brachial artery catheter. He rested one hour between the two studies and exercised to his maximum tolerance on each occasion. On both occasions he stopped exercise because of general fatigue. Resting and exercise ECG readings were normal.

TABLE 3-1. *Selected Respiratory Function Data*

MEASUREMENT	PREDICTED	MEASURED
Age, yr		59
Sex		Male
Height, cm		155
Weight, kg	62	53
Hematocrit, %		46
VC, L	2.90	3.19
IC, L	1.94	2.12
TLC, L	4.51	4.62
FEV_1, L	2.26	2.49
FEV_1/VC, %	78	78
MVV, L/min	112	118
DL_{CO}, ml/min Hg/min	19.9	20.7

TABLE 3-2. *Selected Exercise Data*

MEASUREMENT	PREDICTED	AIR	O_2
Maximum $\dot{V}CO_2$, L/min		2.03	1.93
Maximum $\dot{V}O_2$, L/min	1.53	1.57	
Maximum HR, beats/min	161	192	188
Maximum O_2 pulse, ml/beat	9.5	8.2	
$\Delta\dot{V}O_2/\Delta$WR, ml/min/watt	10.3	9.7	
$\dot{V}O_2$ difference, %	0.0	4.3	
AT, L/min	>0.61	indeterminate	
Blood pressure, mm Hg (rest, max)		100/56,213/88	100/63,231/94
Maximum $\dot{V}E$, L/min		89	72
Exercise breathing reserve, L/min	>15	29	46
Pa_{O_2}, mm Hg (rest, max ex)		102,101	585,586
$P(A-a)_{O_2}$, mm Hg (rest, max ex)		24,25	103,93
$P(a-ET)_{CO_2}$, mm Hg (rest, max ex)		−4,−4	1,−2
VD/VT (rest, heavy ex)		0.19,0.23	0.37,0.26
HCO_3^-, mEq/L (rest, 2 min recov)		23,12	19,14

Table 3-3. *Air Breathing*

TIME min	WORK RATE W	BP mmHg	HR min⁻¹	f	V̇E BTPS	V̇CO₂ —STPD— L/min	V̇O₂	O₂ pulse ml/beat	R	pH	HCO₃⁻ mEq/L	ET —PO₂— mmHg a	A-a	ET —PCO₂— mmHg a	a-ET	V̇E/V̇CO₂	V̇E/V̇O₂	VD/VT
Rest			114	22	12.5	0.24	0.29	2.5	0.83			115		30			44	37	
Rest			118	15	13.6	0.28	0.32	2.7	0.88			114		31			44	38	
Rest		100/ 56	119	11	13.2	0.27	0.27	2.3	1.00	7.48	18	122 102	24	28 24	-4	45	45	0.19
Unloaded			127	21	17.1	0.40	0.63	5.0	0.63			98		34			38	24	
Unloaded			126	23	16.7	0.42	0.63	5.0	0.67			101		35			35	23	
Unloaded		150/ 75	125	25	16.3	0.39	0.42	3.4	0.93	7.41	23	100 93	18	36 37	1	36	34	0.31
1.0	15		130	25	19.2	0.49	0.66	5.1	0.74			103		36			35	26	
2.0	30	163/ 75	140	26	21.9	0.57	0.75	5.4	0.76	7.40	21	103 94	14	37 34	-3	34	26	0.24
3.0	45		145	28	27.6	0.72	0.85	5.9	0.85			107		37			35	30	
4.0	60	194/ 81	145	28	27.2	0.79	0.86	5.9	0.92	7.40	20	107 96	19	39 33	-6	31	29	0.15
5.0	75		161	32	41.4	1.21	1.21	7.5	1.00			112		37			32	32	
6.0	90	194/ 75	171	36	50.8	1.45	1.37	8.0	1.06	7.39	20	115 93	25	36 33	-3	33	35	0.19
7.0	105		182	47	71.0	1.81	1.50	8.2	1.21			120		33			37	45	
8.0	120	213/ 88	192	55	88.6	2.03	1.57	8.2	1.29	7.37	16	126 101	25	33 29	-4	41	53	0.27
Recovery			166	40	60.0	1.43	0.97	5.8	1.47			126		31			40	58	
Recovery		169/ 63	145	34	34.6	0.70	0.46	3.2	1.52	7.33	12	129 122	11	28 24	-4	45	69	0.19

Figure 3-A. *Air Breathing*

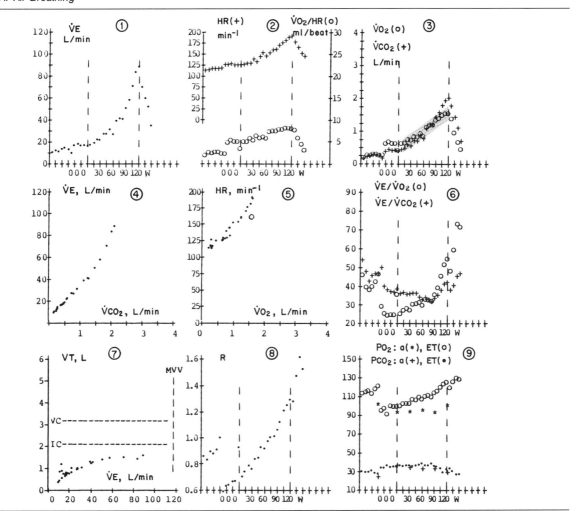

TABLE 3-4. *Oxygen Breathing*

TIME min	WORK RATE W	BP mmHg	HR min⁻¹	f	$\dot{V}_E$ BTPS L/min	$\dot{V}CO_2$ STPD L/min	$\dot{V}O_2$ STPD L/min	O_2 pulse ml/beat	R	pH	HCO_3^- mEq/L	PO_2 ET mmHg	PO_2 a	PO_2 A-a	PCO_2 ET mmHg	PCO_2 a	PCO_2 a-ET	$\dot{V}_E/\dot{V}CO_2$	$\dot{V}_E/\dot{V}O_2$	VD/VT
Rest			120	12	13.2	0.23									23			53		
Rest			123	22	15.9	0.23									22			61		
Rest		100/ 63	119	15	11.4	0.17				7.49	19		585	103	24	25	1	60		0.37
Unloaded			125	44	11.9	0.10									32			82		
Unloaded			121	28	13.9	0.24									35			48		
Unloaded		163/ 81	122	22	12.7	0.28									37			39		
1.0	15		126	22	16.8	0.40									37			37		
2.0	30	181/ 88	134	26	19.4	0.48				7.40	21		591	87	38	35	-3	36		0.27
3.0	45		141	22	22.1	0.64									40			32		
4.0	60	206/ 88	146	25	27.9	0.84				7.38	20		576	103	40	34	-6	31		0.16
5.0	75		156	27	34.8	1.05									40			31		
6.0	90	225/ 91	163	34	43.7	1.28				7.37	20		581	95	40	37	-3	32		0.25
7.0	105		176	42	56.3	1.55									37			34		
8.0	120	231/ 94	188	45	71.7	1.93				7.35	18		586	93	36	34	-2	35		0.26
Recovery			156	29	46.9	1.25									36			36		
Recovery		219/ 75	140	30	32.7	0.69				7.33	14		584	102	30	27	-3	44		0.25

FIGURE 3-B. *Oxygen Breathing*

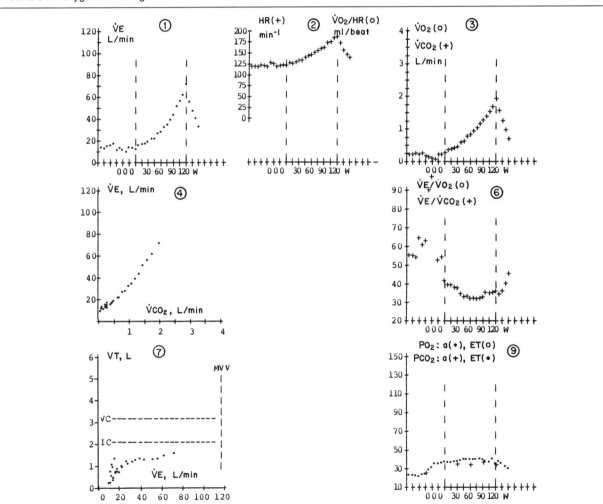

Interpretation

COMMENTS

Resting respiratory function is normal (Table 3-1). The exercise test was repeated with the patient breathing O_2, as part of an experimental study. At rest, the patient acutely hyperventilated while breathing with the mouthpiece; this ceased as soon as the exercise started. The associated relative hypoventilation noted in the transition from rest to unloaded cycling (graph 9 of Figure 3-A) caused a simultaneous marked decrease in R (graph 8 of Figure 3-A). This does not affect the final interpretation but does caution the examiner on the use of the resting bicarbonate values.

ANALYSIS

Flow Chart 1: The maximum $\dot{V}O_2$ is normal (Table 3-2 and Graph 3 of Fig. 3-A). See *Flow Chart 2:* The electrocardiogram, arterial blood gases, and O_2 pulse at maximum $\dot{V}O_2$ are normal *(branchpoint 2.1)*. The subject is not obese *(branchpoint 2.2)*. Thus the cardiorespiratory response to exercise is normal, consistent with this patient's history and clinical findings.

The major difference between the air- and O_2-breathing studies is a significantly reduced exercise ventilation in the latter when performing at the same work rate (Table 3 and 4 and graph 1 of Fig. A and B). Consistent with this is the higher Pa_{CO_2} at maximum exercise during the O_2-breathing study. Arterial oxygen tension was normal (585 mmHg) at rest and remained unchanged throughout exercise during the oxygen breathing study, demonstrating the absence of a significant right-to-left shunt.

CONCLUSION

Normal subject.

Case 4 *Normal woman: Air and oxygen breathing*

Clinical Findings

This 45-year-old housewife was referred for evaluation of dyspnea. She had recently begun to increase her activity and felt that she was shorter of breath than she should be. Physical and laboratory examinations revealed no abnormalities.

Exercise Findings

The patient performed exercise on a cycle ergometer. She pedalled at 60 rpm without added load for 3 minutes. The work rate was then increased 10 watts per minute to her symptom limited maximum. Blood was sampled every second minute and intra-arterial blood pressure was recorded from a percutaneously placed brachial artery catheter. A second incremental exercise test was performed with O_2 breathing, one and one half hours after recovery from the first, with work rate increments of 20 watts per minute. She stopped exercise in each case complaining of general fatigue and shortness of breath. Resting and exercise ECG's were normal.

TABLE 4-1. *Selected Respiratory Function Data*

MEASUREMENT	PREDICTED	MEASURED
Age, yr		45
Sex		Female
Height, cm		165
Weight, kg	64	61
Hematocrit, %		40
VC, L	3.30	3.21
IC, L	2.20	1.99
FEV_1, L	2.68	2.71
FEV_1/VC, %	81	84
MVV, L/min	112	117
DL_{CO}, ml/mm Hg/min	24.1	21.1

TABLE 4-2. *Selected Exercise Data*

MEASUREMENT	PREDICTED	ROOM AIR	O_2
Maximum work rate, watts		130	160
Maximum $\dot{V}O_2$, L/min	1.58	1.71	
Maximum HR, beats/min	175	160	155
Maximum O_2 pulse, ml/beat	9.0	10.7	
$\Delta\dot{V}O_2/\Delta WR$, ml/min/watt	10.3	11.9	
$\dot{V}O_2$ difference, %	0.0	−10.6	
AT, L/min	> 0.63	0.9	
Blood pressure, mm Hg (rest, max)		138/81,194/81	106/75,181/88
Maximum $\dot{V}E$, L/min		70	54
Exercise breathing reserve, L/min	> 15	47	63
Pa_{O_2}, mm Hg (rest, max ex)		105,108	643,552
$P(A−a)_{O_2}$, mm Hg (rest, max ex)		5,16	33,117
$P(a−ET)_{CO_2}$, mm Hg (rest, max ex)		−1,−6	4,−4
VD/VT (rest, heavy ex)		0.21,0.11	0.34,0.18
HCO_3^-, mEq/L (rest, 2 min recov)		25,13	25,20

TABLE 4-3. *Air Breathing*

TIME min	WORK RATE W	BP mmHg	HR min⁻¹	f	V̇E BTPS L/min	V̇CO2 STPD L/min	V̇O2 STPD L/min	O2 pulse ml/beat	R	pH	HCO3⁻ mEq/L	PO2 ET mmHg	PO2 a	PO2 A-a	PCO2 ET mmHg	PCO2 a	PCO2 a-ET	V̇E/V̇CO2	V̇E/V̇O2	VD/VT
Rest	138/ 81									7.42	25		96			40				
Rest		76	16	15.1	0.40	0.41	5.4	0.98			109			38			34	33			
Rest	138/ 75	62	17	6.7	0.17	0.18	2.9	0.94	7.43	25	109	105	5	39	38	-1	31	29	0.21		
Unloaded		77	28	9.8	0.28	0.37	4.8	0.76			99			42			27	20			
Unloaded	144/ 75	77	34	7.4	0.18	0.23	3.0	0.78	7.41	25	97	99	2	44	40	-4	25	19	0.08		
1.0	10		76	19	12.7	0.42	0.51	6.7	0.82			98			44			26	22		
2.0	20	144/ 75	79	29	8.9	0.27	0.33	4.2	0.82	7.41	25	93	100	3	46	40	-6	24	20	0.07
3.0	30		87	16	14.7	0.56	0.68	7.8	0.82			98			45			24	20		
4.0	40	144/ 75	93	20	19.6	0.71	0.82	8.8	0.87	7.39	25	97	95	8	46	42	-4	25	22	0.17
5.0	50		104	23	23.3	0.87	0.93	8.9	0.94			101			45			25	23		
6.0	60	156/ 75	103	18	22.0	0.88	0.92	8.9	0.96			101			47			23	22		
7.0	70		112	17	24.6	1.02	1.01	9.0	1.01			103			47			23	23		
8.0	80	163/ 75	119	19	29.3	1.21	1.19	10.0	1.02	7.37	22	103	101	12	47	38	-9	23	23	0.01
9.0	90		127	22	33.7	1.38	1.30	10.2	1.06			105			47			23	25		
10.0	100	175/ 81	134	23	37.4	1.52	1.38	10.3	1.10			106			47			23	26		
11.0	110		144	28	50.0	1.88	1.60	11.1	1.18			111			43			25	30		
12.0	120		154	34	59.6	2.10	1.71	11.1	1.23			114			41			27	33		
13.0	130	194/ 81	160	38	70.0	2.27	1.64	10.3	1.38	7.31	16	114	108	16	39	33	-6	29	41	0.11
Recovery		132	26	47.5	1.57	0.95	7.2	1.65			123			38			29	48			
Recovery	131/ 63	121	22	28.0	0.84	0.50	4.1	1.68	7.26	13	126	117	13	35	30	-5	31	52	0.07		

FIGURE 4-A. *Air Breathing*

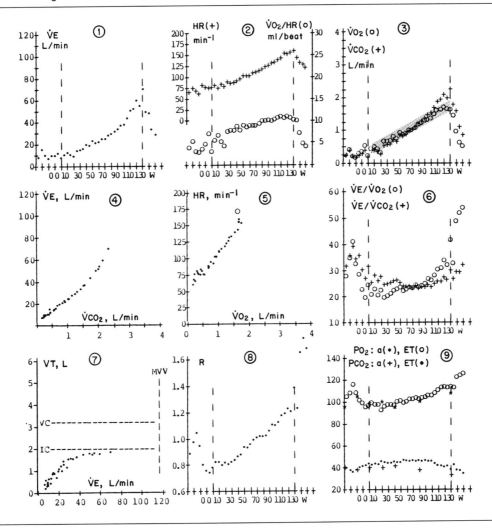

TABLE 4-4. *Oxygen Breathing*

TIME min	WORK RATE W	BP mmHg	HR min⁻¹	f	$\dot{V}E$ BTPS	$\dot{V}CO_2$ STPD L/min	$\dot{V}O_2$ STPD L/min	O_2 pulse ml/beat	R	pH	HCO_3^- mEq/L	PO₂ ET mmHg	PO₂ a mmHg	PO₂ A-a mmHg	PCO₂ ET mmHg	PCO₂ a mmHg	PCO₂ a-ET mmHg	$\dot{V}E/\dot{V}CO_2$	$\dot{V}E/\dot{V}O_2$	VD/VT
Rest			73	15	7.2	0.13									32			46		
Rest		106/ 75	71	15	7.6	0.16				7.44	25		643	33	33	37	4	40		0.34
Unloaded			87	17	10.2	0.31									43			28		
Unloaded		113/ 69	77	24	9.2	0.25				7.39	25		605	67	42	41	-1	29		0.20
1.0	20		90	13	10.0	0.34									44			26		
2.0	40	125/ 69	91	14	11.6	0.43				7.39	26		595	75	48	43	-5	24		0.16
3.0	60		100	16	18.8	0.73									48			24		
4.0	80	144/ 75	112	17	21.7	0.94				7.34	25		601	64	52	48	-4	22		0.15
5.0	100		124	19	27.1	1.18									52			22		
6.0	120	169/ 81	144	25	38.0	1.68				7.29	22		587	79	52	47	-5	21		0.13
7.0	140	175/ 81	155	30	51.4	2.01				7.30	21		564	106	46	43	-3	24		0.17
7.5	160	181/ 88	153	34	53.6	2.06				7.28	20		552	117	48	44	-4	25		0.19
Recovery			143	26	47.4	1.89									48			24		
Recovery			120	22	34.6	1.21									41			27		

FIGURE 4-B. *Oxygen Breathing*

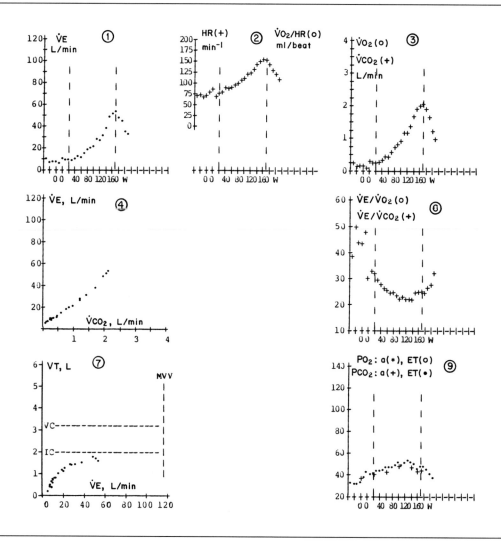

Interpretation

COMMENTS

Resting respiratory function (Table 4-1) and electro-cardiogram are normal.

ANALYSIS

Flow Chart 1: The maximum $\dot{V}O_2$ and anaerobic threshold are normal (Table 4-2). See *Flow Chart 2* for further analysis. There are no ECG abnormalities and arterial blood gas values and VD/VT are normal throughout exercise (Table 4-3) *(branchpoint 2.1)*. The patient is not obese (Table 4-1) *(branchpoint 2.2)*. Thus, this patient has no limitation to exercise for her age and has no physiological evidence for cardiovascular or pulmonary disease.

Pa_{O_2} is also normal during 100% O_2 breathing (Table 4-4), ruling out a significant right-to-left shunt.

Of special note is that the patient was able to exercise to a higher work rate with a slightly lower heart rate during O_2 breathing instead of air breathing. Also, respiratory compensation for the metabolic acidosis (decrease in Pa_{CO_2}) was less evident during the O_2 breathing study.

CONCLUSION

Our final assessment is that this patient was actually normal and her symptoms were the result of anxiety regarding her performance at sports.

CASE 5 *Normal woman*

CLINICAL FINDINGS

This nonsmoking occupational therapist was referred for evaluation of dyspnea. She described the sensation as the inability to take a deep breath. She also noted nervousness, dizziness, and shortness of breath while eating. She was usually active in sports, but also noted shortness of breath in these activities. Physical examination was normal except for resting tachycardia and a ⅖ systolic ejection murmur. Echocardiogram revealed a mitral valve prolapse. There were no dysrhythmias on 24 hour Holter monitoring. Chest roentgenograms, ECG, and respiratory function tests were normal, except for some reduction in expiratory flow rates attributable to reduced effort.

EXERCISE FINDINGS

The patient performed exercise on a cycle ergometer. She pedalled at 60 rpm without added load for 3 minutes. The work rate was then increased 15 watts per minute to her symptom limited maximum. Blood was sampled every second minute and intra-arterial blood pressure was recorded from a percutaneously placed brachial artery catheter. She stopped pedalling at 150 watts complaining of fatigue and a feeling of palpitations. She felt somewhat short of breath. There were no abnormal ST changes or arrhythmia. There was no wheezing or diminution of FEV_1 in the post-exercise period.

TABLE 5-1. *Selected Respiratory Function Data*

MEASUREMENT	PREDICTED	MEASURED
Age, yr		24
Sex		Female
Height, cm		159
Weight, kg	61	51
Hematocrit, %		40
VC, L	3.60	3.50
IC, L	2.40	2.11
TLC, L	4.91	4.71
FEV_1, L	3.01	2.55
FEV_1/VC, %	84	73
MVV, L/min	115	118
DL_{CO}, ml/mm Hg/min	26.5	29.8

TABLE 5-2. *Selected Exercise Data*

MEASUREMENT	PREDICTED	MEASURED
Maximum $\dot{V}O_2$, L/min	1.71	1.62
Maximum HR, beats/min	196	198
Maximum O_2 pulse, ml/beat	8.7	8.2
$\Delta\dot{V}O_2/\Delta WR$, ml/min/watt	10.3	9.1
$\dot{V}O_2$ difference, %	0.0	8.5
AT, L/min	> 0.68	1.0
Blood pressure, mm Hg (rest, max)		135/84,177/87
Maximum $\dot{V}E$, L/min		64
Exercise breathing reserve, L/min	> 15	54
PaO_2, mm Hg (rest, max ex)		95,100
$P(A-a)O_2$, mm Hg (rest, max ex)		14,17
$P(a-ET)_{CO_2}$, mm Hg (rest, max ex)		−1,−3
VD/VT (rest, heavy ex)		0.19,0.16
HCO_3^-, mEq/L (rest, 2 min recov)		25,15

TABLE 5-3

TIME min	WORK RATE W	BP mmHg	HR min⁻¹	f	$\dot{V}E$ BTPS L/min	$\dot{V}CO_2$ STPD L/min	$\dot{V}O_2$ L/min	O_2 pulse ml/beat	R	pH	HCO_3 mEq L	PO₂ ET mmHg	PO₂ a mmHg	PO₂ A-a mmHg	PCO₂ ET mmHg	PCO₂ a mmHg	PCO₂ a-ET mmHg	$\dfrac{\dot{V}E}{\dot{V}CO_2}$	$\dfrac{\dot{V}E}{\dot{V}O_2}$	$\dfrac{VD}{VT}$
Rest		135/ 84								7.47	25	101			35					
Rest			127	11	5.4	0.15	0.19	1.5	0.79			102			38			30	23	
Rest		144/ 84	130	18	11.2	0.32	0.36	2.8	0.89	7.44	25	104	95	14	38	37	−1	30	27	0.19
Rest			126	13	13.7	0.39	0.41	3.3	0.95			105			38			32	31	
Unloaded			139	25	6.8	0.20	0.28	2.0	0.71			93			40			23	17	
Unloaded			132	12	13.8	0.43	0.55	4.2	0.78			98			39			30	23	
Unloaded		141/ 81	132	32	12.5	0.32	0.42	3.2	0.76	7.42	26	97	91	9	40	40	0	31	23	0.23
1.0	15		136	16	14.0	0.46	0.56	4.1	0.82			102			39			27	23	
2.0	30	150/ 84	140	16	19.1	0.63	0.74	5.3	0.85	7.42	25	101	94	10	41	40	−1	28	24	0.22
3.0	45		152	19	18.3	0.64	0.71	4.7	0.90			102			43			26	23	
4.0	60	159/ 84	163	22	20.3	0.74	0.79	4.8	0.94	7.40	25	96	96	11	47	41	−6	25	23	0.14
5.0	75		169	25	25.9	0.97	1.00	5.9	0.97			99			47			24	24	
6.0	90	171/ 81	183	26	35.1	1.28	1.15	6.3	1.11	7.38	23	108	101	12	43	40	−3	26	29	0.15
7.0	105		188	31	39.0	1.43	1.26	6.7	1.13			105			47			25	29	
8.0	120	174/ 87	192	31	42.6	1.60	1.38	7.2	1.16	7.32	21	107	97	16	46	42	−4	25	29	0.17
9.0	135	177/ 87	196	36	52.8	1.89	1.52	7.8	1.24	7.31	19	113	100	17	42	39	−3	26	33	0.15
9.5	150		198	45	64.2	2.11	1.62	8.2	1.30			116			39			29	37	
Recovery			198	36	55.6	1.88	1.48	7.5	1.27			113			42			28	36	
Recovery			186	32	40.3	1.22	0.81	4.4	1.51			121			37			31	46	
Recovery		153/ 78								7.27	15		97			34				

FIGURE 5-A

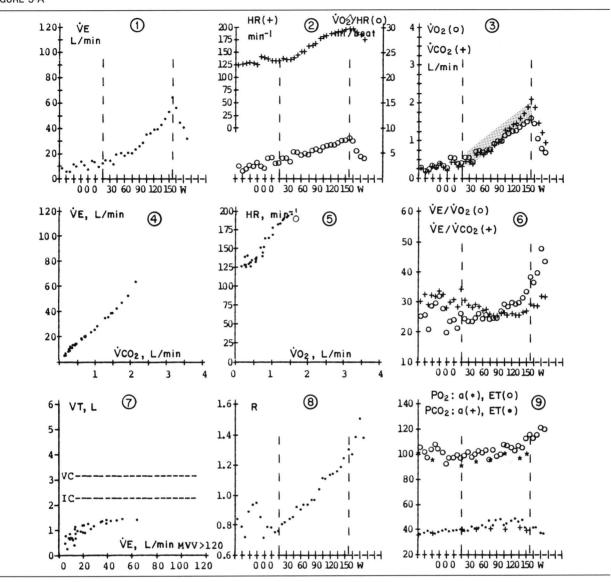

Interpretation

COMMENTS

This young lady, who experienced occasions of dyspnea, has normal lung volumes and flow rates indicating the absence of restrictive or obstructive lung disease (Table 5-1). In addition, her diffusing capacity is normal. Her resting electrocardiogram is also normal.

ANALYSIS

Flow Chart 1: The maximum $\dot{V}O_2$ and anaerobic threshold are normal (Table 5-2). See *Flow Chart 2:* Her electrocardiogram and O_2 pulse at maximum exercise are normal and her arterial blood gases remain normal throughout exercise *(branchpoint 2.1).*

This patient is not obese *(branchpoint 2.2).* This leads to the diagnosis of a normal subject with anxiety. However, she has a marked tachycardia at rest and an appropriate heart rate response to exercise. Hyperthyroidism was ruled out and the tachycardia was not a persistent observation (Holter monitoring) as might be found with vasoregulatory asthenia.

CONCLUSION

Normal young woman with anxiety. However, the sensation of palpitations was not manifest by a cardiac arrhythmia. The patient deserves follow-up for endocrine disorders or other conditions that might account for her symptoms.

CASE 6 *Normal man*

CLINICAL FINDINGS

This 37-year-old shipyard machinist was evaluated because of complaints of dyspnea. He stated that he was unable to play a full game of baseball for the last 6 years and that he gets out of breath and has to stop after climbing 3 to 4 flights on shipboard. He never smoked. He denied cough, chest pain, edema, or other symptoms. Physical, roentgenographic, and laboratory examinations were normal.

EXERCISE FINDINGS

The patient performed exercise on a cycle ergometer. He pedalled at 60 rpm without added load for 3 minutes. The work rate was then increased 25 watts per minute to his symptom limited maximum. Blood was sampled every second minute and intra-arterial blood pressure was recorded from a percutaneously placed brachial artery catheter. He stopped exercise because of general fatigue. Resting and exercise ECG's were normal.

TABLE 6-1. *Selected Respiratory Function Data*

MEASUREMENT	PREDICTED	MEASURED
Age, yr		37
Sex		Male
Height, cm		157
Weight, kg	63	67
Hematocrit, %		45
VC, L	3.30	4.38
IC, L	2.20	2.80
TLC, L	4.52	5.30
FEV_1, L	2.66	3.52
FEV_1/VC, %	81	80
MVV, L/min	127	124
DL_{CO}, ml/mm Hg/min	22.4	29.8

TABLE 6-2. *Selected Exercise Data*

MEASUREMENT	PREDICTED	MEASURED
Maximum $\dot{V}O_2$, L/min	2.34	2.23
Maximum HR, beats/min	183	188
Maximum O_2 pulse, ml/beat	12.8	11.9
$\Delta\dot{V}O_2/\Delta WR$, ml/min/watt	10.3	10.4
$\dot{V}O_2$ difference, %	0.0	−0.5
AT, L/min	> 0.94	1.1
Blood pressure, mm Hg (rest, max)		125/75,188/94
Maximum $\dot{V}E$, L/min		90
Exercise breathing reserve, L/min	> 15	34
Pa_{O_2}, mm Hg (rest, max ex)		84,114
$P(A-a)_{O_2}$, mm Hg (rest, max ex)		7,2
$P(a-ET)_{CO_2}$, mm Hg (rest, max ex)		0,−4
VD/VT (rest, heavy ex)		0.31,0.16
HCO_3^-, mEq/L (rest, 2 min recov)		24,16

TABLE 6-3

TIME min	WORK RATE W	BP mmHg	HR min⁻¹	f	$\dot{V}E$ BTPS L/min	$\dot{V}CO_2$ STPD L/min	$\dot{V}O_2$ STPD L/min	O_2 pulse ml/beat	R	pH	HCO_3^- mEq/L	PO₂ ET mmHg	PO₂ a mmHg	PO₂ A-a mmHg	PCO₂ ET mmHg	PCO₂ a mmHg	PCO₂ a-ET mmHg	$\dot{V}E/\dot{V}CO_2$	$\dot{V}E/\dot{V}O_2$	VD/VT
Rest		125/ 75								7.41	24	103			39					
Rest			78	14	7.5	0.18	0.23	2.9	0.78			107			36			35	27	
Rest			78	13	7.1	0.16	0.20	2.6	0.80			108			35			38	30	
Rest		125/ 81	82	13	6.9	0.17	0.27	3.3	0.63	7.39	24	94	84	7	40	40	0	34	21	0.31
Unloaded			94	28	16.7	0.53	0.76	8.1	0.70			93			42			27	19	
Unloaded			95	31	14.4	0.41	0.57	6.0	0.72			95			44			29	21	
Unloaded		144/ 81	96	28	15.6	0.49	0.61	6.4	0.80	7.37	25	98	91	8	43	43	0	27	22	0.22
1.0	25		102	26	16.6	0.50	0.67	6.6	0.75			96			43			29	21	
2.0	50	150/ 81	117	25	23.5	0.82	1.08	9.2	0.76	7.38	25	95	95	1	44	43	−1	26	20	0.21
3.0	75		127	27	27.7	1.01	1.19	9.4	0.85			99			45			25	21	
4.0	100	181/ 94	141	32	38.6	1.47	1.54	10.9	0.95	7.37	24	102	104	2	45	42	−3	24	23	0.15
5.0	125		162	40	53.5	1.92	1.78	11.0	1.08			110			42			26	28	
6.0	150	188/ 94	176	46	68.8	2.36	2.04	11.6	1.16	7.37	22	112	114	2	42	38	−4	27	32	0.16
7.0	175		188	51	89.7	2.84	2.23	11.9	1.27			118			38			30	38	
Recovery			161	29	47.5	1.66	1.19	7.4	1.39			116			41			27	38	
Recovery		181/100	136	28	37.5	1.08	0.62	4.6	1.74	7.30	16	127	126	2	35	33	−2	33	57	0.18

FIGURE 6-A

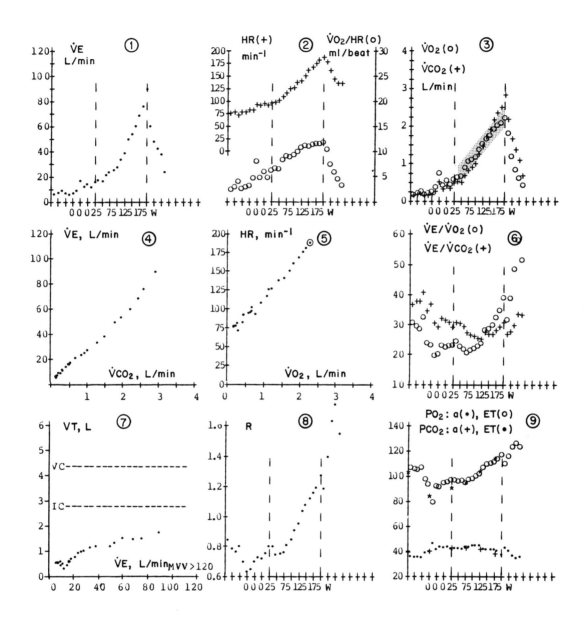

Interpretation

COMMENTS

The results of this patient's resting respiratory function studies are normal (Table 6-1). The resting electrocardiogram is normal.

ANALYSIS

Flow Chart 1: Maximum $\dot{V}O_2$ and the anaerobic threshold are within normal limits (Table 6-2). See

Flow Chart 2: ECG, O_2 pulse at maximum $\dot{V}O_2$ and arterial blood gases are normal *(branchpoint 2.1).* The patient is not obese *(branchpoint 2.2).*

CONCLUSION

Normal 37-year-old man. Symptoms probably relate to anxiety and lack of fitness.

CASE 7 *Exceptionally fit man with mild lung disease*

CLINICAL FINDINGS

This 59-year-old worker had no complaints or history of heart or lung disease. He sustained a gun shot wound to the right chest at age 24 that was not surgically treated. He was exposed to asbestos 20 years previously and smoked 1 package of cigarettes daily for 12 years until 20 years ago. He cycled approximately 50 miles a week. Physical, roentgenographic, and ECG examinations were normal except for evidence of focal, old granulomatous disease and an old rib fracture.

EXERCISE FINDINGS

The patient performed exercise on a cycle ergometer. He pedalled at 60 rpm without added load for 3 minutes. The work rate was then increased 20 watts per minute to his symptom limited maximum. Blood was sampled every second minute and intra-arterial blood pressure was recorded from a percutaneously placed brachial artery catheter. He stopped exercise because of general exhaustion. Exercise ECG's were normal.

TABLE 7-1. *Selected Respiratory Function Data*

MEASUREMENT	PREDICTED	MEASURED
Age, yr		59
Sex		Male
Height, cm		175
Weight, kg	78	93
Hematocrit, %		46
VC, L	4.21	4.34
IC, L	2.79	3.57
TLC, L	6.36	5.86
FEV_1, L	3.58	3.57
FEV_1/VC, %	80	82
MVV, L/min	137	152
DL_{CO}, ml/mm Hg/min	28.2	29.5

TABLE 7-2. *Selected Exercise Data*

MEASUREMENT	PREDICTED	MEASURED
Maximum $\dot{V}O_2$, L/min	2.23	3.40
Maximum HR, beats/min	161	195
Maximum O_2 pulse, ml/beat	13.9	17.4
$\Delta\dot{V}O_2/\Delta WR$, ml/min/watt	10.3	12.7
$\dot{V}O_2$ difference, %	0.0	−18.4
AT, L/min	> 0.89	indeterminate
Blood pressure, mm Hg (rest, max)		125/75,200/88
Maximum $\dot{V}E$, L/min		174
Exercise breathing reserve, L/min	> 15	−22
Pa_{O_2}, mm Hg (rest, max ex)		120,71
$P(A-a)_{O_2}$, mm Hg (rest, max ex)		5,49
$P(a\text{-}ET)_{CO_2}$, mm Hg (rest, max ex)		−4,−13
VD/VT (rest, heavy ex)		0.16,0.05
HCO_3^-, mEq/L (rest, 2 min recov)		25,10

TABLE 7-3

TIME min	WORK RATE W	BP mmHg	HR min⁻¹	f	$\dot{V}E$ BTPS L/min	$\dot{V}CO_2$ STPD L/min	$\dot{V}O_2$ STPD L/min	O_2 pulse ml/beat	R	pH	HCO_3^- mEq/L	PO2 ET mmHg	PO2 a mmHg	PO2 A-a mmHg	PCO2 ET mmHg	PCO2 a mmHg	PCO2 a-ET mmHg	$\dfrac{\dot{V}E}{\dot{V}CO_2}$	$\dfrac{\dot{V}E}{\dot{V}O_2}$	VD VT
Rest		125/ 75								7.45	25	75			36					
Rest			77	17	17.3	0.36	0.28	3.6	1.29			124			29			44	57	
Rest		119/ 75	84	8	14.6	0.36	0.33	3.9	1.09	7.52	21	118	120	5	31	27	−4	39	42	0.16
Unloaded			84	12	21.9	0.65	0.74	8.8	0.88			106			36			32	28	
Unloaded			81	17	26.2	0.68	0.70	8.6	0.97			111			34			36	35	
Unloaded		156/ 81	79	16	23.3	0.65	0.69	8.7	0.94	7.47	22	110	103	15	35	31	−4	34	32	0.17
1.0	20		82	18	23.3	0.70	0.78	9.5	0.90			99			39			31	28	
2.0	40	163/ 81	91	8	24.0	0.87	1.11	12.2	0.78	7.43	24	92	77	28	42	37	−5	27	21	0.13
3.0	60		98	16	24.2	0.90	1.18	12.0	0.76			84			47			25	19	
4.0	80	175/ 81	107	14	36.1	1.38	1.54	14.4	0.90	7.41	24	95	85	24	45	38	−7	25	23	0.10
5.0	100		117	16	43.4	1.72	1.82	15.6	0.95			97			47			24	23	
6.0	120		119	20	56.5	2.08	2.07	17.4	1.00	7.37	21	99	86	27	46	37	−9	26	26	0.11
7.0	140		131	21	61.2	2.33	2.26	17.3	1.03			101			46			26	26	
8.0	160	200/ 88	148	21	69.8	2.65	2.50	16.9	1.06	7.35	18	102	75	43	46	34	−12	26	27	0.01
9.0	180		161	26	82.2	3.11	2.79	17.3	1.11			104			46			26	29	
10.0	200		167	30	90.6	3.40	2.90	17.4	1.17	7.29	16	106	71	49	47	34	−13	26	30	0.02
11.0	220		189	34	117.3	4.01	3.13	16.6	1.28			112			42			29	37	
11.5	240		195	55	174.5	4.75	3.40	17.4	1.40			122			34			36	50	
Recovery		200/ 88	180	35	121.1	3.52	2.68	14.9	1.31	7.26	12	118	83	43	36	29	−7	34	44	0.11
Recovery			159	26	89.2	2.42	1.35	8.5	1.79			125			36			36	64	
Recovery			145	27	67.1	1.50	0.90	6.2	1.67			128			31			43	72	
Recovery		163/ 75								7.20	10		113			26				

FIGURE 7-A

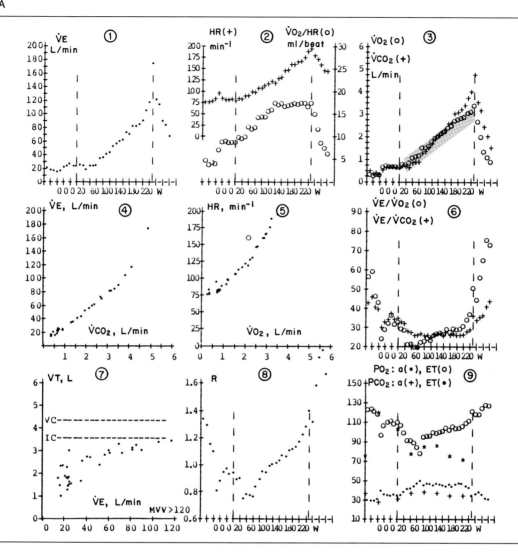

Interpretation

COMMENTS

The results of this patient's respiratory function studies are within normal limits (Table 7-1). The resting electrocardiogram is normal. The respiratory alkalosis at rest, while breathing on the mouthpiece, is acute, developing in anticipation of exercise. It disappears after exercise started. When starting to breathe on the mouthpiece, he hyperventilates to a pH of 7.52, Pa_{CO_2} of 27 mmHg and Pa_{O_2} of 120. The extraordinarily large increase in Pa_{O_2} when starting to breathe on the mouthpiece at rest is probably due to: (1) hypoxemia off the mouthpiece due to microatelectasis associated with obesity (a very common problem in overweight subjects) and (2) the large increase in Pa_{O_2}, which accompanies acute hyperventilation, and a high R.

ANALYSIS

Flow Chart 1: This patient's maximum $\dot{V}O_2$ is markedly above predicted (Table 2). Since he cycled regularly to maintain his fitness, he performed exceedingly well. See *Flow Chart 2:* The electrocardiogram and O_2 pulse (high because of fitness) at maximal exercise are normal, but the blood gases are abnormal *(branchpoint 2.1)*. VD/VT and $P(a-ET)_{CO_2}$ are normal, but $P(A-a)_{O_2}$ at maximum exercise is increased and suggests the presence of mild lung disease *(branchpoint 2.3).*

CONCLUSION

Exceptionally fit man of 59 years with features of mild lung disease.

CASE 8 *Normal man*

CLINICAL FINDINGS

This 74-year-old retired shipyard worker was referred for evaluation and exercise testing because workup at another institution had resulted in a diagnosis of "emphysema" despite no evidence of airway obstruction. The patient had a mild, nonproductive cough, had smoked approximately 35 cigarette pack years, and continued to smoke. He had no other circulatory or respiratory symptoms, except for shortness of breath from climbing two flights of stairs but not from walking for one mile on the level. Physical examination was normal. Exercise testing was performed to help resolve the difference between clinical impressions.

EXERCISE FINDINGS

The patient performed exercise on a cycle ergometer. He pedalled at 60 rpm without added load for 3 minutes. The work rate was then increased 15 watts per minute to his symptom limited maximum. Blood was sampled every second minute and intra-arterial blood pressure was recorded from a percutaneously placed brachial artery catheter. The patient stopped exercise because of shortness of breath. Resting and exercise electrocardiograms were normal.

TABLE 8-1. *Selected Respiratory Function Data*

MEASUREMENT	PREDICTED	MEASURED
Age, yr		74
Sex		Male
Height, cm		169
Weight, kg	73	82
Hematocrit, %		44
VC, L	3.37	4.88
IC, L	2.25	4.12
TLC, L	5.60	6.05
FEV_1, L	2.58	3.96
FEV_1/VC, %	77	81
MVV, L/min	110	107
DL_{CO}, ml/mm Hg/min	21.6	24.8

TABLE 8-2. *Selected Exercise Data*

MEASUREMENT	PREDICTED	MEASURED
Maximum $\dot{V}O_2$, L/min	1.69	1.95
Maximum HR, beats/min	146	132
Maximum O_2 pulse, ml/beat	11.6	14.8
$\Delta\dot{V}O_2/\Delta WR$, ml/min/watt	10.3	10.6
$\dot{V}O_2$ difference, %	0.0	−1.6
AT, L/min	> 0.68	1.3
Blood pressure, mm Hg (rest, max)		150/84,177/79
Maximum $\dot{V}E$, L/min		68
Exercise breathing reserve, L/min	> 15	39
Pa_{O_2}, mm Hg (rest, max ex)		97,101
$P(A-a)_{O_2}$, mm Hg (rest, max ex)		20,16
$P(a-ET)_{CO_2}$, mm Hg (rest, max ex)		3,0
VD/VT (rest, heavy ex)		0.35,0.22
HCO_3^-, mEq/L (rest, 2 min recov)		20,17

TABLE 8-3

TIME min	WORK RATE W	BP mmHg	HR min⁻¹	f	$\dot{V}E$ BTPS L/min	$\dot{V}CO_2$ STPD L/min	$\dot{V}O_2$ STPD L/min	O_2 pulse ml/beat	R	pH	HCO_3^- mEq/L	PO₂ ET mmHg	PO₂ a mmHg	PO₂ A-a mmHg	PCO₂ ET mmHg	PCO₂ a mmHg	PCO₂ a-ET mmHg	$\dot{V}E/\dot{V}CO_2$	$\dot{V}E/\dot{V}O_2$	VD/VT
Rest		150/ 84								7.41	20	103			32					
Rest			73	24	19.7	0.38	0.43	5.9	0.88			117			29			46	41	
Rest		147/ 84	76	27	20.7	0.40	0.44	5.8	0.91	7.42	20	119	97	20	28	31	3	46	42	0.35
Rest			75	30	20.8	0.36	0.37	4.9	0.97			122			26			51	49	
Unloaded			92	31	39.8	0.79	0.78	8.5	1.01			122			26			47	48	
Unloaded			93	26	34.9	0.77	0.84	9.0	0.92			118			29			42	39	
Unloaded		162/ 84	92	20	29.1	0.70	0.80	8.7	0.88	7.42	20	116	103	15	29	29	0	39	34	0.22
1.0	15		92	21	34.8	0.82	0.84	9.1	0.98			117			29			40	39	
2.0	30	159/ 81	90	33	33.7	0.68	0.75	8.3	0.91	7.44	20	117	116	6	28	26	−2	45	41	0.25
3.0	45		99	20	29.7	0.81	1.03	10.4	0.79			106			34			35	27	
4.0	60	168/ 84	104	16	35.6	1.08	1.26	12.1	0.86	7.37	21	105	95	18	36	33	−3	32	27	0.17
5.0	75		114	19	42.8	1.31	1.53	13.4	0.86			106			36			31	27	
6.0	90	186/ 90	115	20	47.9	1.44	1.46	12.7	0.99	7.36	19	109	103	13	37	34	−3	32	32	0.20
7.0	105		122	20	52.2	1.54	1.52	12.5	1.01			110			36			33	33	
8.0	120	177/ 79	132	28	66.1	1.86	1.80	13.6	1.03	7.33	19	115	101	16	34	34	0	34	35	0.25
8.5	135		132	28	67.5	1.98	1.95	14.8	1.02			109			37			33	33	
Recovery			120	20	45.8	1.55	1.60	13.3	0.97			106			40			28	28	
Recovery			106	20	38.8	1.06	0.77	7.3	1.38			121			34			35	48	
Recovery			144	20	25.9	0.61	0.44	3.1	1.39			126			30			40	55	
Recovery		168/ 78								7.31	17	121			31					

FIGURE 8-A

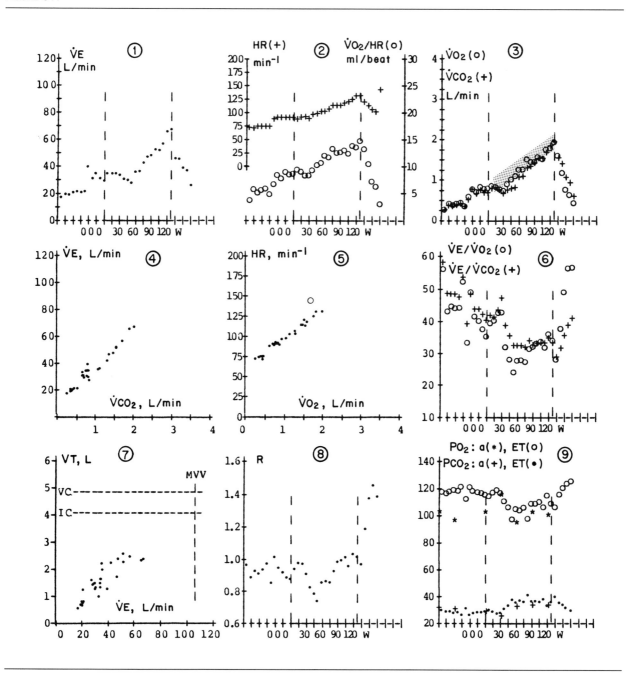

Interpretation

COMMENTS

This patient's resting respiratory function is normal (Table 8-1). The resting electrocardiogram is normal.

ANALYSIS

Flow Chart 1: The maximum $\dot{V}O_2$ and anaerobic threshold are normal (Table 8-2). See *Flow Chart 2:*

The electrocardiogram, O_2 pulse, arterial blood gases, and V_D/V_T are normal *(branchpoint 2.1)*. The patient is not obese *(branchpoint 2.2)*.

CONCLUSION

Normal cardiovascular and respiratory response to exercise. There is no evidence of abnormalities consistent with the diagnosis of "emphysema" given to the patient in a previous examination.

CASE 9 *Normal: Cycle and treadmill*

CLINICAL FINDINGS

This 37-year-old hospital employee was asymptomatic and volunteered for an exercise study. He did not exercise regularly or smoke. Physical examination, chest roentgenograms and resting ECG were normal.

EXERCISE FINDINGS

On two separate days, one month apart, the subject exercised to maximum tolerance using an incremental protocol, first on the cycle and second on the treadmill. He stopped on both occasions because of calf fatigue. There was no arrhythmia or abnormality in the ECG.

TABLE 9-1. *Selected Respiratory Function Data*

MEASUREMENT	PREDICTED	MEASURED
Age, yr		37
Sex		Male
Height, cm		161
Weight, kg	66	53
Hematocrit, %		45
VC, L	3.56	3.21
IC, L	2.37	2.51
TLC, L	4.90	5.01
FEV_1, L	2.87	2.64
FEV_1/VC, %	81	82
MVV, L/min	132	107
DL_{CO}, ml/mm Hg/min	23.1	22.3

TABLE 9-2. *Selected Exercise Data*

MEASUREMENT	PREDICTED		MEASURED	
	cycle	treadmill	cycle	treadmill
Maximum $\dot{V}O_2$, L/min	1.96	2.18	1.87	2.07
Maximum HR, beats/min	183	183	173	183
Maximum O_2 pulse, ml/beat	10.8	11.9	10.8	11.3
$\Delta\dot{V}O_2$/ΔWR, ml/min/watt	10.3		8.4	
$\dot{V}O_2$ difference, %	0.0		13.4	
AT, L/min	> 0.78	> 0.87	1.1	1.1
Maximum $\dot{V}E$, L/min			76	85
Exercise breathing reserve, L/min	> 15	> 15	31	22

TABLE 9-3. *Cycle Ergometry*

TIME min	WORK RATE W	BP mmHg	HR min⁻¹	f	V̇E BTPS	V̇CO₂ —STPD— L/min	V̇O₂	O₂ pulse ml/beat	R	pH	HCO₃ mEq/L	PO₂ ET —mmHg—	PO₂ a	PO₂ A-a	PCO₂ ET —mmHg—	PCO₂ a	PCO₂ a-ET	V̇E/V̇CO₂	V̇E/V̇O₂	VD/VT
Rest			95	14	11.1	0.36	0.42	4.4	0.86			97			45			31	26	
Rest			74	14	7.3	0.19	0.21	2.8	0.90			102			43			39	35	
Unloaded			97	8	11.1	0.44	0.52	5.4	0.85			96			46			25	21	
Unloaded			104	16	15.1	0.56	0.65	6.3	0.86			94			47			27	23	
Unloaded			97	16	14.8	0.55	0.55	5.7	1.00			103			46			27	27	
1.0	25		108	18	16.2	0.57	0.57	5.3	1.00			103			45			28	28	
2.0	50		110	17	17.1	0.67	0.74	6.7	0.91			94			50			26	23	
3.0	75		129	17	19.8	0.85	0.90	7.0	0.94			93			52			23	22	
4.0	100		133	17	22.9	1.07	1.12	8.4	0.96			89			57			21	20	
5.0	125		147	22	35.1	1.64	1.50	10.2	1.09			95			56			21	23	
6.0	150		159	27	44.4	1.94	1.58	9.9	1.23			103			53			23	28	
7.0	175		173	44	75.8	2.79	1.87	10.8	1.49			114			46			27	41	
Recovery			158	30	49.5	1.88	1.29	8.2	1.46			112			49			26	38	
Recovery			140	27	40.1	1.30	0.73	5.2	1.78			121			42			31	55	

FIGURE 9-A. *Cycle Ergometry*

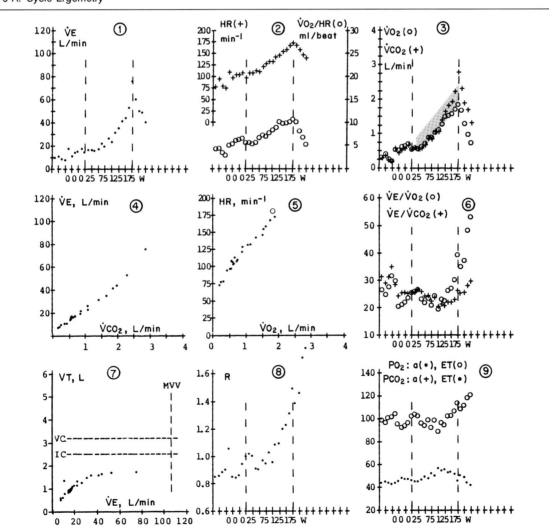

TABLE 9-4. *Treadmill Ergometry*

TIME min	WORK RATE %	BP mmHg	HR min⁻¹	f	V̇E BTPS L/min	V̇CO₂ STPD L/min	V̇O₂ STPD L/min	O₂ pulse ml/beat	R	pH	HCO₃⁻ mEq/L	PO₂ ET mmHg	PO₂ a	PO₂ A-a	PCO₂ ET mmHg	PCO₂ a	PCO₂ a-ET	V̇E/V̇CO₂	V̇E/V̇O₂	VD/VT
Rest			85	19	12.2	0.34	0.37	4.4	0.92			105			40			36	33	
Rest			95	20	13.0	0.34	0.37	3.9	0.92			105			40			38	35	
	0		109	23	19.4	0.62	0.71	6.5	0.87			100			43			31	27	
1.0	3		113	22	22.1	0.77	0.93	8.2	0.83			90			47			29	24	
2.0	6		120	22	25.1	0.94	1.05	8.8	0.90			97			47			27	24	
3.0	9		129	24	30.4	1.17	1.20	9.3	0.98			101			47			26	25	
4.0	12		141	25	35.6	1.43	1.38	9.8	1.04			101			48			25	26	
5.0	15		150	26	39.8	1.59	1.44	9.6	1.10			102			49			25	28	
6.0	18		160	27	47.8	1.98	1.67	10.4	1.19			106			48			24	29	
7.0	21		168	32	59.0	2.33	1.85	11.0	1.26			107			48			25	32	
8.0	24		178	39	71.7	2.69	1.99	11.2	1.35			113			45			27	36	
8.5	27		183	43	84.9	2.97	2.07	11.3	1.43			116			43			29	41	
Recovery			178	28	47.8	1.75	1.26	7.1	1.39			109			49			27	38	
Recovery			171	37	68.3	2.40	1.57	9.2	1.53			116			45			28	44	
Recovery			151	37	49.2	1.41	0.86	5.7	1.64			122			38			35	57	

FIGURE 9-B. *Treadmill Ergometry*

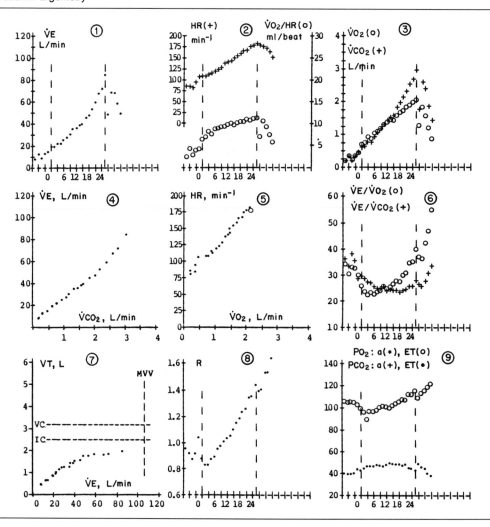

Interpretation

COMMENTS

The results of this subject's resting respiratory function studies are normal (Table 9-1). The resting electrocardiogram is normal. This study is presented to contrast the results when the same subject performed on the cycle and on the treadmill.

ANALYSIS

Flow Chart 1: The maximum $\dot{V}O_2$ and the anaerobic threshold are normal for both cycle and treadmill exercise (Table 9-2). The electrocardiogram and O_2 pulse are normal at maximum work rate *(branchpoint 2.1)*. See *Flow Chart 2:* The subject is not obese *(branchpoint 2.2)*. It should be noted that the maximum $\dot{V}O_2$ is about 10% higher on the treadmill than on the cycle.

CONCLUSION

Normal exercise performance.

CASE 10 *Normal: Immediate effects of cigarette smoking*

CLINICAL FINDINGS

This 27-year-old subject was one of several men who volunteered for a study to investigate the effect of recent cigarette smoking on cardiovascular and respiratory function during exercise. The subject was apparently in excellent general health, but had smoked cigarettes for 10 years. Physical examination, chest x-ray, and ECG were normal.

EXERCISE FINDINGS

Two similar exercise studies were performed six days apart on a cycle ergometer. In the 5 hours before the first study the subject smoked 15 medium tar cigarettes. In the second study, the subject was under observation for five hours without smoking. He breathed oxygen for the first 3 of those 5 hours to reduce the carboxyhemoglobin in his blood. On both occasions he pedalled without added load at 60 rpm for 3 minutes. The work rate was then increased 25 watts every minute to his symptom limited maximum. On both occasions the subject stopped exercise because of fatigue. ECG remained normal. Carboxyhemoglobin levels were 6.1% at the start of the first study and 1.5% at the start of the second study.

TABLE 10-1. *Selected Respiratory Function Data*

MEASUREMENT	PREDICTED	WITH PRIOR smoking	WITHOUT PRIOR smoking
Age, yr		27	
Sex		Male	
Height, cm		168	
Weight, kg	69	83	
Hematocrit, %		47	47
VC, L	4.65	4.18	4.20
IC, L	3.10	3.43	3.43
TLC, L	6.19	6.26	6.68
FEV_1, L	3.79	3.57	3.55
FEV_1/VC, %	81	85	85
MVV, L/min	168	140	163
DL_{CO}, ml/mm Hg/min	31.2	34.7	37.4

TABLE 10-2. *Selected Exercise Data*

MEASUREMENT	PREDICTED	WITH PRIOR smoking	WITHOUT PRIOR smoking
Maximum $\dot{V}O_2$, L/min	2.92	2.55	2.73
Maximum HR, beats/min	193	178	182
Maximum O_2 pulse, ml/beat	15.1	14.3	15.0
$\Delta\dot{V}O_2/\Delta WR$, ml/min/watt	10.3	9.0	9.9
$\dot{V}O_2$ difference, %	0.0	8.4	5.4
AT, L/min	> 1.17	1.03	1.25
Blood pressure, mm Hg (rest, max)		138/84,183/110	132/84,186/105
Maximum $\dot{V}E$, L/min		110	121
Exercise breathing reserve, L/min	> 15	39	42
Pa_{O_2}, mm Hg (rest, max ex)		102,103	109,106
$P(A-a)_{O_2}$, mm Hg (rest, max ex)		5,19	−1,16
$P(a-ET)_{CO_2}$, mm Hg (rest, max ex)		−1,−3	−2,−3
VD/VT (rest, heavy ex)		0.37,0.18	0.28,0.20
HCO_3^-, mEq/L (rest, 2 min recov)		25,14	25,14

TABLE 10-3. *With Prior Smoking*

TIME min	WORK RATE W	BP mmHg	HR min⁻¹	f	V̇E BTPS L/min	V̇CO₂ STPD L/min	V̇O₂ STPD L/min	O₂ pulse ml/beat	R	pH	HCO₃⁻ mEq/L	PO₂ ET mmHg	PO₂ a mmHg	PO₂ A-a mmHg	PCO₂ ET mmHg	PCO₂ a mmHg	PCO₂ a-ET mmHg	V̇E/V̇CO₂	V̇E/V̇O₂	VD/VT
Rest		138/ 84								7.42	24		98			38				
Rest			77	27	13.4	0.27	0.31	4.0	0.87			106			39			41	36	
Rest		138/ 84	77	25	13.2	0.28	0.32	4.2	0.88	7.42	25	107	102	5	40	39	-1	40	35	0.37
Rest			75	25	11.7	0.23	0.26	3.5	0.88			104			41			41	37	
Unloaded			101	20	17.1	0.56	0.65	6.4	0.86			97			43			27	24	
Unloaded			103	21	23.6	0.87	0.96	9.3	0.91			97			45			25	23	
Unloaded		156/ 96	105	23	23.8	0.85	0.92	8.8	0.92	7.39	24	102	98	8	45	41	-4	26	24	0.16
1.0	25		109	21	24.0	0.90	0.99	9.1	0.91			100			44			25	22	
2.0	50	165/ 93	115	23	32.1	1.16	1.17	10.2	0.99	7.38	24	101	95	13	45	42	-3	26	26	0.20
3.0	75		124	25	35.4	1.36	1.33	10.7	1.02			103			46			24	25	
4.0	100	177/ 96	135	26	43.4	1.68	1.53	11.3	1.10	7.36	24	102	94	16	47	43	-4	25	27	0.17
5.0	125		150	30	50.8	2.01	1.88	12.5	1.07			103			48			24	26	
6.0	150	177/ 99	162	36	66.6	2.47	2.09	12.9	1.18	7.33	22	107	95	18	46	42	-4	26	30	0.19
7.0	175		172	43	84.8	2.95	2.34	13.6	1.26			112			43			28	35	
8.0	200		178	62	110.6	3.36	2.55	14.3	1.32	7.32	17	119	103	19	37	34	-3	31	41	0.18
Recovery			164	43	81.4	2.46	1.49	9.1	1.65			123			37			32	52	
Recovery		165/ 84	153	35	53.3	1.46	0.98	6.4	1.49	7.27	14	123	112	14	35	32	-3	34	51	0.21

FIGURE 10-A. *With Prior Smoking*

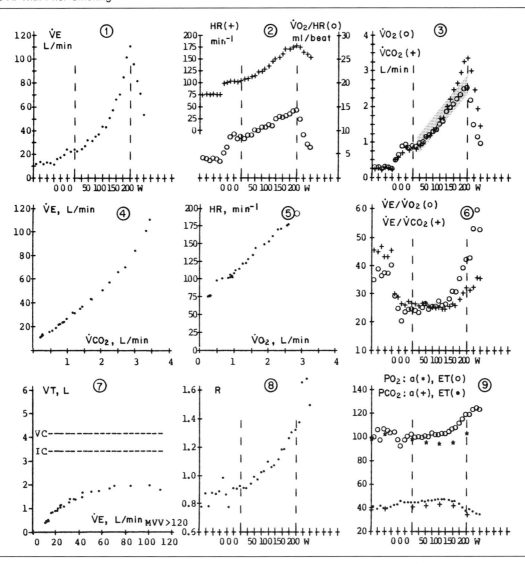

TABLE 10-4. *Without Prior Smoking*

TIME min	WORK RATE W	BP mmHg	HR min⁻¹	f	V̇E BTPS L/min	V̇CO₂ STPD L/min	V̇O₂ L/min	O₂ pulse ml/beat	R	pH	HCO₃ mEq/L	PO₂ ET mmHg	PO₂ a	PO₂ A-a	PCO₂ ET mmHg	PCO₂ a	PCO₂ a-ET	V̇E/V̇CO₂	V̇E/V̇O₂	VD/VT
Rest		129/ 84								7.40	25		99			42				
Rest			67	26	13.8	0.31	0.36	5.4	0.86			105			41			37	32	
Rest		132/ 84	68	20	12.1	0.32	0.35	5.1	0.91	7.43	25	107	109	-1	41	39	-2	33	30	0.28
Rest			68	25	12.5	0.26	0.29	4.3	0.90			107			41			40	36	
Unloaded			97	23	21.0	0.67	0.79	8.1	0.85			101			42			28	24	
Unloaded			97	20	26.0	0.92	0.99	10.2	0.93			97			46			26	25	
Unloaded		141/ 87	92	22	23.8	0.85	0.93	10.1	0.91	7.39	26	95	98	6	48	43	-5	26	24	0.20
1.0	25		100	24	24.0	0.86	1.00	10.0	0.86			97			47			26	22	
2.0	50	153/ 90	105	25	27.0	0.99	1.06	10.1	0.93	7.39	25	100	102	4	46	42	-4	25	24	0.17
3.0	75		117	26	35.8	1.30	1.27	10.9	1.02			103			46			26	26	
4.0	100	168/ 93	126	29	40.6	1.55	1.49	11.8	1.04	7.37	25	102	103	4	48	44	-4	25	26	0.19
5.0	125		139	33	49.0	1.85	1.73	12.4	1.07			105			46			25	27	
6.0	150	177/ 99	150	36	60.4	2.20	1.96	13.1	1.12	7.36	23	106	101	11	46	42	-4	26	29	0.20
7.0	175		166	38	76.8	2.69	2.27	13.7	1.19			110			44			27	32	
8.0	200	186/105	179	52	101.8	3.22	2.55	14.3	1.26	7.35	21	117	107	13	39	36	-3	30	38	0.20
8.5	225		182	64	121.0	3.58	2.73	15.0	1.31	7.32	17	119	106	16	37	34	-3	32	42	0.20
Recovery			179	52	111.9	3.28	2.54	14.2	1.29			118			38			33	42	
Recovery			160	43	74.9	2.18	1.33	8.3	1.64			124			36			33	54	
Recovery		162/ 90								7.26	14		118			33				

FIGURE 10-B. *Without Prior Smoking*

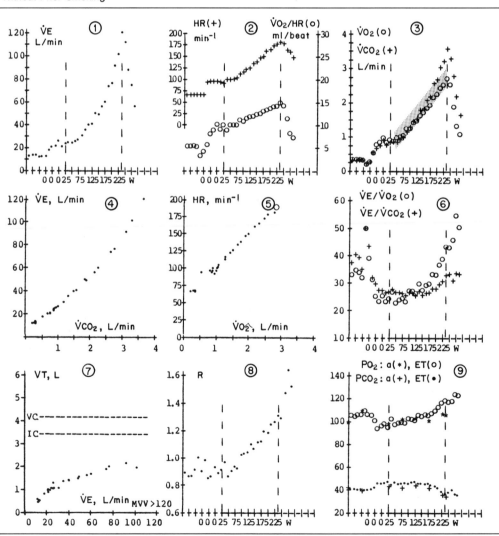

Interpretation

COMMENTS

This study is being presented because it illustrates small but significant effects of acute cigarette smoking on the maximum $\dot{V}O_2$ and the anaerobic threshold. It also illustrates the reproducibility of the cardiac and gas exchange responses to exercise performed on different days, and the effects of obesity.

Results of resting respiratory function studies are normal (Table 10-1). The resting electrocardiogram is normal.

ANALYSIS

Flow Chart 1: The maximum $\dot{V}O_2$ is borderline with prior smoking but clearly normal without prior smoking (Table 10-2). The anaerobic threshold is reduced after smoking but is normal without prior smoking (Table 10-2). See *Flow Chart 2:* The subject is 20% overweight *(branchpoint 2.2).* It should be noted that this obese subject's $\dot{V}O_2$ during unloaded cycling is approximately 0.95 L/min. (Table 10-3 and Graph 3 of Fig. 10-A and 10-B).

Indices other than maximum $\dot{V}O_2$ and *AT* that might reflect the effect of the increased carboxyhemoglobin during exercise are the O_2 pulse and $\Delta\dot{V}O_2/\Delta WR$. These are both reduced following cigarette smoking (Table 10-2). The indices of ventilation/perfusion matching are normal at maximum exercise (see reference 30 in Chapter 4 for a complete report of the acute effects of cigarette smoking on exercise tolerance) in this subject.

CONCLUSION

Cigarette smoking and obesity affecting exercise performance in an otherwise normal subject.

CASE 11 *Normal: Pre- and post-beta-adrenergic blockade*

CLINICAL FINDINGS

This 23-year-old asthmatic student voluntarily participated in a double-blind study evaluating the effect of a beta-adrenergic blocker, pindolol, on exercise induced asthma. He had hay fever and asthma since childhood but was otherwise in excellent health. He was taking no medications. Physical examination, chest x-ray, ECG, and hemogram were normal. He became familiar with the procedures one week prior to the following studies.

EXERCISE FINDINGS

Two similar cycle exercise studies were performed a week apart. After baseline spirometry, 0.4 mg of pindolol or placebo were given over a 20 minute period through a venous catheter. After repeat spirometry, the subject pedalled without added resistance at 60 rpm for 3 minutes and at 60 watts for an additional 3 minutes. Thereafter the work rate was increased 20 watts every minute. On each occasion the subject stopped because of fatigue. ECG pattern remained normal. Repeat spirometry in duplicate or triplicate, performed 2, 7, 12, 17, 22, and 27 minutes post-exercise, did not reveal exercise induced bronchospasm.

TABLE 11-1. *Selected Respiratory Function Data*

MEASUREMENT	PREDICTED	MEASURED
Age, yr		23
Sex		Male
Height, cm		170
Weight, kg	68	64
Hematocrit, %		45
VC, L	4.79	4.86
IC, L	3.21	3.40
TLC, L	6.46	6.72
FEV_1, L	4.04	3.58
FEV_1/VC, %	84	74
MVV, L/min	175	142
DL_{CO}, ml/mm Hg/min	33.2	32.5

TABLE 11-2. *Selected Exercise Data*

MEASUREMENT	PREDICTED	PLACEBO	PINDOLOL
Maximum $\dot{V}O_2$, L/min	2.82	2.57	2.39
Maximum HR, beats/min	197	189	156
Maximum O_2 pulse, ml/beat	14.3	13.6	15.3
$\Delta\dot{V}O_2/\Delta WR$, ml/min/watt	10.3	10.5	9.7
$\dot{V}O_2$ difference, %	0.0	1.3	5.8
AT, L/min	> 1.13	1.5	1.4
Maximum $\dot{V}E$, L/min		94	85
Exercise breathing reserve, L/min	> 15	48	57

TABLE 11-3. *Pre-beta-adrenergic Blockade*

TIME min	WORK RATE W	BP mmHg	HR min⁻¹	f	$\dot{V}E$ BTPS —— L/min	$\dot{V}CO_2$ —STPD—	$\dot{V}O_2$ ——	O_2 pulse ml/beat	R	pH	HCO₃⁻ mEq L	ET	PO_2 a A-a —mmHg—	ET	PCO_2 a a-ET —mmHg—	$\dot{V}E$ $\dot{V}CO_2$	$\dot{V}E$ $\dot{V}O_2$	VD VT
Rest			78	12	8.9	0.19	0.18	2.3	1.06			119		32		47	49	
Rest			85	11	5.6	0.11	0.16	1.9	0.69			107		36		51	35	
Unloaded			99	20	9.1	0.21	0.39	3.9	0.54			92		42		44	23	
Unloaded			93	20	14.0	0.39	0.62	6.7	0.63			90		43		36	23	
Unloaded			98	20	16.9	0.52	0.69	7.0	0.75			101		41		33	25	
1.0	60		122	21	27.3	0.95	1.25	10.2	0.76			99		44		29	22	
2.0	60		128	25	32.9	1.12	1.30	10.2	0.86			105		43		29	25	
3.0	60		129	27	34.9	1.17	1.33	10.3	0.88			108		43		30	26	
4.0	80		133	26	39.7	1.32	1.44	10.8	0.92			108		42		30	28	
5.0	100		138	28	40.1	1.32	1.44	10.4	0.92			108		42		30	28	
6.0	120		154	29	45.4	1.51	1.62	10.5	0.93			110		41		30	28	
7.0	140		160	30	58.0	1.91	2.00	12.5	0.96			104		45		30	29	
8.0	160		168	36	61.0	1.94	2.01	12.0	0.97			111		42		31	30	
9.0	180		177	37	71.3	2.27	2.24	12.7	1.01			115		40		31	32	
10.0	200		189	41	93.8	2.78	2.57	13.6	1.08			119		38		34	36	

FIGURE 11-A. *Pre-beta-adrenergic Blockade*

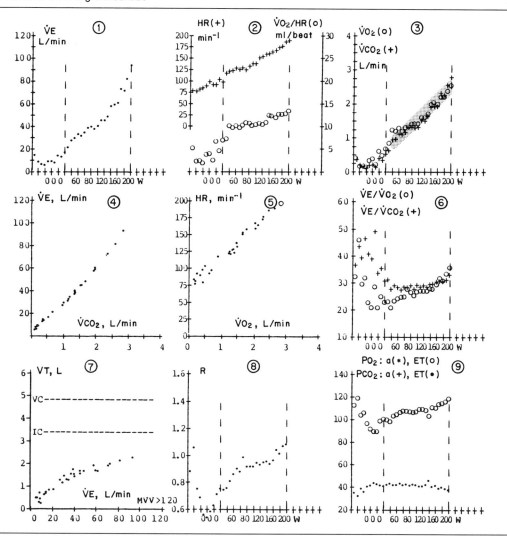

TABLE 11-4. *Post-beta-adrenergic Blockade*

TIME min	WORK RATE W	BP mmHg	HR min⁻¹	f	V̇E BTPS L/min	V̇CO₂ STPD L/min	V̇O₂ STPD L/min	O₂ pulse ml/beat	R	pH	HCO₃⁻ mEq/L	PO₂ ET a A-a mmHg	PCO₂ ET a a-ET mmHg	V̇E/V̇CO₂	V̇E/V̇O₂	VD/VT
Rest			70	24	6.6	0.10	0.16	2.3	0.63			105	39	66	42	
Rest			59	16	8.7	0.20	0.23	3.9	0.87			114	36	43	38	
Unloaded			85	17	13.7	0.43	0.60	7.1	0.72			94	43	32	23	
Unloaded			90	15	9.2	0.27	0.34	3.8	0.79			99	44	34	27	
Unloaded			86	19	15.0	0.49	0.59	6.9	0.83			102	42	31	25	
1.0	60		107	17	20.9	0.76	1.03	9.6	0.74			96	44	28	20	
2.0	60		109	22	27.5	1.00	1.15	10.6	0.87			103	45	28	24	
3.0	60		115	25	30.7	1.12	1.28	11.1	0.88			104	44	27	24	
4.0	80		112	22	30.7	1.11	1.20	10.7	0.93			103	46	28	26	
5.0	100		119	26	33.7	1.25	1.37	11.5	0.91			104	45	27	25	
6.0	120		122	25	40.6	1.55	1.63	13.4	0.95			106	45	26	25	
7.0	140		128	28	48.2	1.78	1.77	13.8	1.01			108	46	27	27	
8.0	160		134	31	52.2	1.95	1.93	14.4	1.01			110	44	27	27	
9.0	180		147	32	63.1	2.37	2.13	14.5	1.11			112	43	27	30	
10.0	200		156	41	85.2	2.92	2.39	15.3	1.22			111	42	29	36	

Figure 11–B. *Post-beta-adrenergic Blockade*

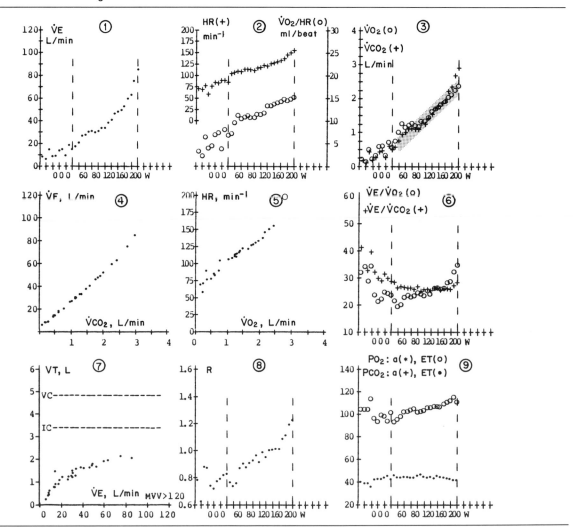

Interpretation

COMMENTS

This study is presented to demonstrate the effect of beta-adrenergic blockade on exercise. The lowest work rate after unloaded cycling is 60 watts, followed by 1 minute increments of 20 watts. This uneven increase in the work rate increment causes the upward distortion in the $\dot{V}O_2$-work rate slope (Graph 3 of Figures 11-A and 11-B). Results of respiratory function testing are normal at the time of study (Table 11-1).

ANALYSIS

Flow Chart 1: The maximum aerobic capacity and *AT* are within normal limits on both pre- and post-beta-adrenergic blockade exercise tests (Table 11-2). See *Flow Chart 2:* The ECG and O_2 pulse at maximum work rate are normal *(branchpoint 2.1).* The large reduction in maximum HR, with slight reduction in maximum $\dot{V}O_2$ and increase in maximum O_2 pulse, is typical of the effect of beta-adrenergic blockade. The chronotropic effect of the beta-blockade increases the time for ventricular filling and results in a larger O_2 pulse at the same work rate.

CONCLUSION

Normal with demonstration of heart rate slowing following beta-adrenergic blockade.

CASE 12 *Normal, with ventilatory chemoreflex insensitivity*

CLINICAL FINDINGS

This 67-year-old retired gentleman worked for 30 years in the shipyards. He never smoked. Three months previously he was found to have hypertension for which he was treated with triamterene and hydrochlorothiazide. He noted shortness of breath after climbing 2 flights of stairs and frequent mild substernal pressure not related to exertion, meals, body position, or stress. Physical, roentgenographic, laboratory, and electrocardiographic examinations were normal.

EXERCISE FINDINGS

The patient performed exercise on a cycle ergometer. He pedalled at 60 rpm without added load for 3 minutes. The work rate was then increased 20 watts per minute to his symptom limited maximum. Blood was sampled every second minute and intra-arterial blood pressure was recorded from a percutaneously placed brachial artery catheter. He stopped exercise with shortness of breath, but without chest pain or pressure. ECG pattern remained normal.

TABLE 12-1. *Selected Respiratory Function Data*

MEASUREMENT	PREDICTED	MEASURED
Age, yr		67
Sex		Male
Height, cm		173
Weight, kg	76	80
Hematocrit, %		48
VC, L	3.82	3.86
IC, L	2.55	2.42
TLC, L	6.06	6.04
FEV_1, L	2.97	3.07
FEV_1/VC, %	78	80
MVV, L/min	124	121
DL_{CO}, ml/mm Hg/min	26.3	32.3

TABLE 12-2. *Selected Exercise Data*

MEASUREMENT	PREDICTED	MEASURED
Maximum $\dot{V}O_2$, L/min	1.96	1.94
Maximum HR, beats/min	153	142
Maximum O_2 pulse, ml/beat	12.8	13.7
$\Delta\dot{V}O_2/\Delta WR$, ml/min/watt	10.3	9.9
$\dot{V}O_2$ difference, %	0.0	2.5
AT, L/min	> 0.78	1.3
Blood pressure, mm Hg (rest, max)		176/92,215/92
Maximum $\dot{V}E$, L/min		56
Exercise breathing reserve, L/min	> 15	65
PaO_2, mm Hg (rest, max ex)		96,81
$P(A-a)O_2$, mm Hg (rest, max ex)		8,22
$P(a-ET)CO_2$, mm Hg (rest, max ex)		1,−6
VD/VT (rest, heavy ex)		0.39,0.23
HCO_3 , mEq/L (rest, 2 min recov)		27,21

TABLE 12-3

TIME min	WORK RATE W	BP mmHg	HR min⁻¹	f	$\dot{V}E$ BTPS L/min	$\dot{V}CO_2$ STPD L/min	$\dot{V}O_2$ STPD L/min	O_2 pulse ml/beat	R	pH	HCO_3 mEq/L	PO₂ ET mmHg	PO₂ a mmHg	PO₂ A-a mmHg	PCO₂ ET mmHg	PCO₂ a mmHg	PCO₂ a-ET mmHg	$\frac{\dot{V}E}{\dot{V}CO_2}$	$\frac{\dot{V}E}{\dot{V}O_2}$	$\frac{VD}{VT}$
Rest		176/ 92								7.41	27	82			43					
Rest			76	19	13.7	0.33	0.38	5.0	0.87			107			38			37	32	
Rest		164/ 92	76	16	9.3	0.20	0.24	3.2	0.83	7.43	26	105	96	8	39	40	1	40	33	0.39
Rest			80	22	11.4	0.25	0.32	4.0	0.78			103			40			38	30	
Unloaded			87	17	15.7	0.54	0.79	9.1	0.68			79			49			26	18	
Unloaded			89	18	11.6	0.42	0.59	6.6	0.71			88			47			24	17	
Unloaded		185/ 92	82	25	15.1	0.47	0.62	7.6	0.76	7.40	27	92	85	10	47	44	−3	28	21	0.25
1.0	20		89	14	14.9	0.54	0.69	7.8	0.78			93			47			25	20	
2.0	40	194/ 89	95	16	20.7	0.73	0.92	9.7	0.79	7.40	27	94	84	12	46	45	−1	26	21	0.26
3.0	60		102	17	25.1	0.92	1.16	11.4	0.79			95			45			26	20	
4.0	80	203/ 89	107	20	30.0	1.10	1.31	12.2	0.84	7.40	27	98	85	16	46	43	−3	26	22	0.21
5.0	100		115	22	37.4	1.38	1.54	13.4	0.90			100			46			26	23	
6.0	120		127	26	47.2	1.74	1.87	14.7	0.93			93			51			26	24	
7.0	140	215/ 92	140	29	43.6	1.65	1.61	11.5	1.02	7.35	26	96	81	22	54	48	−6	25	26	0.26
7.5	160		142	27	55.5	2.13	1.94	13.7	1.10			105			47			25	27	
Recovery			132	29	49.0	1.80	1.58	12.0	1.14			105			49			26	29	
Recovery			113	24	35.4	1.09	0.70	6.2	1.56			121			40			31	48	
Recovery		209/ 92								7.37	21		115			38				

FIGURE 12-A

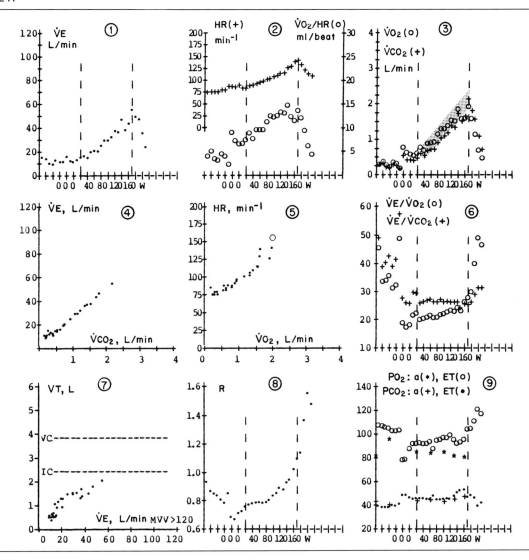

Interpretation

COMMENTS

Results of the resting respiratory function studies are normal (Table 12-1). The resting electrocardiogram is normal.

ANALYSIS

Flow Chart 1: The maximum $\dot{V}_{O_2}$ and anaerobic threshold are normal (Table 12-2). See *Flow Chart 2:* The exercise electrocardiogram, arterial blood gases, V_D/V_T and O_2 pulse at maximum $\dot{V}_{O_2}$ are normal *(branchpoint 2.1).* The patient is not obese *(branchpoint 2.2).* It should be noted that while the arterial CO_2 tension is normal at rest, the increase in ventilation lagged the increase in CO_2 production, causing arterial P_{CO_2} to rise gradually during exercise (Graph 9, Fig. 12-A and Table 12-3). This is occasionally seen when the ventilatory chemoreflex is relatively insensitive. Because the CO_2 stores are increasing in the body as a consequence of the rising Pa_{CO_2}, CO_2 output does not rise as steeply as it otherwise might, particularly above the anaerobic threshold. Thus, $\dot{V}_E/\dot{V}_{CO_2}$ at the termination of work is not increased over that at the *AT* (Graph 6, Fig. 12-A) and there is no steepening in the $\dot{V}_E$-work rate relationship (Graph 1 and 4, Fig. 12-A).

CONCLUSION

Normal cardiovascular and respiratory function in a patient likely to have a relatively insensitive ventilatory chemoreflex.

CASE 13 *Poor effort with acute hyperventilation and anxiety in a moderately obese man*

CLINICAL FINDINGS

This 56-year-old shipyard worker complained of progressive dyspnea on exertion, evident when climbing two flights of stairs. He also noted anterior chest pain with exertion, relieved by rest, associated with dyspnea and diaphoresis but not with palpitations, lightheadedness, syncope or numbness. He stopped smoking 20 years ago after 20 pack years. He took no medications but was told he had hypertension several years ago. Physical examination and resting ECG were normal. Chest x-ray showed mild pleural thickening bilaterally.

EXERCISE FINDINGS

After percutaneous insertion of a brachial artery catheter, while being positioned on the cycle ergometer, the patient became lightheaded and syncopal. The patient was placed on a guerney in the reverse Trendelenburg position. Continuous monitoring revealed a transient sinus bradycardia as low as 25 with normal blood pressure. The bradycardia lasted only a few minutes. After 15 minutes he felt well and was able to exercise. He pedalled at 60 rpm without added load for 3 minutes. The work rate was then increased 15 watts every minute. Blood was sampled every second minute and intra-arterial blood pressure was recorded from the brachial artery catheter. Mild chest pain began at 45 watts; exercise was stopped at 90 watts because of the patient's continuing and increasing chest pain, which was typical of his usual symptom. There were no ST abnormalities nor was there arrhythmia during or after exercise.

TABLE 13-1. *Pre-exercise Data Summary*

MEASUREMENT	PREDICTED	MEASURED
Age, yr		56
Sex		Male
Height, cm		172
Weight, kg	75	98
Hematocrit, %		46
VC, L	4.10	3.16
IC, L	2.74	2.55
TLC, L	6.17	4.77
FEV_1, L	3.23	2.78
FEV_1/VC, %	79	88
MVV, L/min	137	98
DL_{CO}, ml/mm Hg/min	26.3	20.9

TABLE 13-2. *Post-exercise Data Summary*

MEASUREMENT	PREDICTED	MEASURED
Maximum $\dot{V}O_2$, L/min	2.25	1.51
Maximum HR, beats/min	164	130
Maximum O_2 pulse, ml/beat	13.7	11.6
$\Delta\dot{V}O_2/\Delta WR$, ml/min/watt	10.3	9.3
$\dot{V}O_2$ difference, %	0.0	4.6
AT, L/min	> 0.90	indeterminate
Blood pressure, mm Hg (rest, max)		168/96,228/111
Maximum $\dot{V}E$, L/min		79
Exercise breathing reserve, L/min	> 15	19
Pa_{O_2}, mm Hg (rest, max ex)		112,100
$P(A-a)_{O_2}$, mm Hg (rest, max ex)		21,25
$P(a-ET)_{CO_2}$, mm Hg (rest, max ex)		2,0
VD/VT (rest, heavy ex)		0.30,0.27
HCO_3^-, mEq/L (rest, 2 min recov)		25,20

TABLE 13-3

TIME min	WORK RATE W	BP mmHg	HR min⁻¹	f	$\dot{V}E$ BTPS —L/min—	$\dot{V}CO_2$ —STPD— L/min	$\dot{V}O_2$ —STPD— L/min	O_2 pulse ml/beat	R	pH	HCO_3^- mEq/L	PO₂ ET mmHg	PO₂ a mmHg	PO₂ A-a mmHg	PCO₂ ET mmHg	PCO₂ a mmHg	PCO₂ a-ET mmHg	$\dfrac{\dot{V}E}{\dot{V}CO_2}$	$\dfrac{\dot{V}E}{\dot{V}O_2}$	VD VT
Rest		168/ 96								7.47	25	88			34					
Rest			66	26	27.9	0.49	0.34	5.2	1.44			131			22			52	76	
Rest		156/ 87	64	29	23.8	0.38	0.26	4.1	1.46	7.59	22	134	112	21	21	23	2	56	82	0.30
Rest			64	27	27.9	0.39	0.26	4.1	1.50			135			18			66	98	
Rest			65	25	16.6	0.26	0.28	4.3	0.93			126			23			56	52	
Unloaded			90	61	38.6	0.68	0.68	7.6	1.00			123			26			49	49	
Unloaded			93	46	37.5	0.77	0.80	8.6	0.96			117			30			44	42	
Unloaded		207/108	90	49	40.4	0.84	0.85	9.4	0.99	7.50	23	120	102	18	29	30	1	43	43	0.30
1.0	15		97	55	51.1	0.99	0.89	9.2	1.11			123			27			47	52	
2.0	30	210/108	103	61	55.4	1.05	0.98	9.5	1.07	7.52	22	123	106	18	27	27	0	48	51	0.30
3.0	45		108	59	56.0	1.15	1.16	10.7	0.99			120			28			44	44	
4.0	60	216/108	120	59	63.2	1.35	1.31	10.9	1.03	7.49	22	121	102	20	28	29	1	43	44	0.29
5.0	75		126	56	71.8	1.58	1.43	11.3	1.10			123			28			42	47	
6.0	90	228/111	129	56	71.3	1.65	1.37	10.6	1.20	7.46	20	124	100	25	29	29	0	40	49	0.24
Recovery			119	49	48.2	1.09	0.99	8.3	1.10			118			32			40	44	
Recovery										7.45	20		103			29				

FIGURE 13-A

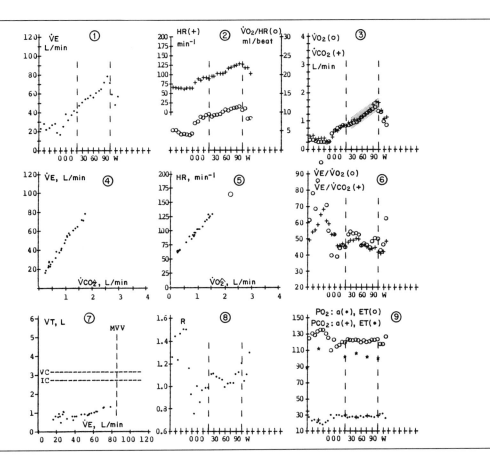

Interpretation

COMMENTS

Resting respiratory function studies reveal the patient to have a mild restrictive defect of the type generally seen with obesity (normal inspiratory capacity, but reduced expiratory reserve volume) (Table 13-1). The patient is, in fact, 23 kg overweight. Resting electrocardiogram is normal. As the patient was getting ready to cycle, he became light-headed and hypotensive. His blood pressure decreased and he developed a marked bradycardia consistent with a vasovagal reaction. When placed in a supine position, the patient's pulse and blood pressure became normal and he resumed his position on the cycle ergometer for testing. However, he acutely hyperventilated at rest, demonstrating a marked respiratory alkalosis (Table 13-3).

ANALYSIS

Flow Chart 1: The maximum $\dot{V}O_2$ is reduced and the anaerobic threshold is indeterminate (Table 13-2). See *Flow Chart 5:* The indices of ventilation/perfusion mismatching (V_D/V_T, $P(A-a)_{O_2}$ and $P(a-ET)_{CO_2}$) at the maximum work rate are normal (Table 13-3) *(branchpoint 5.1)*, heart rate reserve is high *(branchpoint 5.2)*, breathing reserve is normal *(branchpoint 5.5)*, and $\Delta\dot{V}O_2/\Delta WR$ is normal *(branchpoint 5.8)*. The analytical steps taken indicate that this patient's low maximum $\dot{V}O_2$ is due to poor effort, possibly secondary to apprehension. However, this patient does have significant obesity and hypertension. Re-evaluation is in order when the patient is less anxious.

CONCLUSION

Poor effort with acute resting hyperventilation and anxiety in a moderately obese man. The combination of high heart rate reserve and normal breathing reserve without objective evidence of either myocardial, pulmonary vascular, peripheral vascular, or underlying lung disease, suggests that this patient's reduced maximum oxygen uptake, and perhaps symptom of dyspnea, is psychogenic. The pre-exercise vasovagal reaction and the acute hyperventilation in the anticipation of exercise are consistent with this interpretation.

CASE 14 *Poor effort*

CLINICAL FINDINGS

This 59-year-old shipyard worker was made aware of an abnormality in his chest x-ray 1 year prior to evaluation. Retrospectively, he felt that he had some shortness of breath for 2 years when jogging or climbing stairs. He smoked cigarettes for 20 years, until age 35. Results of physical, laboratory, and roentgenographic examinations were normal except for prostatic enlargement and extensive pleural calcification.

EXERCISE FINDINGS

The patient performed exercise on a cycle ergometer. He pedalled at 60 rpm without added load for 3 minutes. The work rate was then increased 20 watts per minute to his symptom limited maximum. Blood was sampled every second minute and intra-arterial blood pressure was recorded from a percutaneously placed brachial artery catheter. The patient pedalled irregularly during the test. He stopped pedalling complaining of shortness of breath and leg fatigue, and stated he could go no further. Resting and exercise ECG were normal.

TABLE 14-1. *Selected Respiratory Function Data*

MEASUREMENT	PREDICTED	MEASURED
Age, yr		59
Sex		Male
Height, cm		173
Weight, kg	76	72
Hematocrit, %		44
VC, L	3.65	3.05
IC, L	2.44	2.44
TLC, L	5.57	4.93
FEV_1, L	2.87	2.49
FEV_1/VC, %	79	82
MVV, L/min	121	110
DL_{CO}, ml/mm Hg/min	22.6	24.6

TABLE 14-2. *Selected Exercise Data*

MEASUREMENT	PREDICTED	MEASURED
Maximum $\dot{V}O_2$, L/min	2.07	1.08
Maximum HR, beats/min	161	110
Maximum O_2 pulse, ml/beat	12.9	9.8
AT, L/min	> 0.83	indeterminate
Blood pressure, mm Hg (rest, max)		135/78,144/78
Maximum $\dot{V}E$, L/min		30
Exercise breathing reserve, L/min	> 15	80
Pa_{O_2} mm Hg (rest, max ex)		98,96
$P(A-a)_{O_2}$, mm Hg (rest, max ex)		0,10
$P(a-ET)_{CO_2}$, mm Hg (rest, max ex)		0,−3
VD/VT (rest, heavy ex)		0.35,0.36
HCO_3^-, mEq/L (rest, 2 min recov)		25,23

TABLE 14-3

TIME min	WORK RATE W	BP mmHg	HR min⁻¹	f	V̇E BTPS L/min	V̇CO₂ STPD L/min	V̇O₂ STPD L/min	O₂ pulse ml/beat	R	pH	HCO₃⁻ mEq/L	PO₂ ET mmHg	PO₂ a mmHg	PO₂ A-a mmHg	PCO₂ ET mmHg	PCO₂ a mmHg	PCO₂ a-ET mmHg	V̇E/V̇CO₂	V̇E/V̇O₂	VD/VT
Rest		135/ 78								7.51	24	118			30					
Rest			76	14	4.9	0.11	0.15	2.0	0.73			96			39			34	25	
Rest		132/ 78	78	20	11.2	0.26	0.36	4.6	0.72	7.41	25	95	98	0	40	40	0	37	26	0.35
Rest			83	18	12.3	0.32	0.41	4.9	0.78			99			39			34	26	
Unloaded			90	29	17.6	0.42	0.57	6.3	0.74			100			39			36	27	
Unloaded			90	32	21.9	0.49	0.53	5.9	0.92			102			40			39	36	
Unloaded		144/ 78	87	26	23.5	0.55	0.50	5.7	1.10	7.43	24	115	104	13	35	36	1	39	43	0.35
1.0	20		95	20	14.3	0.41	0.50	5.3	0.82			95			40			31	25	
2.0	40	144/ 78	101	36	25.0	0.58	0.68	6.7	0.85	7.41	24	98	96	10	42	39	−3	38	32	0.36
2.5	60		110	25	29.7	0.89	1.08	9.8	0.82			91			44			31	26	
Recovery		150/ 78	97	25	26.2	0.67	0.65	6.7	1.03	7.41	23	110	102	12	37	37	0	36	37	0.32
Recovery			88	38	16.0	0.32	0.33	3.8	0.97			105			40			40	39	
Recovery			84	30	14.5	0.27	0.28	3.3	0.96			110			37			44	43	
Recovery			88	16	11.0	0.25	0.27	3.1	0.93			113			35			39	36	
Recovery		132/ 84								7.41	23		94			38				

FIGURE 14-A

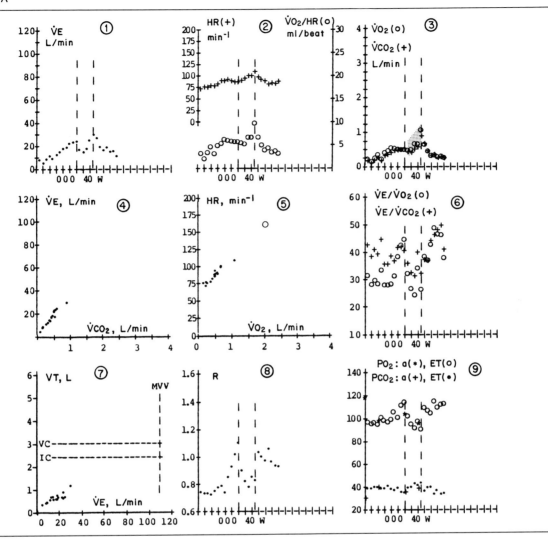

Interpretation

COMMENTS

Resting respiratory function (Table 14–1) is within normal limits.

ANALYSIS

Flow Chart 1: The maximum $\dot{V}O_2$ is significantly reduced and the anaerobic threshold is indeterminate (Table 14-2). See *Flow Chart 5:* While the resting V_D/V_T is normal, it does not decrease appropriately during exercise. However, only light exercise was performed, and the lack of a decrease might be spurious owing to the low tidal volume, tachypnea, and work rate performed (Table 3). Because $P(a–ET)_{CO_2}$ and $P(A–a)_{O_2}$ are normal *(branchpoint 5.1)*, we conclude that the indices of ventilation relative to perfu-

sion are normal. Heart rate reserve *(branchpoint 5.2)* is high and the breathing reserve *(branchpoint 5.5)* is also high (Table 14-3). The $\Delta\dot{V}O_2/\Delta WR$ *(branchpoint 5.8)* cannot be measured because of the brevity of exercise. There is no exercise hypertension. These findings place the patient in the diagnostic category of poor effort. The following findings are consistent with this diagnosis: 1) the normal exercise electrocardiogram, 2) R of only 0.82 at the maximum $\dot{V}O_2$, 3) minimal decline in HCO_3^- induced by the exercise (Table 14-3), and the previously mentioned high heart rate reserve, high breathing reserve, normal blood gases, and normal indices of ventilation/perfusion mismatching.

CONCLUSION

Poor effort.

CASE 15 *Mitral insufficiency*

CLINICAL FINDINGS

This 43-year-old electronics assembler had rheumatic fever at age 10. In the last 6 months she developed increasing dyspnea and orthopnea, with intermittent atrial fibrillation and pleural effusion, requiring repeated hospitalizations. There was no evidence of mitral stenosis or coronary artery disease on catheterization, angiography, or echocardiography. At the time of exercise study she had a sinus rhythm, findings of mitral regurgitation with left atrial and left ventricular enlargement, but no pleural effusion or dependent edema. Her medications were digoxin, furosemide, and potassium chloride.

EXERCISE FINDINGS

The patient performed exercise on a cycle ergometer. She pedalled at 60 rpm without added load for 3 minutes. The work rate was then increased 5 watts per minute to her symptom limited maximum. She stopped cycling because of general fatigue. There were no ST segment changes or arrhythmia.

TABLE 15-1. *Selected Respiratory Function Data*

MEASUREMENT	PREDICTED	MEASURED
Age, yr		43
Sex		Female
Height, cm		160
Weight, kg	61	56
Hematocrit, %		40
VC, L	2.88	2.03
IC, L	1.92	1.49
TLC, L	4.33	3.32
FEV_1, L	2.36	1.81
FEV_1/VC, %	82	89
MVV, L/min	90	90
DL_{CO}, ml/mm Hg/min	21.7	23.5

TABLE 15-2. *Selected Exercise Data*

MEASUREMENT	PREDICTED	MEASURED
Maximum $\dot{V}O_2$, L/min	1.49	0.79
Maximum HR, beats/min	177	186
Maximum O_2 pulse, ml/beat	8.4	4.2
$\Delta\dot{V}O_2/\Delta WR$, ml/min/watt	10.3	5.6
$\dot{V}O_2$ difference, %	0.0	21.5
AT, L/min	>0.60	0.55
Maximum $\dot{V}E$, L/min		31
Exercise breathing reserve, L/min	>15	59

TABLE 15-3.

TIME min	WORK RATE W	BP mmHg	HR min⁻¹	f	$\dot{V}E$ BTPS L/min	$\dot{V}CO_2$ STPD L/min	$\dot{V}O_2$ STPD L/min	O_2 pulse ml/beat	R	pH	HCO₃⁻ mEq L	ET PO₂ mmHg	a PO₂	A-a	ET PCO₂ mmHg	a	a-ET	$\dot{V}E/\dot{V}CO_2$	$\dot{V}E/\dot{V}O_2$	VD/VT
Rest		102	26	11.0	0.21	0.26	2.5	0.81			108			35			52	42	
Rest		102	25	10.9	0.22	0.27	2.6	0.81			112			34			50	40	
Unloaded		138	24	13.8	0.33	0.45	3.3	0.73			106			35			42	31	
Unloaded		140	26	16.2	0.44	0.57	4.1	0.77			103			38			37	28	
Unloaded		140	24	15.5	0.43	0.53	3.8	0.81			104			38			36	29	
1.0	5	138	26	16.4	0.43	0.49	3.6	0.88			109			36			38	33	
2.0	10	143	27	16.9	0.41	0.46	3.2	0.89			110			35			41	37	
3.0	15	148	26	16.6	0.41	0.48	3.2	0.85			111			35			40	34	
4.0	20	158	27	17.8	0.46	0.54	3.4	0.85			110			35			39	33	
5.0	25	155	25	17.1	0.47	0.56	3.6	0.84			108			37			36	31	
6.0	30	175	28	21.0	0.58	0.64	3.7	0.91			110			37			36	33	
7.0	35	179	27	21.9	0.64	0.68	3.8	0.94			111			37			34	32	
8.0	40	181	30	23.7	0.66	0.70	3.9	0.94			111			37			36	34	
9.0	45	179	29	25.6	0.74	0.76	4.2	0.97			112			37			35	34	
10.0	50	186	33	30.5	0.84	0.79	4.2	1.06			116			36			36	39	
Recovery		152	35	27.2	0.69	0.60	3.9	1.15			120			33			39	45	
Recovery		138	32	21.1	0.50	0.48	3.5	1.04			114			36			42	44	

FIGURE 15-A.

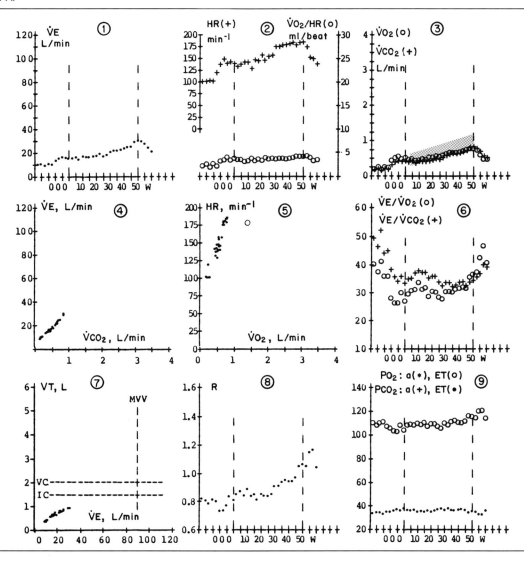

Interpretation

COMMENTS

Respiratory function at rest is compatible with a restrictive defect but the diffusing capacity (DL_{CO}) is normal (Table 15-1).

ANALYSIS

Flow Chart 1: The maximum $\dot{V}O_2$ and anaerobic threshold are low (Table 15-2). See *Flow Chart 4.* The breathing reserve is high *(branchpoint 4.1).* The ventilatory equivalent for CO_2 is slightly elevated at the anaerobic threshold. By referring to the insert in figure 3-13 and the PET_{CO_2} values in Table 15-3, the slightly elevated $\dot{V}E/\dot{V}CO_2$ appears to be due to a mild degree of hyperventilation of the pulmonary

blood flow, rather than an increase in VD/VT *(branchpoint 4.3).* This indicates that the abnormality is an O_2-flow problem of nonpulmonary origin. The hematocrit is normal *(branchpoint 4.4).* The striking finding is the low and flat O_2 pulse throughout exercise (Graph 2, Fig. 15-A) *(branchpoint 4.6)* leading to the diagnosis of heart disease. The steep heart rate-$\dot{V}O_2$ relationship (Graph 5, Fig. 15-A), low heart rate reserve and low $\Delta\dot{V}O_2/\Delta WR$ confirm the diagnosis of heart disease. The very low and unchanging O_2 pulse suggests that the patient's effective stroke volume is low and the arterial-mixed venous O_2 difference is maximized at a very low work rate.

CONCLUSION

Valvular heart disease, as suggested by the patient's history, causing marked exercise intolerance.

CASE 16 *Mitral stenosis: Pre- and post- beta-adrenergic blockade*

CLINICAL FINDINGS

This 57-year-old former receptionist had rheumatic fever at age 16. She had orthopnea during pregnancy at age 24. She was otherwise well except for gradually increasing dyspnea of 6 years duration and exertional dull substernal aching radiating to the jaw and left arm of 3 months duration. Examination revealed a grade II pre-systolic murmur, and an opening snap. The mitral valve area was mildly decreased and the left atrium was moderately dilated. Coronary arteriography was normal. The second exercise study was performed 17 months after the first while the patient was receiving propranolol 3 times daily. At that time she complained of increasing dyspnea, even at rest, associated with lightheadedness, sweating, numbness of the fingers, and perioral tingling.

EXERCISE FINDINGS

On both occasions the patient exercised on a cycle ergometer to her symptom limited maximum. She pedalled at 60 rpm without added load for 3 minutes. During the first test the work rate was increased 10 watts per minute, and during the second test (17 months later), it was increased 5 watts per minute. Blood was sampled every second minute and intra-arterial blood pressure was recorded from a percutaneously placed brachial artery catheter. Resting ECG's showed left atrial enlargement and sinus rhythm; there were no abnormal ST segment changes, nor arrhythmia during exercise. She stopped exercise in both studies complaining of leg fatigue, not dyspnea or chest pain.

TABLE 16-1. *Selected Respiratory Function Data*

MEASUREMENT	PREDICTED	BEFORE BLOCKADE	AFTER BLOCKADE
Age, yr		57	59
Sex		Female	
Height, cm		166	
Weight, kg	65	67	
Hematocrit, %		40	
VC, L	3.10	3.16	2.73
IC, L	2.07	2.26	2.19
TLC, L	5.15	5.01	4.62
FEV_1, L	2.48	2.58	2.26
FEV_1/VC, %	80	82	83
MVV, L/min	93	96	81
DL_{CO}, ml/mm Hg/min	21.9	20.3	18.7

TABLE 16-2. *Selected Exercise Data*

MEASUREMENT	PREDICTED	BEFORE BLOCKADE	AFTER BLOCKADE
Maximum $\dot{V}O_2$, L/min	1.40	0.74	0.91
Maximum HR, beats/min	162	120	108
Maximum O_2 pulse, ml/beat	8.6	6.2	8.4
$\Delta\dot{V}O_2/\Delta WR$, ml/min/watt	10.3		7.4
$\dot{V}O_2$ difference, %	0.0		9.1
AT, L/min	>0.56	indeterminate	indeterminate
Blood pressure, mm Hg (rest, max)		128/62,164/83	153/72,168/78
Maximum $\dot{V}E$, L/min		43	47
Exercise breathing reserve, L/min	>15	53	34
Pa_{O_2}, mm Hg (rest, max ex)		97,125	87,122
$P(A-a)_{O_2}$, mm Hg (rest, max ex)		10,2	11,5
$P(a-ET)_{CO_2}$, mm Hg (rest, max ex)		0,−1	3,0
VD/VT (rest, heavy ex)		0.26,0.25	0.28,0.19
HCO_3^-, mEq/L (rest, 2 min recov)		24,18	24,18

TABLE 16-3. *Pre-beta-adrenergic Blockade*

TIME min	WORK RATE W	BP mmHg	HR min⁻¹	f	VE BTPS	VCO2 STPD	VO2 STPD	O2 pulse	R	pH	HCO3⁻ mEq/L	PO2 ET	PO2 a	PO2 A-a	PCO2 ET	PCO2 a	PCO2 a-ET	VE/VCO2	VE/VO2	VD/VT
Rest		128/ 62								7.40	24	100			39					
Rest			65	18	8.2	0.16	0.24	3.7	0.67			105			32			42	28	
Rest			59	15	7.1	0.13	0.20	3.4	0.65			104			32			45	29	
Rest		140/ 77	65	17	9.6	0.21	0.30	4.6	0.70	7.43	21	107	97	10	32	32	0	39	27	0.26
Unloaded			82	12	13.0	0.32	0.39	4.8	0.82			113			31			37	31	
Unloaded			83	25	17.1	0.38	0.42	5.1	0.90			116			30			39	36	
Unloaded		146/ 80	82	33	14.5	0.29	0.33	4.0	0.88	7.47	20	116	118	1	29	28	-1	40	35	0.19
1.0	10		95	36	30.3	0.56	0.53	5.6	1.06			120			28			49	51	
2.0	20	152/ 80	108	45	31.9	0.52	0.50	4.6	1.04	7.50	21	125	123	1	25	27	2	54	56	0.36
3.0	30		114	43	42.2	0.77	0.68	6.0	1.13			125			26			50	57	
4.0	40	164/ 83	120	49	42.9	0.81	0.74	6.2	1.09	7.49	19	124	125	2	26	25	-1	48	52	0.25
Recovery			88	29	25.9	0.53	0.51	5.8	1.04			121			29			44	46	
Recovery		149/ 71	77	20	16.2	0.32	0.29	3.8	1.10	7.42	18	123	126	-2	29	28	-1	45	50	0.29

FIGURE 16-A. *Pre-beta-adrenergic Blockade*

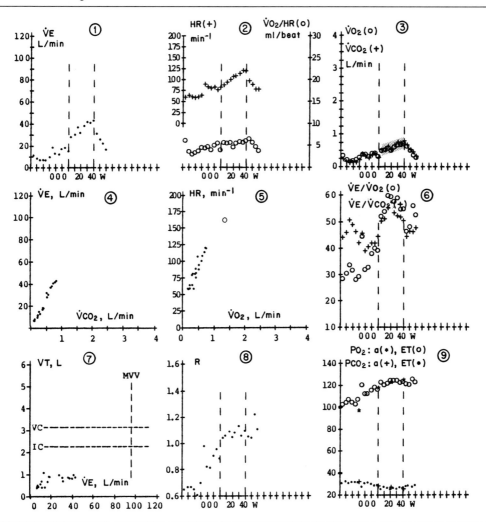

TABLE 16-4. *Post-beta-adrenergic Blockade*

TIME min	WORK RATE W	BP mmHg	HR min⁻¹	f	V̇E BTPS	V̇CO₂ STPD	V̇O₂ STPD	O₂ pulse	R	pH	HCO₃⁻ mEq/L	PO₂ ET	PO₂ a	PO₂ A-a	PCO₂ ET	PCO₂ a	PCO₂ a-ET	V̇E/V̇CO₂	V̇E/V̇O₂	VD/VT
Rest		153/ 72								7.48	22	109			30					
Rest			60	19	4.9	0.06	0.09	1.5	0.67			99			36			55	36	
Rest			62	12	6.7	0.18	0.31	5.0	0.58			91			38			31	18	
Rest		159/ 72	59	13	7.5	0.19	0.28	4.7	0.68	7.41	24	100	87	11	35	38	3	34	23	0.28
Unloaded			86	28	19.2	0.46	0.50	5.8	0.92			114			31			36	34	
Unloaded			88	22	27.1	0.67	0.68	7.7	0.99			116			30			38	37	
Unloaded		162/ 78	84	24	29.4	0.68	0.68	8.1	1.00	7.50	21	121	122	1	27	27	0	40	40	0.19
1.0	5		79	37	42.5	0.78	0.70	8.9	1.11			127			23			50	56	
2.0	10	168/ 78	90	35	40.1	0.76	0.74	8.3	1.03	7.52	20	125	120	6	24	25	1	49	50	0.27
3.0	15		95	33	39.1	0.76	0.76	8.0	1.00			123			25			48	48	
4.0	20	171/ 81	99	45	38.4	0.74	0.79	8.0	0.94	7.49	20	115	113	9	29	27	-2	47	44	0.28
5.0	25	168/ 78	100	37	39.8	0.80	0.83	8.3	0.96	7.51	19	120	123	2	27	24	-3	46	44	0.20
6.0	30	168/ 78	103	38	40.9	0.82	0.85	8.3	0.96	7.51	18	123	133	-7	24	23	-1	46	44	0.17
7.0	35	168/ 78	108	41	46.8	0.90	0.91	8.4	0.99	7.50	18	125	122	5	23	23	0	48	48	0.20
Recovery			84	34	32.5	0.66	0.71	8.5	0.93			121			25			45	42	
Recovery		156/ 72	79	28	26.0	0.53	0.53	6.7	1.00	7.49	18	124	128	-2	25	24	-1	45	45	0.18

FIGURE 16-B. *Post-beta-adrenergic Blockade*

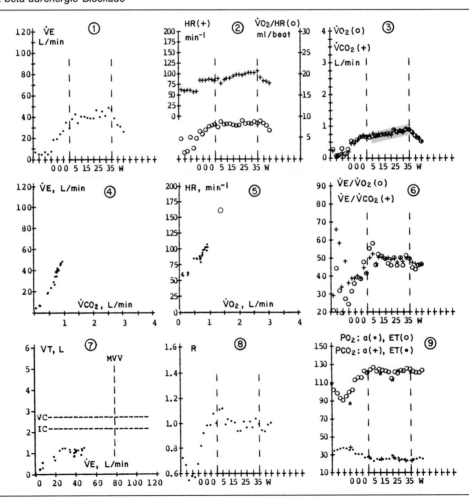

Interpretation

COMMENTS

Resting pulmonary function is normal on both occasions of study (Table 16-1). The electrocardiogram is normal except for evidence of left atrial enlargement. This case is presented because it illustrates the abnormalities of mitral stenosis and changes in O_2 pulse with propranolol. Also, it is presented because the development of respiratory alkalosis during exercise is unusual.

ANALYSIS

During exercise, the maximum $\dot{V}O_2$ is decreased and the anaerobic threshold is indeterminate (Table 16-2). See *Flow Chart 5*. The indices of distribution of ventilation relative to perfusion are normal at maximum exercise, making lung disease and pulmonary vascular disease unlikely diagnoses *(branchpoint 5.1)*. The heart rate reserve was high but since the patient was taking a β-adrenergic blocking drug this is an unreliable index for separating heart diseases from other disorders *(branchpoint 5.2)*. If considered to have a normal heart rate reserve and normal hematocrit (branchpoint 5.4), then heart disease is the likely primary disorder. Consistent with heart disease as the primary diagnosis is the low O_2 pulse that fails to rise as the work rate increases.

Commonly, an anticipatory respiratory alkalosis occurs at rest, but disappears with the start of exercise. The respiratory alkalosis in response to exercise as observed in this patient on both study occasions is unusual and probably abnormal.

In the post-propranolol study (Fig. 16-B), after an initial elevation, $\dot{V}E$ remains relatively unchanged (Graph 1, Fig. 16-B) while R remains high (Graph 8, Fig. 16-B) and Pa_{CO_2} falls further as work rate is increased (Graph 9, Fig. 16-B and Table 16-4). The further hyperventilation of the arterial blood (decrease in Pa_{CO_2}) without an increase in $\dot{V}E$ probably results from an inordinately small pulmonary blood flow increase in response to increasing work rate. This also accounts for the shallow $\dot{V}O_2$ response as work rate is increased (Graph 3, Fig. 16-B) and the low flat O_2-pulse response (Graph 2, Fig. 16-B).

CONCLUSION

Mitral stenosis with and without beta-adrenergic blockade. A very rare occurrence of exercise-induced respiratory alkalosis.

CASE 17 *Coronary artery disease*

CLINICAL FINDINGS

This 58-year-old man has been exposed to asbestos, sand blasting, and 35 pack years of cigarettes. On questioning, he admitted to a grinding chest pain, originating in the midback and radiating around the left chest into the substernal area. The pain was brought on when walking on cold days, was relieved in a few minutes by rest, and was not previously treated or diagnosed. He denied shortness of breath. A physical examination revealed no evidence of peripheral vascular disease, heart murmurs, or abnormal heart sounds. Resting 12-lead ECG was within normal limits.

EXERCISE FINDINGS

The patient performed exercise on a cycle ergometer. He pedalled at 60 rpm without added load for 3 minutes. The work rate was then increased 20 watts per minute to his symptom limited maximum. Blood was sampled every second minute and intra-arterial blood pressure was recorded from a percutaneously placed brachial artery catheter. The patient stopped exercise because of interscapular pain and right anterior chest pain. The ECG showed a 2 mm ST segment depression in leads 2, 3, AVF, and V3 through V6 during exercise but returned to normal after 9 minutes of recovery. The chest pain resolved within 1 minute after cessation of exercise.

TABLE 17-1. *Selected Respiratory Function Data*

MEASUREMENT	PREDICTED	MEASURED
Age, yr		58
Sex		Male
Height, cm		173
Weight, kg	76	82
Hematocrit, %		41
VC, L	4.09	4.04
IC, L	2.73	3.39
TLC, L	6.20	5.93
FEV_1, L	3.21	3.43
FEV_1/VC, %	79	85
MVV, L/min	135	155
DL_{CO}, ml/mm Hg/min	25.5	25.9

TABLE 17-2. *Selected Exercise Data*

MEASUREMENT	PREDICTED	MEASURED
Maximum $\dot{V}O_2$, L/min	2.22	1.47
Maximum HR, beats/min	162	146
Maximum O_2 pulse, ml/beat	13.7	10.3
$\Delta\dot{V}O_2/\Delta WR$, ml/min/watt	10.3	7.2
$\dot{V}O_2$ difference, %	0.0	19.4
AT, L/min	>0.89	0.8
Blood pressure, mm Hg (rest, max)		174/81,222/99
Maximum $\dot{V}E$, L/min		75
Exercise breathing reserve, L/min	>15	80
Pa_{O_2}, mm Hg (rest, max ex)		87,115
$P(A-a)_{O_2}$, mm Hg (rest, max ex)		18,10
$P(a-ET)_{CO_2}$, mm Hg (rest, max ex)		-3,-6
V_D/V_T (rest, heavy ex)		0.21,0.12
HCO_3^-, mEq/L (rest, 2 min recov)		22,16

TABLE 17-3.

TIME min	WORK RATE W	BP mmHg	HR min⁻¹	f	$\dot{V}E$ BTPS L/min	$\dot{V}CO_2$ STPD L/min	$\dot{V}O_2$ STPD L/min	O_2 pulse ml/beat	R	pH	HCO_3^- mEq L	PO2 ET mmHg	PO2 a mmHg	PO2 A-a mmHg	PCO2 ET mmHg	PCO2 a mmHg	PCO2 a-ET mmHg	$\dot{V}E$ $\dot{V}CO_2$	$\dot{V}E$ $\dot{V}O_2$	VD VT
Rest										7.42	22	91			35					
Rest			74	11	9.5	0.25	0.29	3.9	0.86			109			35			34	29	
Rest			77	10	9.5	0.27	0.37	4.8	0.73	7.41	22	98	87	18	38	35	-3	32	23	0.21
Unloaded			95	11	15.7	0.48	0.64	6.7	0.75			96			40			31	23	
Unloaded			95	15	18.0	0.53	0.64	6.7	0.83			103			38			32	26	
Unloaded		174/ 81	89	13	16.6	0.52	0.63	7.1	0.83	7.41	22	99	90	18	39	36	-3	30	25	0.18
1.0	20		93	13	13.1	0.40	0.49	5.3	0.82			98			40			30	25	
2.0	40	192/ 84	104	15	19.4	0.66	0.83	8.0	0.80	7.40	22	95	86	19	42	37	-5	27	22	0.14
3.0	60		112	13	23.0	0.82	0.93	8.3	0.88			98			43			27	23	
4.0	80	204/ 90	123	20	33.4	1.09	1.14	9.3	0.96	7.39	23	104	97	14	41	38	-3	29	28	0.21
5.0	100		134	21	40.5	1.37	1.38	10.3	0.99			100			44			28	28	
6.0	120	222/ 99	143	25	59.6	1.70	1.41	9.9	1.21	7.42	19	117	115	10	35	29	-6	34	41	0.12
7.0	140		146	32	75.1	1.92	1.45	9.9	1.32			119			35			38	50	
Recovery			105	22	48.0	1.48	1.12	10.7	1.32			115			39			31	41	
Recovery		210/ 72	97	21	37.0	1.09	0.77	7.9	1.42	7.34	16	119	119	7	37	31	-6	32	46	0.13
Recovery			86	19	29.2	0.83	0.55	6.4	1.51			122			35			33	50	

FIGURE 17-A.

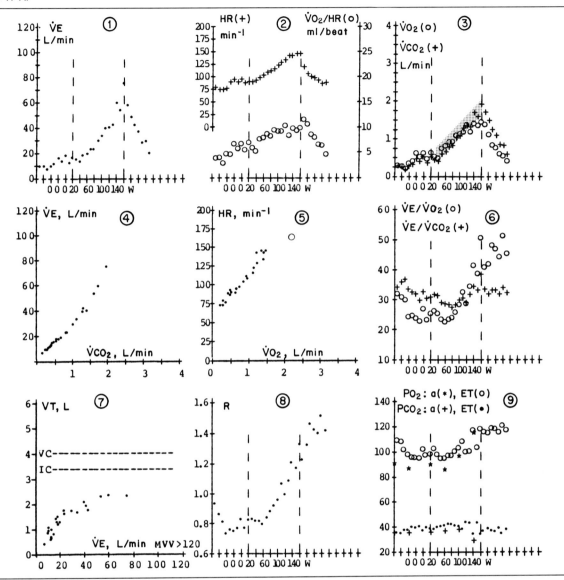

Interpretation

COMMENTS

Resting respiratory function is normal (Table 17-1).

ANALYSIS

Flow Chart 1: The patient has a reduced maximum $\dot{V}O_2$ and anaerobic threshold (Table 17-2). See *Flow Chart 4.* The breathing reserve is high *(branchpoint 4.1).* $\dot{V}E/\dot{V}CO_2$ at the anaerobic threshold is normal *(branchpoint 4.3).* This suggests that the patient has an O_2 flow problem of a nonpulmonary origin, which is confirmed by both a normal $P(A-a)_{O_2}$ and $P(a-ET)_{CO_2}$ at all levels of exercise (Table 17-3). The hematocrit is normal *(branchpoint 4.4)* and the O_2 pulse (Graph 2, Fig. 17-A) reaches a low-value plateau at

sub-maximal exercise *(branchpoint 4.6).* This leads to the diagnosis of heart disease. The patient has chest pain, ST segment changes in the electrocardiogram, and the failure for $\dot{V}O_2$ to rise during the last two minutes of exercise (Graph 3, Fig. 17-A), findings consistent with the diagnosis of ischemic heart disease. It should be noted that these changes occurred at a heart rate above 140 beats per minute. Thus, if the exercise test was not continued past this heart rate, the symptom of chest pain and electrocardiographic evidence of ischemia may not have been noted.

CONCLUSION

Myocardial ischemia secondary to coronary artery disease.

CASE 18 *Coronary artery disease*

CLINICAL FINDINGS

This 61-year-old retired shipyard worker complained of breathing difficulties that he could not quantify or describe well. He denied shortness of breath but stated that he stopped using stairs because of a "peculiar feeling in his chest." He also complained of a stabbing substernal and right flank pain not associated with exertion or stress and neck pain, associated with movement of the head attributed to degenerative cervical spine arthritis. He never smoked cigarettes. Examination revealed psoriasis and normal blood pressure, heart sounds, and peripheral pulses. He had bilateral pleural plaques on chest x-ray. He also had ECG findings suggestive of left ventricular hypertrophy.

EXERCISE FINDINGS

The patient performed exercise on a cycle ergometer. He pedalled at 60 rpm without added load for 3 minutes. The work rate was then increased 20 watts per minute to his symptom limited maximum. Blood was sampled every second minute and intra-arterial blood pressure was recorded from a percutaneously placed brachial artery catheter. The patient stopped exercise because of shortness of breath and tired thighs. He denied chest pain. The ECG developed slight ST segment depression in leads 2, 3, AVF, V5, and V6 at 120 watts of exercise that gradually became more prominent with a maximum ST depression of 5 mm at the cessation of exercise (180 watts). A rare, unifocal, premature ventricular contraction was noted. The ECG returned to baseline after 14 minutes of recovery.

TABLE 18-1. *Selected Respiratory Function Data*

MEASUREMENT	PREDICTED	MEASURED
Age, yr		61
Sex		Male
Height, cm		176
Weight, kg	78	70
Hematocrit, %		39
VC, L	4.23	3.95
IC, L	2.82	2.60
TLC, L	6.47	6.01
FEV$_1$, L	3.32	3.25
FEV$_1$/VC, %	78	82
MVV, L/min	137	121
DL$_{CO}$, ml/mm Hg/min	25.5	33.3

TABLE 18-2. *Selected Exercise Data*

MEASUREMENT	PREDICTED	MEASURED
Maximum $\dot{V}O_2$ L/min	1.99	1.90
Maximum HR, beats/min	159	180
Maximum O$_2$ pulse, ml/beat	12.5	10.6
$\Delta\dot{V}O_2/\Delta$WR, ml/min/watt	10.3	8.8
$\dot{V}O_2$ difference, %	0.0	10.5
AT, L/min	>0.80	0.75
Blood pressure, mm Hg (rest, max)		144/75,246/108
Maximum $\dot{V}E$, L/min		86
Exercise breathing reserve, L/min	>15	35
Pa$_{O_2}$, mm Hg (rest, max ex)		87,103
P(A–a)$_{O_2}$, mm Hg (rest, max ex)		5,15
P(a–ET)$_{CO_2}$, mm Hg (rest, max ex)		2,–1
VD/VT (rest, heavy ex)		0.48,0.26
HCO$_3^-$, mEq/L (rest, 2 min recov)		26,20

TABLE 18-3.

TIME min	WORK RATE W	BP mmHg	HR min⁻¹	f	$\dot{V}E$ BTPS L/min	$\dot{V}CO_2$ STPD L/min	$\dot{V}O_2$ STPD L/min	O$_2$ pulse ml/beat	R	pH	HCO$_3^-$ mEq L	PO$_2$ ET mmHg	PO$_2$ a mmHg	PO$_2$ A-a mmHg	PCO$_2$ ET mmHg	PCO$_2$ a mmHg	PCO$_2$ a-ET mmHg	$\dot{V}E$/$\dot{V}CO_2$	$\dot{V}E$/$\dot{V}O_2$	VD/VT
Rest	144/ 75									7.48	26	106			36					
Rest			67	16	9.1	0.19	0.27	4.0	0.70			101			37			41	29	
Rest	150/ 75		70	14	7.6	0.13	0.20	2.9	0.65	7.44	28	97	87	5	39	41	2	49	32	0.48
Rest			70	15	13.2	0.28	0.40	5.7	0.70			91			42			43	30	
Unloaded			88	17	13.2	0.34	0.52	5.9	0.65			90			42			35	23	
Unloaded			86	17	14.2	0.39	0.59	6.9	0.66			89			43			33	22	
Unloaded	171/ 78		88	17	15.0	0.43	0.63	7.2	0.68	7.41	29	90	83	4	45	46	1	31	21	0.36
1.0	20		93	19	17.9	0.52	0.68	7.3	0.76			95			44			31	24	
2.0	40	192/ 78	102	17	24.3	0.85	1.03	10.1	0.83	7.40	29	94	83	11	45	48	3	27	22	0.31
3.0	60		105	22	26.9	0.92	1.05	10.0	0.88			97			46			27	24	
4.0	80	216/ 87	127	25	36.1	1.26	1.29	10.2	0.98	7.40	28	101	94	9	47	46	–1	27	26	0.29
5.0	100		136	28	37.4	1.35	1.30	9.6	1.04			102			48			26	27	
6.0	120	231/ 96	150	33	50.8	1.77	1.50	10.0	1.18	7.39	26	108	98	12	46	45	–1	27	32	0.28
7.0	140		168	34	63.3	2.13	1.74	10.4	1.22			111			44			28	35	
8.0	160	234/ 99	178	34	76.0	2.53	1.90	10.7	1.33	7.38	23	117	103	15	41	40	–1	29	38	0.24
8.5	180	246/108	180	47	85.5	2.62	1.85	10.3	1.42			118			41			31	44	
Recovery			171	35	71.3	2.46	1.90	11.1	1.29			114			43			28	36	
Recovery			143	30	47.5	1.53	1.03	7.2	1.49			116			43			29	44	
Recovery		192/ 78								7.30	20		107			41				

FIGURE 18-A.

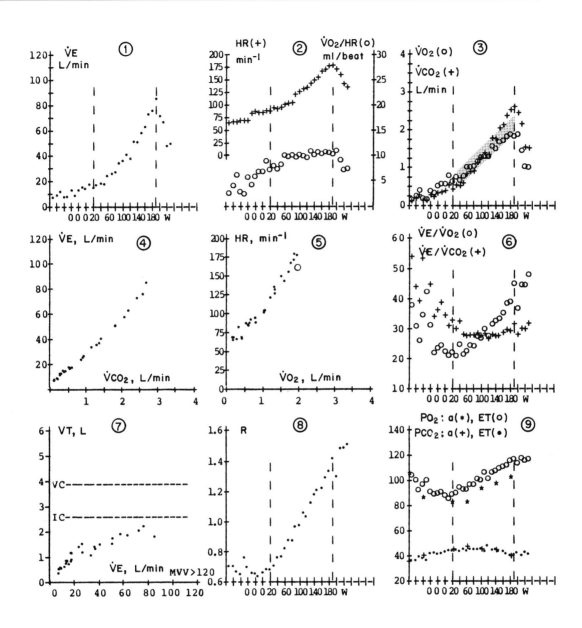

Interpretation

COMMENTS

Resting respiratory function (Table 18-1) and electrocardiogram are normal.

ANALYSIS

Flow Chart 1: The patient has a normal maximum $\dot{V}O_2$ but a low anaerobic threshold (Table 18-2). See *Flow Chart 2:* The ECG is abnormal and the O_2 pulse at maximum exercise is reduced and reaches a plateau value at about 80 watts (Graph 2, Fig. 18-A)

(branchpoint 2.1). The indices of ventilation/perfusion matching are normal (branchpoint 2.3). The low anaerobic threshold, the low O_2-pulse, the steep heart rate-$\dot{V}O_2$ relationship and the low $\Delta\dot{V}O_2/\Delta WR$ (Table 18-2) indicate that the ST segment changes are functionally significant, i.e., consistent with coronary artery disease.

CONCLUSION

Myocardial ischemia secondary to coronary artery disease, despite the absence of chest pain or reduced maximum oxygen uptake.

CASE 19 *Cardiomyopathy*

CLINICAL FINDINGS

This 41-year-old former brickworker, woodworker, sandblaster, and security guard has been placed on disability for a back injury 9 years ago. Hypertension was diagnosed 6 years ago. He started complaining of dyspnea and a productive cough 3 years ago. He was diagnosed as having "probable pulmonary asbestosis" and "asthmatic bronchitis" 2 years ago. He denied smoking but had repeated hospitalizations for alcoholism. He was being treated with propranolol, hydrochlorothiazide, oxtriphylline, and potassium supplementation. Auscultation of the heart and lungs was entirely normal, as were posteroanterior, lateral, and oblique chest roentgenograms.

EXERCISE FINDINGS

The patient performed exercise on a cycle ergometer. He pedalled at 60 rpm without added load for 3 minutes. The work rate was then increased 20 watts per minute to his symptom limited maximum. Blood was sampled every second minute and intra-arterial blood pressure was recorded from a percutaneously placed brachial artery catheter. Resting ECG was normal. He stopped exercise with complaints of shortness of breath, a feeling that he was "going to faint," and leg "tiredness." One interpolated ventricular contraction occurred during exercise, but exercise and recovery ECG were otherwise normal.

TABLE 19-1. *Selected Respiratory Function Data*

MEASUREMENT	PREDICTED	MEASURED
Age, yr		41
Sex		Male
Height, cm		170
Weight, kg	74	78
Hematocrit, %		44
VC, L	3.95	4.00
IC, L	2.63	3.30
TLC, L	5.58	5.28
FEV_1, L	3.16	3.43
FEV_1/VC, %	80	86
MVV, L/min	137	118
DL_{CO}, ml/mm Hg/min	25.8	24.7

TABLE 19-2. *Selected Exercise Data*

MEASUREMENT	PREDICTED	MEASURED
Maximum $\dot{V}O_2$, L/min	2.58	1.75
Maximum HR, beats/min	179	150
Maximum O_2 pulse, ml/beat	14.4	11.7
$\Delta\dot{V}O_2/\Delta WR$, ml/min/watt	10.3	8.3
$\dot{V}O_2$ difference, %	0.0	14.3
AT, L/min	>1.03	0.8
Blood pressure, mm Hg (rest, max)		132/87,204/108
Maximum $\dot{V}E$, L/min		78
Exercise breathing reserve, L/min	>15	40
PaO_2, mm Hg (rest, max ex)		87,117
$P(A-a)O_2$, mm Hg (rest, max ex)		4,3
$P(a-ET)CO_2$, mm Hg (rest, max ex)		2,−2
VD/VT (rest, heavy ex)		0.36,0.23
HCO_3^-, mEq/L (rest, 2 min recov)		27,17

TABLE 19-3.

TIME min	WORK RATE W	BP mmHg	HR min⁻¹	f	$\dot{V}E$ BTPS L/min	$\dot{V}CO_2$ STPD L/min	$\dot{V}O_2$ STPD L/min	O_2 pulse ml/beat	R	pH	HCO_3 mEq/L	PO₂ ET mmHg	PO₂ a mmHg	PO₂ A-a mmHg	PCO₂ ET mmHg	PCO₂ a mmHg	PCO₂ a-ET mmHg	$\dot{V}E/\dot{V}CO_2$	$\dot{V}E/\dot{V}O_2$	VD/VT
Rest		132/ 87								7.39	27	88			45					
Rest			74	21	8.3	0.19	0.25	3.4	0.76			99			42			35	26	
Rest		126/ 84	71	17	6.4	0.14	0.19	2.7	0.74	7.39	27	96	87	4	44	46	2	35	26	0.36
Rest			73	20	7.4	0.17	0.22	3.0	0.77			99			43			33	26	
Unloaded			86	34	12.5	0.35	0.45	5.2	0.78			95			44			28	21	
Unloaded			84	19	12.9	0.41	0.55	6.5	0.75			93			46			27	20	
Unloaded		138/ 84	85	21	13.8	0.45	0.54	6.4	0.83	7.37	27	99	88	8	45	47	2	27	22	0.27
1.0	20		86	22	15.7	0.54	0.62	7.2	0.87			100			46			26	22	
2.0	40	147/ 90	97	25	20.3	0.72	0.79	8.1	0.91	7.38	28	101	94	4	46	48	2	25	23	0.26
3.0	60		105	25	23.6	0.90	0.89	8.5	1.01			103			47			24	24	
4.0	80	159/ 90	115	27	31.2	1.20	1.05	9.1	1.14	7.36	26	107	103	5	48	47	−1	24	27	0.22
5.0	100		121	25	38.3	1.45	1.18	9.8	1.23			109			48			25	31	
6.0	120	192/105	129	31	46.2	1.71	1.30	10.1	1.32	7.35	24	112	111	3	46	44	−2	25	33	0.22
7.0	140		144	32	57.0	2.06	1.50	10.4	1.37			115			44			26	36	
8.0	160	204/108	150	40	77.6	2.48	1.75	11.7	1.42	7.34	20	118	117	3	41	39	−2	30	42	0.25
Recovery			129	34	45.8	1.43	1.02	7.9	1.40			115			43			30	42	
Recovery		150/ 78	124	36	30.1	0.87	0.66	5.3	1.32	7.28	17	116	116	3	41	38	−3	31	41	0.24

FIGURE 19-A.

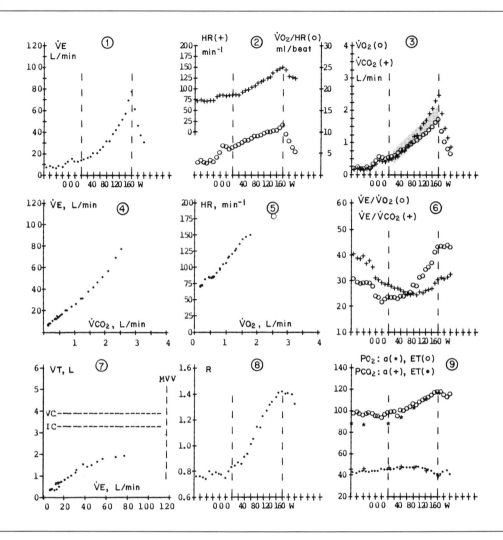

Interpretation

COMMENTS

Resting pulmonary function (Table 19-1) and electrocardiogram are normal.

ANALYSIS

Flow Chart 1: The maximum $\dot{V}O_2$ and anaerobic threshold are reduced (Table 19-2). See *Flow Chart 4:* The ventilatory equivalent at the anaerobic threshold *(branchpoint 4.3)* and the indices of ventilation/perfusion matching are normal. These findings indicate that this patient does not have primary lung or pulmonary vascular disease, but does have a nonlung disease O_2 flow problem. Since the hematocrit is normal *(branchpoint 4.4),* this is most likely due to cardiovascular disease. The exercise electrocardiogram is essentially normal throughout exercise. His

$\Delta\dot{V}O_2/\Delta WR$ is low and he has a low but rising O_2 pulse at maximum work rate (Graph 2 of Fig. 19-A). The patient's blood pressure response to exercise and heart rate reserve are normal (Table 19-2) and the patient did not have leg pain with exercise, making peripheral vascular disease unlikely. Since propranolol, itself, one of this patient's medications, ordinarily gives a high O_2 pulse during exercise, the finding of a low O_2 pulse at maximum exercise supports the diagnosis of primary heart disease. (Pulmonary vascular disease already ruled out.)

CONCLUSION

Cardiovascularly limited, 41-year-old chronically alcoholic man. Pulmonary vascular, peripheral vascular, and coronary artery disease were shown to be unlikely causes of the limitation. Two dimensional echocardiography with exercise supported the diagnosis of cardiomyopathy.

CASE 20 *Cardiomyopathy, hypertrophic type*

CLINICAL FINDINGS

This 65-year-old real estate broker was referred for evaluation of exertional dyspnea of one year duration. She noted dyspnea without chest pain when walking one half block on the level or climbing less than one flight of stairs. She denied asthma but had smoked cigarettes until 6 years previously. She was treated 2 decades ago for hyperthyroidism. Workup elsewhere revealed mild airway obstruction, hypertension, and normal thyroid status. Cardiac catheterization showed 40% stenosis of one coronary artery; echocardiogram was interpreted as normal; and a wall motion study showed a left ventricular ejection fraction of 72%, decreasing slightly during exercise. Medications were clonidine, triamterene, and hydrochlorothiazide. Examination was normal except for systemic hypertension, mild obesity, and a variable systolic murmur at the third left interspace near the sternum. Resting ECG showed left ventricular hypertrophy.

EXERCISE FINDINGS

The patient performed cycle ergometer exercise on two occasions. During the first study, the murmur was loud, her O_2 pulse declined as exercise progressed, and she was more hypertensive and became symptomatic with minimal exercise. Two weeks later she returned for the second study shortly after taking clonidine. She had less hypertension and a barely audible systolic murmur. She pedalled at 60 rpm without added load for 3 minutes. The work rate was then increased 10 watts per minute to her symptom limited maximum. Blood was sampled every second minute and intra-arterial blood pressure recorded from a percutaneously placed brachial artery catheter. The patient stopped exercise because of overall fatigue and shortness of breath. Less than 1 mm of downsloping ST segment depression developed in leads 1, AVL, and V6, while an increasing number of atrial and ventricular premature contractions developed near the end of exercise. A recording of brachial artery pressure is shown.

TABLE 20-1. *Selected Respiratory Function Data*

MEASUREMENT	PREDICTED	MEASURED
Age, yr		65
Sex		Female
Height, cm		164
Weight, kg	64	69
Hematocrit, %		40
VC, L	2.86	2.78
IC, L	1.91	2.30
TLC, L	4.93	5.45
FEV$_1$, L	2.26	1.88
FEV$_1$/VC, %	79	67
MVV, L/min	85	67
DL$_{CO}$, ml/mm Hg/min	21.0	19.3

TABLE 20-2. *Selected Exercise Data*

MEASUREMENT	PREDICTED	FIRST STUDY	SECOND STUDY
Maximum V̇O$_2$, L/min	1.25	0.88	1.15
Maximum HR, beats/min	155	142	148
Maximum O$_2$ pulse, ml/beat	8.1	5.8	7.8
ΔV̇O$_2$/ΔWR, ml/min/watt	10.3		6.3
V̇O$_2$ difference, %	0.0		19.9
AT, L/min	>0.5	indeterminate	indeterminate
Blood pressure, mm Hg (rest, max)		168/80,243/102	159/69,240/79
Maximum V̇E, L/min		54	65
Exercise breathing reserve, L/min	>15	13	2
Pa$_{O_2}$, mm Hg (rest, max ex)			84,109
P(A−a)$_{O_2}$, mm Hg (rest, max ex)			20,16
P(a−ET)$_{CO_2}$, mm Hg (rest, max ex)			5,2
VD/VT (rest, heavy ex)			0.34,0.32
HCO$_3^-$, mEq/L (rest, 2 min recov)			26,22

TABLE 20-3. *Second Study*

TIME min	WORK RATE W	BP mmHg	HR min⁻¹	f	V̇E BTPS L/min	V̇CO₂ STPD L/min	V̇O₂ STPD L/min	O₂ pulse ml/beat	R	pH	HCO₃⁻ mEq/L	PO₂ ET mmHg	PO₂ a mmHg	PO₂ A-a mmHg	PCO₂ ET mmHg	PCO₂ a mmHg	PCO₂ a-ET mmHg	V̇E/V̇CO₂	V̇E/V̇O₂	VD/VT
Rest		159/ 69								7.46	26	79			37					
Rest			83	20	8.9	0.17	0.19	2.3	0.89			114			30			42	38	
Unloaded			92	33	17.6	0.35	0.43	4.7	0.81			111			30			42	34	
Unloaded		184/ 75	101	38	23.1	0.51	0.66	6.5	0.77	7.47	26	108	84	20	32	37	5	39	30	0.34
Unloaded			110	58	41.2	0.74	0.69	6.3	1.07			120			28			49	52	
1.0	10		110	66	36.3	0.66	0.70	6.4	0.94			120			27			46	44	
2.0	20	201/ 90	112	63	40.4	0.75	0.75	6.7	1.00	7.52	24	123	103	17	25	30	5	47	47	0.33
3.0	30		119	62	40.4	0.73	0.75	6.3	0.97			121			25			48	47	
4.0	40	193/ 73	122	64	42.0	0.83	0.88	7.2	0.94	7.51	25	120	101	17	27	31	4	44	42	0.32
5.0	50		128	60	47.1	0.97	1.00	7.8	0.97			119			28			43	42	
6.0	60	220/ 73	132	53	47.0	1.00	1.01	7.7	0.99	7.49	24	118	93	21	30	31	1	43	42	0.31
7.0	70		138	48	46.0	1.04	1.04	7.5	1.00			115			32			40	40	
8.0	80	240/ 79	148	51	65.5	1.36	1.15	7.8	1.18	7.49	22	124	109	16	27	29	2	45	53	0.32
Recovery			126	40	50.8	1.15	1.00	7.9	1.15			124			28			41	47	
Recovery		261/ 92	118	43	34.3	0.78	0.75	6.4	1.04	7.42	22	120	106	11	29	34	5	39	41	0.32

FIGURE 20-A. *Second Study*

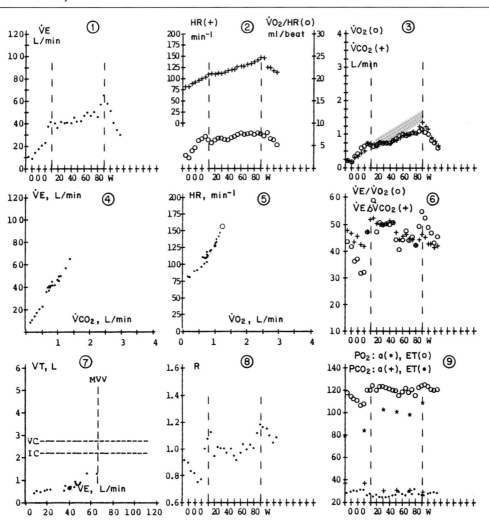

FIGURE 20-B.

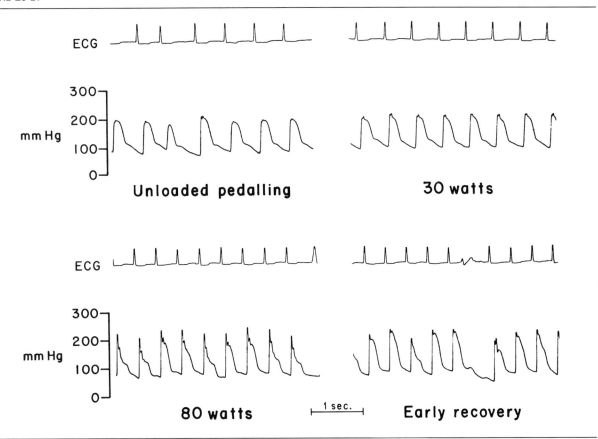

Four tracings of ECG (upper) and brachial artery blood pressure (lower) during and immediately after cycle ergometer exercise: (1) Unloaded pedalling, (2) 30 watts, (3) 80 watts, and (4) early recovery. Each tracing is 4 seconds in duration. Note premature contractions at unloaded pedalling and early recovery and their effect on the contour of the following pulse.

Interpretation

COMMENTS

The results of the resting respiratory function studies are compatible with mild airflow obstruction. A resting ECG is normal except for left ventricular hypertrophy. Her left ventricular ejection fraction at rest is 72%.

ANALYSIS

Flow Chart 1: The maximum oxygen uptake is reduced in the first study and is low normal in the second study; the anaerobic threshold is indeterminate (Table 20-2). See *Flow Chart 5:* Addressing the question of *branchpoint 5.1,* V_D/V_T and $P(a - ET)_{CO_2}$ are mildly abnormal, but $P(A-a)_{O_2}$ is normal throughout exercise (Table 20-2 and 20-3). Taking the abnormal branch of *branchpoint 5.1,* we address the question of the breathing reserve *(branchpoint 5.3).* In this

patient, it is slightly reduced due, in part, to her lung disease and, to a greater degree, to the hyperventilation that she develops during exercise. Because the abnormalities in ventilation/perfusion mismatching are borderline, the heart rate reserve is normal, and she does not develop a respiratory acidosis at maximal exercise, obstructive lung disease is probably not the primary limiting disorder.

The prominent abnormality is a low $\Delta\dot{V}_{O_2}/\Delta WR$, with a low O_2 pulse that fails to increase with increasing work rate (Fig. 20-A and Table 20-2). Therefore, it seems more likely that this patient has a cardiovascular defect. Thus, taking the left branch of *branchpoint 5.1* and addressing the question of *branchpoint 5.2,* the heart rate reserve is normal. The hematocrit is normal *(branchpoint 5.4).* At this point we should conclude that this patient has a heart disease limiting her exercise performance. To support this diagnosis are the observations that her $\dot{V}_{O_2}$ does not rise normally in response to increasing work rate

(Graph 3, Fig. 20-A), the O_2 pulse is flat (Graph 2, Fig. 20-A), and her heart rate becomes steeper with increasing $\dot{V}O_2$ (Graph 5, Fig. 20-A). On her more symptomatic test (not shown here), not only was her limitation greater, but her O_2 pulse actually decreased with increasing work rate.

The directly recorded arterial pressures are quite unusual and provide the clue to her cardiac diagnosis. The systolic arterial pressure wave becomes notched with increasing work rate and remains so during the early recovery period (Figure 20-B), characteristic of idiopathic hypertrophic subaortic stenosis. Premature ventricular contractions in recovery were followed by heart beats with a reduced, rather than increased, systolic and pulse pressure, demonstrating the increased ventricular outflow obstruction under conditions that cause the force of contraction to increase.

CONCLUSION

Cardiomyopathy of the idiopathic hypertrophic subaortic stenotic type limited exercise performance.

CASE 21 *Peripheral vascular disease*

CLINICAL FINDINGS

This 59-year-old former shipyard worker retired 5 years previously due to a back injury. He complained of dyspnea when walking 2 blocks. He smoked 46 pack years of cigarettes until stopping 24 years ago. He had a productive evening cough. He was treated with radioactive iodine for hyperthyroidism 24 years ago and is now on levo-thyroxine therapy. Chest roentgenograms showed mild bilateral pleural thickening with normal cardiovascular shadows.

EXERCISE FINDINGS

The patient performed exercise on a cycle ergometer. He pedalled at 60 rpm without added load for 3 minutes. The work rate was then increased 20 watts per minute to his symptom limited maximum. Blood was sampled every second minute and intra-arterial blood pressure was recorded from a percutaneously placed brachial artery catheter. Resting ECG was normal except for PR interval of 0.22 sec and notched P waves in V2 and V3. The patient stopped exercising because of bilateral thigh cramping. There were no abnormal ST changes or arrhythmias.

TABLE 21-1. *Selected Respiratory Function Data*

MEASUREMENT	PREDICTED	MEASURED
Age, yr		59
Sex		male
Height, cm		170
Weight, kg	74	76
Hematocrit, %		44
VC, L	3.50	3.64
IC, L	2.34	2.73
TLC, L	5.35	5.55
FEV_1, L	2.75	2.80
FEV_1/VC, %	79	77
MVV, L/min	118	110
DL_{CO}, ml/mm Hg/min	22.8	24.5

TABLE 21-2. *Selected Exercise Data*

MEASUREMENT	PREDICTED	MEASURED
Maximum $\dot{V}O_2$, L/min	2.12	1.46
Maximum HR, beats/min	161	117
Maximum O_2 pulse, ml/beat	13.2	12.5
$\Delta\dot{V}O_2/\Delta WR$, ml/min/watt	10.3	7.7
$\dot{V}O_2$ difference, %	0.0	16.7
AT, L/min	>0.85	0.7
Blood pressure, mm Hg (rest, max)		128/74,182/86
Maximum $\dot{V}E$, L/min		96
Exercise breathing reserve, L/min	>15	14
Pa_{O_2}, mm Hg (rest, max ex)		90,126
$P(A-a)_{O_2}$, mm Hg (rest, max ex)		−2,1
$P(a-ET)_{CO_2}$, mm Hg (rest, max ex)		0,−1
VD/VT (rest, heavy ex)		0.27,0.27
HCO_3^-, mEq/L (rest, 2 min recov)		21,14

TABLE 21-3.

TIME min	WORK RATE W	BP mmHg	HR min⁻¹	f	$\dot{V}E$ BTPS L/min	$\dot{V}CO_2$ STPD L/min	$\dot{V}O_2$ STPD L/min	O_2 pulse ml/beat	R	pH	HCO_3^- mEq/L	PO₂ ET mmHg	PO₂ a mmHg	PO₂ A-a mmHg	PCO₂ ET mmHg	PCO₂ a mmHg	PCO₂ a-ET mmHg	$\dot{V}E$/$\dot{V}CO_2$	$\dot{V}E$/$\dot{V}O_2$	VD/VT
Rest		128/74								7.37	21	103			38					
Rest			63	17	6.2	0.13	0.18	2.9	0.72			100			36			36	26	
Rest		128/74	60	12	5.8	0.14	0.25	4.2	0.56	7.36	21	89	90	−2	38	38	0	34	19	0.27
Rest			57	9	5.0	0.13	0.19	3.3	0.68			100			36			32	22	
Unloaded			72	14	8.9	0.27	0.35	4.9	0.77			99			39			29	22	
Unloaded			72	11	13.5	0.43	0.57	7.9	0.75			99			38			29	22	
Unloaded		143/77	76	13	19.7	0.61	0.75	9.9	0.81	7.35	22	94	95	8	41	40	−1	30	25	0.28
1.0	20		79	13	21.7	0.68	0.72	9.1	0.94			108			38			30	29	
2.0	40	146/77	86	14	22.6	0.75	0.86	10.0	0.87	7.36	21	104	109	0	40	37	−3	28	25	0.17
3.0	60		89	19	31.5	0.99	0.98	11.0	1.01			106			40			30	31	
4.0	80	164/80	97	26	45.9	1.30	1.08	11.1	1.20	7.35	20	114	115	3	37	37	0	34	40	0.29
5.0	100		103	29	56.5	1.54	1.21	11.7	1.27			117			36			35	45	
6.0	120	182/86	114	38	78.7	1.85	1.36	11.9	1.36	7.39	17	125	126	1	30	29	−1	41	56	0.26
6.5	140		117	43	95.7	2.04	1.46	12.5	1.40			127			27			45	63	
Recovery			108	47	76.9	1.62	1.22	11.3	1.33			127			27			45	60	
Recovery			94	43	59.4	1.15	0.68	7.2	1.69			131			26			48	82	
Recovery			96	42	48.9	0.84	0.50	5.2	1.68			133			23			54	91	
Recovery			86	43	43.4	0.66	0.38	4.4	1.74			135			21			60	105	
Recovery		113/59								7.36	14		137			25				

FIGURE 21-A.

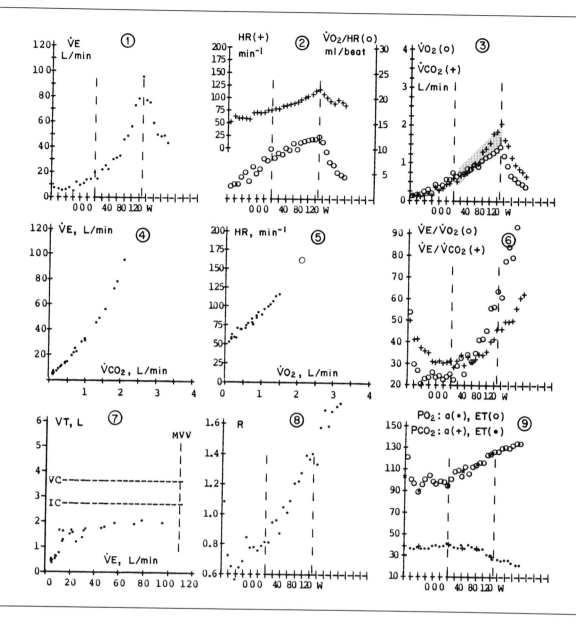

Interpretation

COMMENTS

Respiratory function at rest is normal (Table 21-1). The ECG is normal, except for a prolonged PR interval.

ANALYSIS

Flow Chart 1: Maximum $\dot{V}O_2$ and the anaerobic threshold are reduced (Table 21-2). See *Flow Chart 4.* The breathing reserve is borderline normal *(branchpoint 4.1).* Because the blood gas indices of ventilation/perfusion matching are normal, the diagnoses under the normal breathing reserve branch are

considered. The ventilatory equivalent for CO_2 at the anaerobic threshold is normal *(branchpoint 4.3)* suggesting a non-lung disease O_2 flow problem. The hematocrit is normal *(branchpoint 4.4).* The O_2 pulse is not low at the patient's maximum work rate (Table 21-2) *(branchpoint 4.6).* This observation suggests that the diagnosis is peripheral vascular disease. Findings of a high heart rate reserve, leg pain and a shallow slope for $\Delta\dot{V}O_2/\Delta WR$ and increased $\dot{V}O_2$ difference at maximal work rate (Table 21-2) support this diagnosis.

CONCLUSION

Exercise limited by peripheral vascular disease.

CASE 22 *Hypertensive cardiovascular disease and carboxyhemoglobinemia*

CLINICAL FINDINGS

This 46-year-old current shipyard worker was referred for evaluation of shortness of breath. He complained of chronic cough and sputum production of 8 to 10 years duration. He dated the shortness of breath to a hospitalization for a leg fracture 6 years ago. He previously abused alcohol, but his history of cigarette smoking was contradictory. Physical examination revealed a smooth liver edge 5 cm below the right costal margin without other evidence of liver disease. There were no physical signs of cardiovascular or pulmonary disease. Chest roentgenogram showed small bilateral pleural plaques. ECG showed a left anterior hemiblock.

EXERCISE FINDINGS

The patient performed exercise on a cycle ergometer. He pedalled at 60 rpm without added load for 3 minutes. The work rate was then increased 20 watts per minute to his symptom limited maximum. Blood was sampled every second minute and intra-arterial blood pressure was recorded from a percutaneously placed brachial artery catheter. He stopped exercise complaining of shortness of breath and exhaustion. Carboxyhemoglobin level was 7.5% at the start of exercise, suggesting that the patient had recently smoked. There was no chest pain or abnormal ECG changes.

TABLE 22-1. *Selected Respiratory Function Data*

MEASUREMENT	PREDICTED	MEASURED
Age, yr		46
Sex		Male
Height, cm		161
Weight, kg	67	70
Hematocrit, %		43
VC, L	3.32	3.23
IC, L	2.22	2.24
TLC, L	4.77	4.77
FEV_1, L	2.65	2.62
FEV_1/VC, %	80	81
MVV, L/min	122	104
DL_{CO}, ml/mm Hg/min	22.3	22.1

TABLE 22-2. *Selected Exercise Data*

MEASUREMENT	PREDICTED	MEASURED
Maximum $\dot{V}O_2$, L/min	2.24	1.17
Maximum HR, beats/min	174	144
Maximum O_2 pulse, ml/beat	12.9	8.1
$\Delta\dot{V}O_2/\Delta WR$, ml/min/watt	10.3	7.6
$\dot{V}O_2$ difference, %	0.0	14.7
AT, L/min	>0.90	0.8
Blood pressure, mm Hg (rest, max)		168/108,228/126
Maximum $\dot{V}E$, L/min		45
Exercise breathing reserve, L/min	>15	59
Pa_{O_2}, mm Hg (rest, max ex)		93,101
$P(A-a)_{O_2}$, mm Hg (rest, max ex)		12,21
$P(a-ET)_{CO_2}$, mm Hg (rest, max ex)		0,-2
VD/VT (rest, heavy ex)		0.25,0.18
HCO_3^-, mEq/L (rest, 2 min recov)		23,18

TABLE 22-3.

TIME min	WORK RATE W	BP mmHg	HR min⁻¹	f	V̇E BTPS	V̇CO₂ —STPD—	V̇O₂ L/min	O₂ pulse ml/beat	R	pH	HCO₃⁻ mEq/L	PO₂ ET	PO₂ a	PO₂ A-a	PCO₂ ET	PCO₂ a	PCO₂ a-ET	V̇E/V̇CO₂	V̇E/V̇O₂	VD/VT
Rest		168/108								7.44	23	95			34					
Rest			92	18	8.7	0.20	0.27	2.9	0.74			102			36			36	27	
Rest		168/108	95	16	9.1	0.22	0.30	3.2	0.73	7.41	22	104	93	12	35	35	0	35	26	0.25
Rest			99	16	11.1	0.28	0.36	3.6	0.78			108			34			35	27	
Unloaded			108	15	15.6	0.44	0.57	5.3	0.77			104			35			33	25	
Unloaded			109	22	18.8	0.50	0.57	5.2	0.88			112			33			34	30	
Unloaded		186/111	106	21	19.1	0.53	0.62	5.8	0.85	7.45	22	110	101	12	34	33	-1	33	28	0.18
1.0	20		113	20	20.8	0.58	0.67	5.9	0.87			110			33			33	29	
2.0	40		124	22	23.2	0.68	0.91	7.3	0.75			103			36			31	23	
3.0	60		130	29	27.8	0.81	0.90	6.9	0.90			106			38			31	28	
4.0	80	225/123	142	25	38.3	1.17	1.13	8.0	1.04	7.41	21	113	100	17	36	34	-2	31	32	0.17
4.5	100		144	28	42.4	1.25	1.17	8.1	1.07			113			36			32	34	
Recovery		228/126	149	31	45.3	1.35	1.07	7.2	1.26	7.40	21	117	101	21	36	34	-2	32	40	0.18
Recovery			123	24	38.1	1.00	0.76	6.2	1.32			121			33			36	47	
Recovery		183/111	118	26	32.7	0.70	0.45	3.8	1.56	7.41	18	131	120	9	26	29	3	43	68	0.29

FIGURE 22-A.

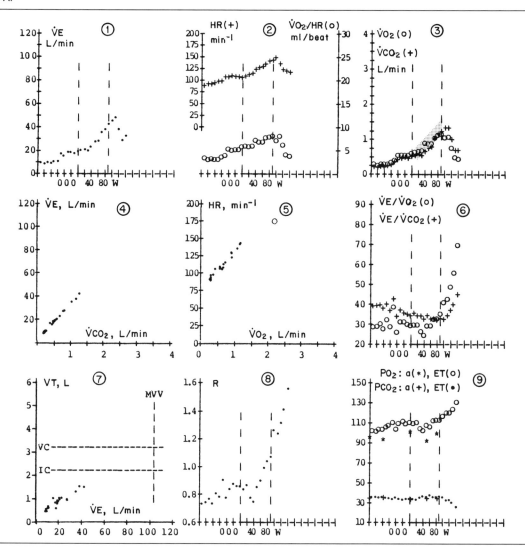

Interpretation

COMMENTS

Respiratory function at rest is normal (Table 22-1). Resting ECG is consistent with a left anterior hemiblock.

ANALYSIS

Flow Chart 1: The maximum $\dot{V}O_2$ and anaerobic threshold are reduced during exercise (Table 22-2). See *Flow Chart 4:* The breathing reserve is high (Table 22-2) *(branchpoint 4.1).* The ventilatory equivalent for CO_2 at the anaerobic threshold is normal (see Fig. 3-13) and the indices of distribution of ventilation relative to perfusion are normal *(branchpoint 4.3),* supporting the diagnosis of an O_2 flow problem of nonpulmonary origin. The hemato-

crit is normal *(branchpoint 4.4).* The O_2 pulse is low at the reduced maximum work rate. $\Delta\dot{V}O_2/\Delta WR$ is significantly decreased. The patient did not experience chest pain and his electrocardiogram remained normal throughout the exercise test. He has resting and exercise hypertension.

CONCLUSION

The patient evidently has exercise intolerance secondary to cardiovascular disease. This is possibly secondary to combined peripheral vascular dysfunction with systemic hypertension, and failure of the heart to respond adequately to the increased after-load. However, the reduced O_2 capacity of the blood and shift to the left of the oxyhemoglobin dissociation curve, caused by the elevated carboxyhemoglobin concentration, may also contribute to the patient's circulatory dysfunction.

CASE 23 *Circulatory disease: Heart and peripheral vascular, with anemia and carboxyhemoglobinemia*

CLINICAL FINDINGS

This 54-year-old male bartender was referred for pre-operative study to evaluate his exercise capacity. He occasionally had calf pain at rest and always after walking one block. He smoked at least 60 pack years but denied cardiac or respiratory symptoms. The right iliac and superficial femoral arteries were demonstrated to be obstructed on angiography. He was moderately anemic (Hematocrit = 34) with occult blood in the stool.

EXERCISE FINDINGS

The patient performed exercise on a cycle ergometer. He pedalled at 60 rpm without added load for 3 minutes. The work rate was then increased 15 watts per minute to his symptom limited maximum. Blood was sampled every second minute and intra-arterial blood pressure was recorded from a percutaneously placed brachial artery catheter. Resting and exercise ECG's were normal. He stopped exercise due to severe leg pain, which was more prominent on the left. Carboxyhemoglobin was 5.6% in his resting arterial blood.

TABLE 23-1. *Selected Respiratory Function Data*

MEASUREMENT	PREDICTED	MEASURED
Age, yr		59
Sex		Male
Height, cm		168
Weight, kg	72	60
Hematocrit, %		34
VC, L	3.94	3.84
IC, L	2.63	3.64
TLC, L	5.86	7.16
FEV_1, L	3.12	3.07
FEV_1/VC, %	79	80
MVV, L/min	136	110
DL_{CO}, ml/mm Hg/min	23.0	22.9

TABLE 23-2. *Selected Exercise Data*

MEASUREMENT	PREDICTED	MEASURED
Maximum $\dot{V}O_2$, L/min	1.84	0.82
Maximum HR, beats/min	161	141
Maximum O_2 pulse, ml/beat	11.4	5.8
$\Delta\dot{V}O_2/\Delta WR$, ml/min/watt	10.3	6.2
$\dot{V}O_2$ difference, %	0.0	19.7
AT, L/min	> 0.74	0.6
Blood pressure, mm Hg (rest, max)		168/72,255/114
Maximum $\dot{V}E$, L/min		60
Exercise breathing reserve, L/min	> 15	50
Pa_{O_2}, mm Hg (rest, max ex)		94,117
$P(A-a)_{O_2}$, mm Hg (rest, max ex)		20,11
$P(a-ET)_{CO_2}$, mm Hg (rest, max ex)		3,2
VD/VT (rest, heavy ex)		0.44,0.35
HCO_3^-, mEq/L (rest, 2 min recov)		20,16

TABLE 23-3.

TIME min	WORK RATE W	BP mmHg	HR min⁻¹	f	$\dot{V}E$ BTPS L/min	$\dot{V}CO_2$ STPD L/min	$\dot{V}O_2$ STPD L/min	O_2 pulse ml/beat	R	pH	HCO_3^- mEq/L	ET PO₂ mmHg	a PO₂	A-a PO₂	ET PCO₂ mmHg	a PCO₂	a-ET PCO₂	$\frac{\dot{V}E}{\dot{V}CO_2}$	$\frac{\dot{V}E}{\dot{V}O_2}$	VD/VT
Rest		168/ 72								7.43	20		90			31				
Rest			94	15	14.3	0.25	0.29	3.1	0.86			117			28			52	45	
Rest		168/ 72	95	14	11.6	0.19	0.23	2.4	0.83	7.42	20	116	94	20	28	31	3	55	45	0.44
Rest			92	16	11.1	0.19	0.23	2.5	0.83			115			29			51	42	
Unloaded			108	20	17.9	0.31	0.35	3.2	0.89			119			27			52	46	
Unloaded			110	20	20.5	0.38	0.43	3.9	0.88			117			28			50	44	
Unloaded		231/ 93	111	21	22.3	0.46	0.52	4.7	0.88	7.43	20	117	97	20	28	30	2	45	39	0.33
1.0	15		116	24	27.1	0.57	0.61	5.3	0.93			120			27			44	41	
2.0	30	245/102	121	24	32.3	0.68	0.69	5.7	0.99	7.43	19	121	106	15	27	29	2	45	44	0.31
3.0	45		128	31	40.1	0.78	0.72	5.6	1.08			124			26			48	52	
4.0	60	255/114	141	38	59.7	1.02	0.82	5.8	1.24	7.44	17	128	117	11	24	26	2	55	69	0.38
Recovery			113	25	38.6	0.74	0.61	5.4	1.21			127			25			49	60	
Recovery		258/102	107	26	31.7	0.59	0.46	4.3	1.28	7.39	16	127	117	11	26	27	1	50	64	0.34

Figure 23-A.

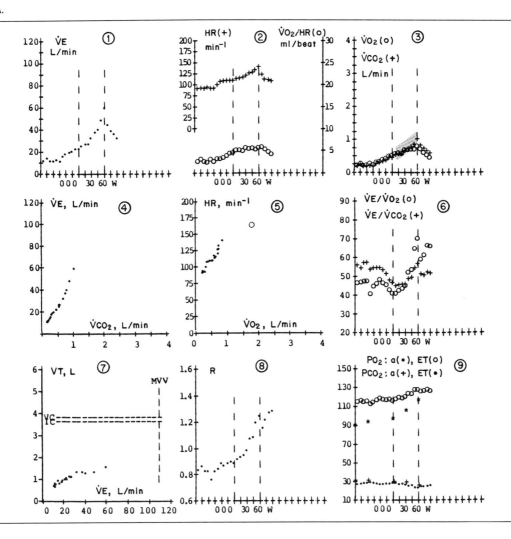

Interpretation

Comments

The resting respiratory function is normal, including the diffusing capacity (Table 23-1).

Analysis

Flow Chart 1: Maximum $\dot{V}O_2$ and anaerobic threshold are reduced during exercise testing (Table 23-2). See *Flow Chart 4* for further analysis. The breathing reserve is high *(branchpoint 4.1)*. This patient has a combination of abnormalities that fit the major diagnoses leading from both branches of *branchpoint 4.3*. Mildly elevated values of V_D/V_T and $P(a - ET)_{CO_2}$, and normal $P(A-a)_{O_2}$ and Pa_{O_2} at maximal exercise suggest mild ventilation-perfusion mismatching such as might be seen in the case of minimal disease involving pulmonary circulation (right branch of *branch-point 4.3*). However, the low $\Delta\dot{V}O_2/\Delta WR$, high $\dot{V}O_2$ difference and flat O_2-pulse suggest an O_2 flow problem of nonpulmonary origin (left branch of *branchpoint 4.3*). While these major abnormalities point to a dominant cardiovascular disturbance, the patient's anemia and carboxyhemoglobinemia *(branchpoint 4.4)* may contribute to the abnormality in peripheral oxygenation. The steep heart rate vs. $\dot{V}O_2$ relationship and low O_2 pulse noted with increasing work rate is consistent with either a cardiac abnormality, anemia, or a combination of both disorders.

Conclusion

While the patient has ischemic peripheral vascular disease as documented by angiography and reflected by his leg pain in response to exercise, the flat O_2 pulse pattern as work rate is increased and the steep heart rate response to exercise suggest that heart disease, the patient's anemia, and carboxyhemoglobinemia are also major factors contributing to exercise limitation.

CASE 24 *Emphysema, severe*

CLINICAL FINDINGS

This 65-year-old man had a long history of asbestos exposure and heavy cigarette smoking. He was being treated with aminophylline, inhaled bronchodilators, and home oxygen therapy. He was also receiving chlorothiazide for treatment of hypertension. He stopped smoking 12 years previously. Resting ECG suggested left atrial enlargement.

EXERCISE FINDINGS

The patient performed exercise on a cycle ergometer. He first pedalled at 60 rpm, without added load, for 3 minutes. The work rate was then increased 10 watts per minute to his symptom limited maximum. Blood was sampled every second minute and intra-arterial blood pressure was recorded from a brachial artery catheter. There were no abnormal ST segment changes at rest or during exercise. He stopped exercise complaining of shortness of breath.

TABLE 24-1. *Selected Respiratory Function Data*

MEASUREMENT	PREDICTED	MEASURED
Age, yr		65
Sex		Male
Height, cm		170
Weight, kg	74	99
Hematocrit, %		53
VC, L	3.72	2.17
IC, L	2.48	1.31
TLC, L	5.85	8.22
FEV_1, L	2.89	0.56
FEV_1/VC, %	78	26
MVV, L/min	123	31
DL_{CO}, ml/mm Hg/min	25.1	13.2

TABLE 24-2. *Selected Exercise Data*

MEASUREMENT	PREDICTED	MEASURED
Maximum $\dot{V}O_2$, L/min	1.96	0.90
Maximum HR, beats/min	155	129
Maximum O_2 pulse, ml/beat	12.6	7.0
$\Delta\dot{V}O_2/\Delta WR$, ml/min/watt	10.3	8.9
$\dot{V}O_2$ difference, %	0.0	6.0
AT, L/min	> 0.79	indeterminate
Blood pressure, mm Hg (rest, max)		175/94,256/138
Maximum $\dot{V}E$, L/min		28
Exercise breathing reserve, L/min	>15	3
Pa_{O_2}, mm Hg (rest, max ex)		56,46
$P(A-a)_{O_2}$, mm Hg (rest, max ex)		39,55
$P(a-ET)_{CO_2}$, mm Hg (rest, max ex)		−1,6
VD/VT (rest, heavy ex)		0.40,0.41
HCO_3^-, mEq/L (rest, 2 min recov)		28,27

TABLE 24-3.

TIME min	WORK RATE W	BP mmHg	HR min⁻¹	f	$\dot{V}E$ BTPS	$\dot{V}CO_2$ —STPD— L/min	$\dot{V}O_2$	O_2 pulse ml/beat	R	pH	HCO_3^- mEq L	PO_2 ET	a	A-a —mmHg—	PCO_2 ET	a	a-ET —mmHg—	$\dot{V}E$ $\dot{V}CO_2$	$\dot{V}E$ $\dot{V}O_2$	VD VT
Rest		175/ 94	102	15	11.1	0.28	0.36	3.5	0.78	7.41	28	87	56	39	46	45	−1	35	27	0.40
Unloaded			110	23	17.5	0.42	0.52	4.7	0.81			92			44			37	30	
1.0	10		112	24	19.4	0.51	0.62	5.5	0.82			97			41			34	28	
2.0	20	225/113	119	27	21.3	0.57	0.69	5.8	0.83	7.40	29	97	49	45	42	48	6	33	28	0.41
3.0	30		125	29	24.0	0.66	0.78	6.2	0.85			95			44			33	28	
4.0	40	250/131	129	31	25.8	0.72	0.83	6.4	0.87	7.37	28	92	47	49	47	48	1	32	28	0.40
4.5	50	256/138	129	33	26.2	0.73	0.85	6.6	0.86	7.37	28	93	46	48	44	50	6	32	27	0.41
Recovery			122	34	28.0	0.79	0.90	7.4	0.88			95			45			32	28	
Recovery			115	32	23.5	0.62	0.70	6.1	0.89			98			43			34	30	
Recovery			107	27	20.8	0.54	0.59	5.5	0.92			95			47			34	31	
Recovery		194/ 94								7.38	27		49			46				

FIGURE 24-A.

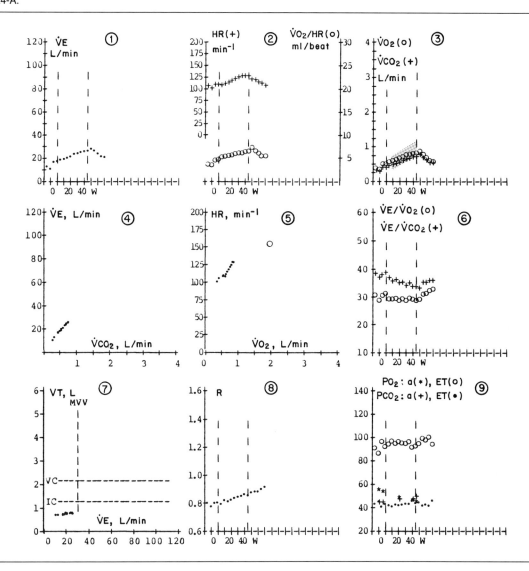

Interpretation

COMMENTS

This patient clearly has evidence of very severe obstructive lung disease (Table 24-1). His resting electrocardiogram suggests left atrial enlargement.

ANALYSIS

Flow Chart 1. The maximum oxygen uptake is significantly reduced but the anaerobic threshold is indeterminate, possibly because of the low maximum $\dot{V}O_2$ achieved (Table 24-2). See *Flow Chart 5.* The indices of ventilation-perfusion mismatching (V_D/V_T, $P(A-a)O_2$ and $P(a - ET)CO_2$) are abnormal *(branchpoint 5.1)*. The breathing reserve *(branchpoint 5.3)* is reduced. The respiratory rate (f) at maximum $\dot{V}O_2$ is 33 *(branchpoint 5.7)*. The diagnosis resulting from this analysis of exercise responses is obstructive lung disease (compatible with the results of this patient's resting respiratory function tests). Confirmatory observations consistent with this diagnosis are mild respiratory acidosis that develops as work rate is increased and a high heart rate reserve.

CONCLUSION

This patient, while having ECG evidence for left atrial enlargement, clearly is limited by his obstructive lung disease and not by cardiac dysfunction. The presence of a high heart rate reserve and absence of a ventilatory reserve, along with the development of mild respiratory acidosis at this patient's maximum $\dot{V}O_2$, support the conclusion that this patient is ventilatory limited.

Case 25 *Emphysema and bronchitis, severe: Effect of oxygen breathing*

Clinical Findings

This 62-year-old retired accountant had a long history of heavy cigarette smoking but stopped 4 years previously. He had a chronic cough and shortness of breath. He gradually increased his activity by physical training and rode his bicycle many miles daily. There was no history of congestive failure. He took oral aminophylline but no other medications. He participated in a study evaluating the effects of oxygen supplementation.

Exercise Findings

The patient performed exercise on a cycle ergometer. He pedalled at 60 rpm without added load for 3 minutes while breathing humidified compressed air. The work rate was then increased 10 watts per minute to his symptom limited maximum. Blood was sampled every second minute and intra-arterial blood pressure was recorded from a percutaneously placed brachial artery catheter. He stopped exercise complaining of shortness of breath. Following 30 minutes of rest he was given humidified 100% O_2 to breathe while the exercise study was repeated. He again stopped exercise complaining of shortness of breath. 12 lead ECG showed no ST segment changes or arrhythmia.

MEASUREMENT	PREDICTED	MEASURED
Age, yr		62
Sex		Male
Height, cm		173
Weight, kg	76	78
Hematocrit, %		51
VC, L	4.30	1.67
IC, L	2.87	1.22
TLC, L	6.87	8.30
FEV_1, L	3.40	0.54
FEV_1/VC, %	79	32
MVV, L/min	131	32
DL_{CO}, ml/mm Hg/min	30.9	18.5

TABLE 25-2. *Selected Exercise Data*

MEASUREMENT	PREDICTED	ROOM AIR	100% O_2
Maximum WR, watts		80	120
Maximum $\dot{V}O_2$, L/min	2.11	0.96	
Maximum HR, beats/min	158	140	165
Maximum O_2 pulse, ml/beat	13.4	6.9	
$\Delta\dot{V}O_2/\Delta WR$, ml/min/watt	10.3	8.3	
$\dot{V}O_2$ difference, %	0.0	12.3	
AT, L/min	> 0.84	indeterminate	
Blood pressure, mm Hg (rest, max)		169/106,250/125	144/94,234/119
Maximum $\dot{V}E$, L/min		32	40
Exercise breathing reserve, L/min	> 15	0	−8
Pa_{O_2}, mm Hg (rest, max ex)		78,53	587,583
$P(A-a)_{O_2}$, mm Hg (rest, max ex)		21,51	74,66
$P(a-ET)_{CO_2}$, mm Hg (rest, max ex)		6,5	8,3
VD/VT (rest, heavy ex)		0.42,0.37	0.49,0.40
HCO_3, mEq/L (rest, 2 min recov)		25,24	26,22

TABLE 25-3. *Air Breathing*

TIME min	WORK RATE W	BP mmHg	HR min⁻¹	f	V̇E BTPS L/min	V̇CO₂ STPD L/min	V̇O₂ STPD L/min	O₂ pulse ml/beat	R	pH	HCO₃⁻ mEq/L	PO₂ ET	PO₂ a	PO₂ A-a	PCO₂ ET	PCO₂ a	PCO₂ a-ET	V̇E/V̇CO₂	V̇E/V̇O₂	VD/VT
Rest			109	21	8.7	0.17	0.19	1.7	0.89			94			46			41	37	
Rest			117	20	9.8	0.22	0.24	2.1	0.92			102			42			37	34	
Rest		169/106	115	19	9.1	0.20	0.22	1.9	0.91	7.35	25	102	78	21	42	47	6	37	34	0.42
Unloaded			117	25	13.4	0.31	0.37	3.2	0.84			97			44			36	30	
Unloaded			121	23	14.2	0.35	0.40	3.3	0.88			96			45			35	31	
Unloaded		181/100	117	24	15.3	0.39	0.44	3.8	0.89	7.35	27	99	71	25	43	49	6	34	30	0.42
1.0	10		121	25	14.9	0.38	0.42	3.5	0.90			98			43			33	30	
2.0	20	187/106	124	25	16.3	0.42	0.48	3.9	0.88	7.35	27	97	68	27	43	49	6	34	29	0.41
3.0	30		128	22	18.6	0.56	0.64	5.0	0.88			94			46			30	26	
4.0	40	213/113	130	24	21.1	0.64	0.72	5.5	0.89	7.35	26	94	61	36	47	43	1	30	27	0.36
5.0	50		136	28	23.9	0.72	0.77	5.7	0.94			96			46			30	28	
6.0	60	225/119	135	28	25.6	0.81	0.86	6.4	0.94	7.35	26	96	57	42	48	49	1	29	27	0.35
7.0	70		138	32	29.0	0.91	0.94	6.3	0.97			95			48			29	28	
8.0	80	250/125	124	37	32.2	1.02	0.85	6.9	1.20	7.32	27	93	53	51	48	53	5	28	34	0.39
Recovery			102	26	25.2	0.83	0.79	7.7	1.05			97			50			28	29	
Recovery		213/106	117	22	17.8	0.52	0.47	4.0	1.11	7.30	24	103	89	15	47	50	3	31	34	0.39
Recovery			110	20	19.4	0.63	0.58	5.3	1.09			183			50			28	30	

FIGURE 25-A. *Air Breathing*

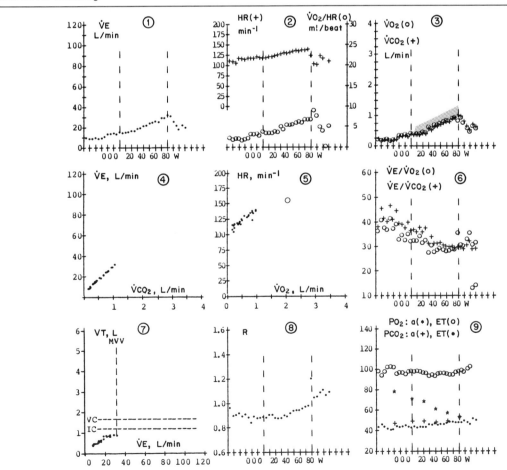

TABLE 25-4. *Oxygen Breathing*

TIME min	WORK RATE W	BP mmHg	HR min⁻¹	f	V̇E BTPS L/min	V̇CO₂ STPD L/min	V̇O₂ STPD L/min	O₂ pulse ml/beat	R	pH	HCO₃ mEq/L	PO₂ ET mmHg	PO₂ a mmHg	PO₂ A-a mmHg	PCO₂ ET mmHg	PCO₂ a mmHg	PCO₂ a-ET mmHg	V̇E/V̇CO₂	V̇E/V̇O₂	VD/VT
Rest			113	21	8.3	0.13									40			50		
Rest			111	26	10.6	0.17									39			49		
Rest		144/ 94	113	19	8.6	0.16				7.35	26		587	77	41	49	8	44		0.49
Unloaded			114	22	7.9	0.14									49			43		
Unloaded			108	20	9.6	0.22									49			36		
Unloaded		181/106	114	21	10.5	0.24				7.29	28		587	67	50	59	9	36		0.50
1.0	10		114	21	11.2	0.31									52			30		
2.0	20	194/106	112	22	14.8	0.45				7.30	27		584	72	52	57	5	29		0.42
3.0	30		119	23	18.1	0.57									53			28		
4.0	40	200/106	123	24	19.9	0.65				7.29	27		580	74	54	59	5	27		0.42
5.0	50		130	24	22.2	0.75									53			27		
6.0	60	206/100	132	26	23.6	0.78				7.29	27		595	60	55	58	3	27		0.41
7.0	70		138	29	25.8	0.91									57			26		
8.0	80	213/106	144	29	29.8	1.07				7.27	27		601	50	57	62	5	26		0.42
9.0	90		150	28	31.5	1.21									58			24		
10.0	100	231/106	155	29	34.2	1.33				7.24	27		606	43	60	64	4	24		0.40
11.0	110	234/119	159	39	35.4	1.40				7.23	26		583	66	62	64	2	23		0.37
12.0	120		165	37	40.1	1.64									66			23		
Recovery			141	26	32.1	1.38									62			22		
Recovery		214/100	138	28	27.6	0.97				7.21	22		587	69	54	57	3	26		0.38

FIGURE 25-B. *Oxygen Breathing*

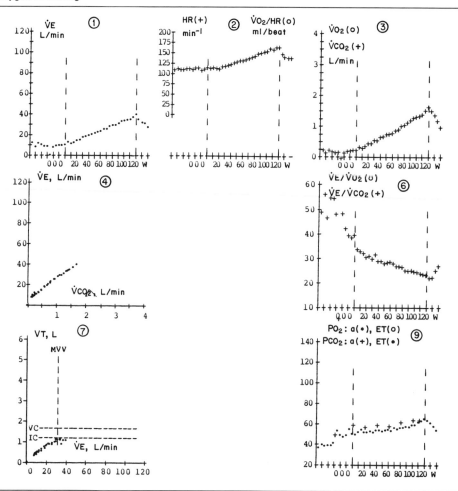

Interpretation

COMMENTS

Resting respiratory function studies indicate that this patient has severe obstructive lung disease (Table 25-1); he also had significant systemic hypertension at rest.

ANALYSIS

Flow Chart 1. Maximum $\dot{V}O_2$ is moderately severely reduced and the anaerobic threshold is indeterminate (Table 25-2). See *Flow Chart 5.* The indices of ventilation-perfusion mismatching (VD/VT, $P(a - ET)_{CO_2}$ and $P(A-a)_{O_2}$) are abnormal *(branchpoint 5.1).* The breathing reserve is zero *(branchpoint 5.3)* indicating that the patient's exercise limitation is a result of lung disease. The breathing frequency (f) is less than 50 at the maximum work rate *(branchpoint 5.7)* consistent with the diagnosis of lung disease of the obstructive type. Other abnormal findings are an obstructive expiratory flow pattern (not shown), arterial oxygen tension, and $P(A-a)_{O_2}$ that were normal at rest but becomes abnormal with exercise, a high heart rate reserve, and a respiratory acidosis at the maximum $\dot{V}O_2$.

As a result of breathing 100% O_2, the patient was able to increase his maximal work rate by 40 watts and the maximum heart rate by 25 beats per minute (i.e., from 140 during air breathing to 165 during 100% oxygen breathing). These results demonstrate that the increased heart rate reserve, during the air breathing test, results from his ventilatory limitation. It should also be noted that the maximum exercise ventilation increases during oxygen breathing at the maximum work rate from 32 L/min, the value of his resting MVV, to 40 L/min.

The increased work rate achieved during O_2 breathing is primarily the result of depression in the ventilatory response to exercise. Consequently, the patient develops a more significant respiratory acidosis as compared to the air breathing test (increase in Pa_{CO_2} of 6 mm Hg above rest during air breathing, as compared to 15 mm Hg for oxygen breathing). Pa_{O_2} remains above 580 mm Hg when breathing oxygen, indicating that no significant right-to-left shunt develops during exercise. Bicarbonate does not decrease in either study until two minutes after the exercise was terminated, because of the rising Pa_{CO_2} during exercise.

CONCLUSION

Exercise performance is limited by severe obstructive lung disease. Oxygen breathing results in an increased work capacity, despite a normal resting Pa_{O_2}.

CASE 26 *Chronic bronchitis, moderate*

CLINICAL FINDINGS

This 69-year-old former shipyard worker first noted dyspnea on exertion 16 years ago, later accompanied by cough, sputum production and frequent wheezing. He had been receiving bronchodilators and antibiotics intermittently for 16 years. Physical examination revealed obesity, bilaterally decreased breath sounds, and fine expiratory wheezes. There was no evidence of cardiovascular disease. Chest x-ray study revealed moderate pleural thickening bilaterally and scattered parenchymal calcifications compatible with inactive granulomatous disease. The heart was not enlarged. ECG was compatible with left atrial enlargement and left ventricular hypertrophy. He admitted to a 15 pack year history of cigarette smoking.

EXERCISE FINDINGS

The patient performed exercise on a cycle ergometer. He first pedalled at 60 rpm, without added load, for 3 minutes. The work rate was then increased 10 watts per minute to his symptom limited maximum. Blood was sampled every second minute and intra-arterial blood pressure was recorded from a percutaneously placed brachial artery catheter. The patient stopped exercising complaining of shortness of breath and chest tightness. There were no ST segment changes or arrhythmia.

TABLE 26-1. *Selected Respiratory Function Data*

MEASUREMENT	PREDICTED	MEASURED
Age, yr		69
Sex		Male
Height, cm		166
Weight, kg	70	98
Hematocrit, %		45
VC, L	3.31	2.91 (2.15*)
IC, L	2.21	2.35 (1.89*)
TLC, L	5.38	7.32
FEV$_1$, L	2.55	1.47 (1.30*)
FEV$_1$/VC, %	77	51 (60*)
MVV, L/min	112	56 (44*)
DL$_{CO}$, ml/mm Hg/min	22.6	26.0

*on day of exercise study

TABLE 26-2. *Selected Exercise Data*

MEASUREMENT	PREDICTED	MEASURED
Maximum $\dot{V}O_2$, L/min	1.77	1.50
Maximum HR, beats/min	151	125
Maximum O$_2$ pulse, ml/beat	11.7	12.0
$\Delta\dot{V}O_2/\Delta WR$, ml/min/watt	10.3	10.4
$\dot{V}O_2$ difference, %	0.0	−0.5
AT, L/min	>0.7	1.3
Blood pressure, mm Hg (rest, max)		142/72,234/99
Maximum $\dot{V}E$, L/min		55
Exercise breathing reserve, L/min	>15	1
Pa$_{O_2}$, mm Hg (rest, max ex)		73,87
P(A−a)$_{O_2}$, mm Hg (rest, max ex)		32,22
P(a − ET)$_{CO_2}$, mm Hg (rest, max ex)		6,0
VD/VT (rest, heavy ex)		0.40,0.35
HCO$_3^-$, mEq/L (rest, 2 min recov)		26,22

TABLE 26-3.

TIME min	WORK RATE W	BP mmHg	HR min⁻¹	f	$\dot{V}E$ BTPS	$\dot{V}CO_2$ STPD	$\dot{V}O_2$ STPD	O$_2$ pulse ml/beat	R	pH	HCO$_3^-$ mEq/L	PO$_2$ ET	PO$_2$ a	PO$_2$ A-a	PCO$_2$ ET	PCO$_2$ a	PCO$_2$ a-ET	$\dot{V}E$/$\dot{V}CO_2$	$\dot{V}E$/$\dot{V}O_2$	VD/VT
Rest		142/ 72								7.40	26	75			43					
Rest			76	18	10.7	0.27	0.36	4.7	0.75			100			39			34	26	
Rest		156/ 81	77	21	12.8	0.27	0.31	4.0	0.87	7.42	25	110	73	32	34	40	6	41	35	0.40
Rest			80	22	12.9	0.24	0.28	3.5	0.86			110			34			46	39	
Unloaded			98	50	28.0	0.53	0.66	6.7	0.80			108			34			45	36	
Unloaded			101	43	31.8	0.79	0.89	8.8	0.89			99			42			36	32	
Unloaded		198/ 83	105	47	34.6	0.76	0.85	8.1	0.89	7.40	26	106	82	22	39	42	3	40	36	0.43
1.0	10		103	53	37.6	0.85	0.93	9.0	0.91			107			38			39	36	
2.0	20	204/ 87	107	47	34.5	0.82	0.91	8.5	0.90	7.37	25	106	84	17	40	45	5	37	34	0.43
3.0	30		109	50	39.8	0.95	1.05	9.6	0.90			105			39			37	34	
4.0	40	204/ 87	110	46	42.2	1.11	1.28	11.6	0.87	7.38	24	106	80	23	38	42	4	34	30	0.37
5.0	50		114	44	38.7	1.02	1.16	10.2	0.88			103			41			34	30	
6.0	60	219/ 90	120	54	48.3	1.24	1.34	11.2	0.93	7.38	23	107	87	22	39	39	0	35	33	0.34
7.0	70	234/ 99	125	51	55.0	1.43	1.50	12.0	0.95			110			38			35	34	
Recovery			117	41	47.1	1.30	1.30	11.1	1.00			112			37			34	34	
Recovery			110	51	45.1	0.98	0.94	8.5	1.04			113			36			42	43	
Recovery		204/ 84								7.37	22		95			39				

FIGURE 26-A.

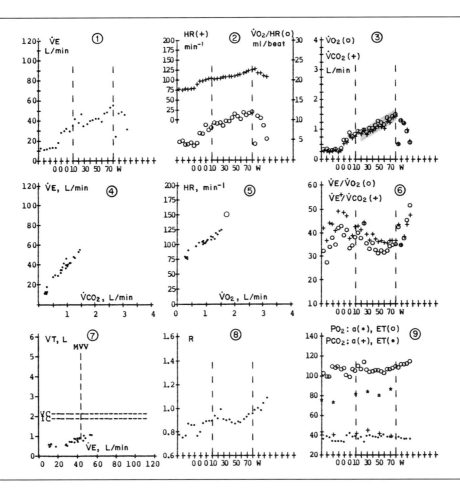

Interpretation

COMMENTS

Respiratory function studies indicate that this patient has a moderate obstructive defect (Table 26-1). The ECG is interpreted to demonstrate left ventricular hypertrophy and left atrial enlargement.

ANALYSIS

Flow Chart 1. Maximum $\dot{V}_{O_2}$ is borderline and anaerobic threshold is normal. See *Flow Chart 3.* The breathing reserve is low *(branchpoint 3.1)* indicating that this patient has lung disease. Confirming this diagnosis is the finding that the indices of ventilation-perfusion matching (V_D/V_T, $P(A-a)_{O_2}$ and $P(a-ET)_{CO_2}$) are abnormal and the heart rate reserve is high.

The actual maximum work rate performed by the patient is quite low, despite a borderline reduced maximum $\dot{V}_{O_2}$, because he has an exceptionally high oxygen cost for unloaded cycling ($\dot{V}_{O_2}=.85$ l/min). This is most likely due to his obesity (added metabolic cost of moving his lower extremities). The fall in $P(A-a)_{O_2}$ and rise in Pa_{O_2}, when changing activity from rest to exercise, suggest that the resting hypoxemia in this patient is attributable to obesity-related basilar micro-atelectasis at rest which disappears with the increased ventilation accompanying exercise.

The elevated dead space fraction of the tidal volume (V_D/V_T) and high metabolic cost of exercise caused by obesity, combined with mechanical limitation to breathe caused by moderate obstructive lung disease are all likely contributors to the patient's exertional dyspnea. Evidence against primary heart disease causing this patient's symptom is the absence of myocardial ischemia on the 12-lead ECG and the high heart rate reserve at maximum exercise.

CONCLUSION

Exertional dyspnea secondary to moderate obstructive lung disease and obesity.

CASE 27 *Chronic bronchitis and obesity*

CLINICAL FINDINGS

This 50-year-old shipyard worker was referred for evaluation. He had a 65 pack year history of smoking and complained of shortness of breath and frequent chest colds with cough and sputum production for the last 7 years. He had been told that he had border-line hypertension but took no medications for this or his pulmonary symptoms. Examination was normal except for obesity, blood pressure of 140/100, and expiratory wheezes on forced expiration. Chest roentgenograms showed focal pleural plaques.

EXERCISE FINDINGS

The patient performed exercise on a cycle ergometer. He pedalled at 60 rpm without added load for 3 minutes. The work rate was then increased 20 watts per minute to his symptom limited maximum. Blood was sampled every second minute and intra-arterial blood pressure was recorded from a percutaneously placed brachial artery catheter. Resting carboxyhemoglobin level was 9.4%. He stopped exercise complaining of shortness of breath. After exercise, while sitting quietly on the cycle, he became lightheaded and hypotensive. He was put in the supine position and his legs elevated; this provided immediate relief of his lightheadedness and return of his systemic blood pressure to pre-exercise levels. Resting, exercise, and recovery ECGs showed no abnormalities.

TABLE 27-1. *Selected Respiratory Function Data*

MEASUREMENT	PREDICTED	BEFORE BRONCHODILATOR	AFTER BRONCHODILATOR
Age, yr		50	
Sex		Male	
Height, cm		174	
Weight, kg	77	113	
Hematocrit, %		45	
VC, L	4.40	3.95	4.36
IC, L	2.94	3.30	3.75
TLC, L	6.44	6.08	
FEV_1, L	3.49	2.53	2.96
FEV_1/VC, %	79	64	
MVV, L/min	147	96	101
DL_{CO}, ml/mm Hg/min	28.6	30.6	

TABLE 27-2. *Selected Exercise Data*

MEASUREMENT	PREDICTED	MEASURED
Maximum $\dot{V}O_2$, L/min	2.47	1.84
Maximum HR, beats/min	170	131
Maximum O_2 pulse, ml/beat	14.5	14.3
$\Delta\dot{V}O_2/\Delta WR$, ml/min/watt	10.3	10.2
$\dot{V}O_2$ difference, %	0.0	0.7
AT, L/min	> 0.99	1.0
Blood pressure, mm Hg (rest, max)		131/88,206/106
Maximum $\dot{V}E$, L/min		93
Exercise breathing reserve, L/min	> 15	3
PaO_2, mm Hg (rest, max ex)		73,97
$P(A-a)O_2$, mm Hg (rest, max ex)		34,23
$P(a-ET)CO_2$, mm Hg (rest, max ex)		7,3
VD/VT (rest, heavy ex)		0.41,0.31

TABLE 27-3.

TIME min	WORK RATE W	BP mmHg	HR min⁻¹	f	$\dot{V}E$ BTPS L/min	$\dot{V}CO_2$ STPD L/min	$\dot{V}O_2$ STPD L/min	O_2 pulse ml/beat	R	pH	HCO₃⁻ mEq/L	PO₂ ET mmHg	PO₂ a mmHg	PO₂ A-a mmHg	PCO₂ ET mmHg	PCO₂ a mmHg	PCO₂ a-ET mmHg	$\dot{V}E/\dot{V}CO_2$	$\dot{V}E/\dot{V}O_2$	VD/VT
Rest		131/ 88								7.41	23	71			37					
Rest			69	16	12.6	0.28	0.39	5.7	0.72			109			31			40	29	
Rest		138/ 88	69	18	14.0	0.28	0.35	5.1	0.80	7.38	21	112	73	34	29	36	7	45	36	0.41
Unloaded			71	25	20.9	0.46	0.65	9.2	0.71			107			31			41	29	
Unloaded			73	24	24.6	0.55	0.69	9.5	0.80			110			31			41	33	
Unloaded		150/ 88	72	26	23.7	0.52	0.66	9.2	0.79	7.39	22	108	74	30	32	38	6	41	33	0.41
1.0	20		76	27	27.0	0.62	0.78	10.3	0.79			109			32			40	32	
2.0	40	156/ 88	81	27	30.2	0.74	0.92	11.4	0.80	7.42	21	109	74	35	32	34	2	38	30	0.30
3.0	60		88	30	41.5	1.05	1.14	13.0	0.92			113			32			37	34	
4.0	80	169/ 94	101	31	47.8	1.28	1.33	13.2	0.96	7.36	20	111	91	21	36	37	1	35	34	0.32
5.0	100		110	35	64.4	1.68	1.54	14.0	1.09			117			33			37	40	
6.0	120	200/100	124	39	78.3	2.02	1.72	13.9	1.17	7.35	19	120	97	23	32	34	3	37	44	0.30
7.0	140	206/106	131	45	87.3	2.18	1.81	13.8	1.20			108			42			38	46	
Recovery		113/ 63	94	31	71.9	1.63	1.22	13.0	1.34			124			29			43	57	
Recovery		75/ 31	46	34	62.7	1.09	0.71	15.4	1.54			133			22			55	84	

FIGURE 27-A.

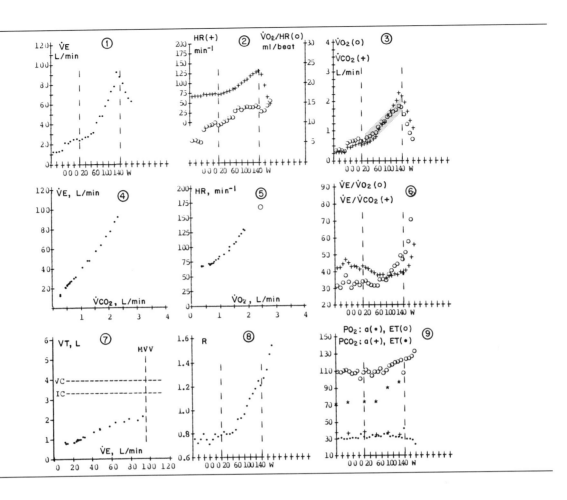

Interpretation

COMMENTS

Resting respiratory function studies reveal mild airflow obstruction that improves following treatment with an aerosolized bronchodilator (Table 27-1). The patient is 36 kg overweight. His resting carboxyhemoglobin is 9.4% (normal < 2.0%). The patient's resting electrocardiogram is normal. This case is presented because of the orthostasis that the patient developed when stopping exercise; this phenomenon is occasionally observed when heavy, upright exercise is abruptly terminated. To avoid this, we usually ask the patient who exercised hard to continue very light exercise (unloading cycling or slow walking) after completing the maximum work rate.

ANALYSIS

Flow Chart 1: The maximum $\dot{V}O_2$ is significantly reduced but the anaerobic threshold is normal. See *Flow Chart 3:* The breathing reserve is low *(branchpoint 3.1).* The combination of a low maxi-

mum $\dot{V}O_2$ and normal *AT* with low breathing reserve suggests that the pathology limiting the patient is that of lung disease. All four items in the diagnostic box supporting the diagnosis of lung disease are either abnormal or close to being abnormal, i.e. high V_D/V_T, $P(a-ET)_{CO_2}$, $P(A-a)_{O_2}$, and heart rate reserve at maximum $\dot{V}O_2$ (Tables 27-2 and 27-3). Breathing frequency (f) is less than 50 at the maximum $\dot{V}O_2$ *(branchpoint 3.2),* supporting the primary diagnosis of obstructive lung disease. The mild airflow obstruction, however, is probably not the only phenomenon contributing to this patient's symptom of exertional dyspnea. He is obese, and, consequently, requires more oxygen to do a given amount of external work than normal. Furthermore, he had a high blood level of carbon monoxide, and this will significantly reduce the arterial oxygen content and impair O_2 unloading in the tissue capillaries. There is no evidence of cardiovascular limitation.

CONCLUSION

Mild airflow obstruction, obesity, and cigarette smoking induced exercise limitation.

CASE 28 *Chronic bronchitis, mild*

CLINICAL FINDINGS

This 55-year-old shipyard worker complained of dyspnea after walking one flight of stairs or a few blocks on a level surface. He had morning cough several months of each year and noted occasional retrosternal pain unrelated to exertion or emotional upset. He had 35 pack years of smoking until stopping 12 years ago. He exercised regularly. The physical examination was normal except for mild obesity. Chest x-ray studies showed bilateral pleural thickening in the mid lung zones and old granulomatous disease in the right upper lobe. Resting ECG was normal.

EXERCISE FINDINGS

The patient performed exercise on a cycle ergometer. He first pedalled at 60 rpm, without added load, for 3 minutes. The work rate was then increased 20 watts per minute to his symptom limited maximum. Blood was sampled every second minute and intra-arterial blood pressure was recorded from a percutaneously placed brachial artery catheter. The patient stopped exercise because of "exhaustion." ECG remained normal throughout exercise.

TABLE 28-1. *Selected Respiratory Function Data*

MEASUREMENT	PREDICTED	MEASURED
Age, yr		54
Sex		Male
Height, cm		174
Weight, kg	77	88
Hematocrit, %		45
VC, L	4.28	3.59
IC, L	2.86	3.12
TLC, L	6.38	6.15
FEV_1, L	3.39	2.40
FEV_1/VC, %	79	67
MVV, L/min	142	112
DL_{CO} ml/mm Hg/min	28.8	29.8

TABLE 28-2. *Selected Exercise Data*

MEASUREMENT	PREDICTED	MEASURED
Maximum $\dot{V}O_2$, L/min	2.33	2.66
Maximum HR, beats/min	166	169
Maximum O_2 pulse, ml/beat	14.0	15.7
$\Delta\dot{V}O_2/\Delta WR$, ml/min/watt	10.3	9.9
$\dot{V}O_2$, difference, %	0.0	2.4
AT, L/min	> 0.92	1.2
Blood pressure, mm Hg (rest, max)		141/93,225/117
Maximum $\dot{V}E$, L/min		86
Exercise breathing reserve, L/min	> 15	26
Pa_{O_2}, mm Hg (rest, max ex)		73,97
$P(A-a)_{O_2}$, mm Hg (rest, max ex)		34,23
$P(a-ET)_{CO_2}$, mm Hg (rest, max ex)		7,3
VD/VT (rest, heavy ex)		0.41,0.31
HCO_3^-, mEq/L (rest, 2 min recov)		26,16

TABLE 28-3.

TIME min	WORK RATE W	BP mmHg	HR min⁻¹	f	$\dot{V}E$ BTPS L/min	$\dot{V}CO_2$ STPD L/min	$\dot{V}O_2$ STPD L/min	O_2 pulse ml/beat	R	pH	HCO_3^- mEq/L	PO_2 ET mmHg	PO_2 a mmHg	PO_2 A-a mmHg	PCO_2 ET mmHg	PCO_2 a mmHg	PCO_2 a-ET mmHg	$\dfrac{\dot{V}E}{\dot{V}CO_2}$	$\dfrac{\dot{V}E}{\dot{V}O_2}$	VD VT
Rest		141/ 93								7.42	26		77		41					
Rest		141/ 90	76	20	10.5	0.23	0.27	3.6	0.85			107			38			38	32	
Rest			78	19	10.2	0.22	0.27	3.5	0.81	7.40	26	104	81	18	38	43	5	39	32	0.41
Rest			77	24	10.4	0.21	0.26	3.4	0.81			102			39			40	32	
Rest			78	17	10.0	0.24	0.29	3.7	0.83			104			38			36	30	
Unloaded			94	21	15.2	0.46	0.62	6.6	0.74			95			42			29	22	
Unloaded			88	20	18.2	0.59	0.72	8.2	0.82			95			43			28	23	
Unloaded		162/ 99	94	19	19.4	0.62	0.75	8.0	0.83	7.39	26	98	83	17	41	43	2	29	24	0.27
1.0	20		98	22	19.6	0.63	0.81	8.3	0.78			93			43			28	22	
2.0	40	174/ 96	102	20	24.3	0.82	1.02	10.0	0.80	7.37	27	97	91	5	42	45	3	28	22	0.28
3.0	60		107	23	30.9	1.05	1.25	11.7	0.84			94			42			28	23	
4.0	80	174/ 93	110	25	36.1	1.25	1.39	12.6	0.90	7.37	25	100	95	8	43	43	0	27	24	0.25
5.0	100		117	26	40.1	1.39	1.46	12.5	0.95			98			46			27	26	
6.0	120	204/ 99	127	25	48.7	1.76	1.80	14.2	0.98	7.36	24	94	92	14	49	43	-6	26	26	0.23
7.0	140		132	29	55.4	2.00	1.92	14.5	1.04			103			46			26	28	
8.0	160	210/105	143	32	63.7	2.24	2.09	14.6	1.07	7.35	23	105	93	16	45	43	-2	27	29	0.25
9.0	180		152	33	68.8	2.52	2.35	15.5	1.07			104			47			26	28	
10.0	200	228/114	164	38	85.7	2.89	2.55	15.5	1.13	7.33	21	108	91	22	43	41	-2	29	32	0.25
10.5	220	225/117	169	38	86.0	2.97	2.66	15.7	1.12	7.31	20	108	92	21	44	40	-4	28	31	0.22
Recovery			166	32	78.5	2.74	2.27	13.7	1.21			111			42			28	33	
Recovery			148	28	58.3	1.85	1.18	8.0	1.57			116			42			30	47	
Recovery		183/ 96								7.27	16		119			35				

FIGURE 28-A.

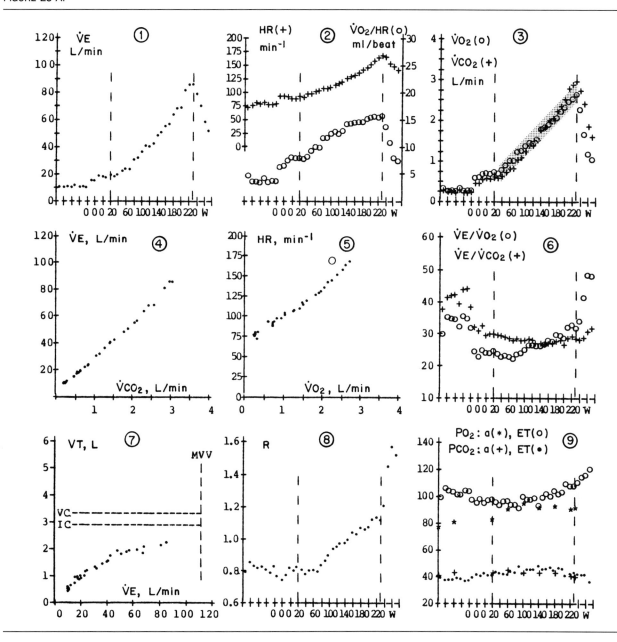

Interpretation

COMMENTS

Resting respiratory function is compatible with mild airflow obstruction (Table 28-1). The resting electrocardiogram is normal.

ANALYSIS

Flow Chart 1: The maximum oxygen uptake and anaerobic threshold are normal (Table 28-2). See *Flow Chart 2:* Arterial blood gases and ECG at maxi-

mum $\dot{V}O_2$ are normal *(branchpoint 2.1).* The patient is about 14% overweight *(branchpoint 2.2).* This is not a serious obesity problem but does contribute toward the additional metabolic cost of work. The patient also has mild airflow obstruction, however, causing a characteristic obstructive pattern at high exercise levels.

CONCLUSION

Normal exercise performance in mildly obese man with airflow obstruction.

CASE 29 *Bullous emphysema: Pre- and postbullectomy*

CLINICAL FINDINGS

This 50-year-old computer technician retired approximately 10 years prior to initial evaluation because of progressive dyspnea. He denied cough, sputum production, wheezing, or chest pain. There was no family history of lung disease. Chest x-ray studies showed large bullous lesions in the right mid and upper lung fields. Flow rates did not improve following four breaths of nebulized isoproterenol. Perfusion scan demonstrated no perfusion in the right mid and upper hemithorax or at the left apex. Alpha-1 antitrypsin levels were normal. One month after the first exercise test the patient's right upper lobe and portions of the right middle lobe were resected. The resected lung showed bullous and centriacinar emphysema with patchy atelectasis; a small squamous cell scar carcinoma was found in the upper lobe. He continued to smoke heavily.

EXERCISE FINDINGS

Preoperatively, the patient performed exercise on a cycle ergometer breathing room air, and following a 90 minute rest, breathing 100% oxygen. Three months postoperatively only an air breathing study was performed. On each occasion he pedalled at 60 rpm, on an unloaded cycle, for 2, 3, or 4 minutes. The work rate was then increased 20 watts every minute. Blood was sampled every second minute and intra-arterial blood pressure was recorded from a percutaneous branchial artery catheter. Resting ECG's were normal. Preoperatively the patient stopped exercise because of dyspnea without an exercise induced abnormality in the ECG. He stopped during the postoperative test because of dyspnea and pressure-like right-sided chest pain. There were multifocal, back-to-back, and salvos of premature ventricular contractions at the end of exercise and for two minutes of recovery without abnormal ST segment changes.

TABLE 29-1. *Selected Respiratory Function Data*

MEASUREMENT	PREDICTED	PREOPERATIVE	POSTOPERATIVE
Age, yr		50	
Sex		Male	
Height, cm		170	
Weight, kg	74	71	
Hematocrit, %		46	
VC, L	3.89	3.01	3.57
IC, L	2.59	2.03	2.46
TLC, L	5.69	7.05	5.56
FEV_1, L	3.09	1.93	2.44
FEV_1/VC, %	79	64	68
MVV, L/min	131	90	110
DL_{CO}, ml/mm Hg/min	26.5	10.0	13.0

TABLE 29-2. *Selected Exercise Data*

MEASUREMENT	PREDICTED	PREOPERATIVE	POSTOPERATIVE
Maximum $\dot{V}O_2$, L/MIN	2.30	0.99	1.06
Maximum HR, beats/min	170	144	144
Maximum O_2 pulse, ml/beat	13.5	7.5	8.0
$\Delta \dot{V}O_2/\Delta WR$, ml/min/watt	10.3	5.1	5.8
$\dot{V}O_2$ difference, %	0.0	33.4	28.8
AT, L/min	> 0.92	0.6	0.7
Blood pressure, mm Hg (rest, max)		144/90,187/100	144/88,238/94
Maximum $\dot{V}E$, L/min		84	80
Exercise breathing reserve, L/min	> 15	6	30
Pa_{O_2}, mm Hg (rest, max ex)		67,54	74,74
$P(A-a)_{O_2}$, mm Hg (rest, max ex)		47,72	34,52
$P(a-ET)_{CO_2}$, mm Hg (rest, max ex)		4,8	4,3
VD/VT (rest, heavy ex)		0.39,0.47	0.40,0.41
HCO_3^-, mEq/L (rest, 2 min recov)		21,14	22,14

TABLE 29-3. *Pre-bullectomy Study*

TIME min	WORK RATE W	BP mmHg	HR min⁻¹	f	V̇E BTPS L/min	V̇CO₂ STPD L/min	V̇O₂ STPD L/min	O₂ pulse ml/beat	R	pH	HCO₃⁻ mEq/L	PO₂ ET mmHg	PO₂ a	PO₂ A-a	PCO₂ ET mmHg	PCO₂ a	PCO₂ a-ET	V̇E/V̇CO₂	V̇E/V̇O₂	VD/VT
Rest										7.41	21		63			34				
Rest			69	17	10.3	0.16	0.20	2.9	0.80			117			26			55	44	
Rest			70	19	10.7	0.18	0.22	3.1	0.82			117			27			50	41	
Rest		144/ 90	69	15	10.1	0.17	0.21	3.0	0.81	7.41	19	119	67	47	26	30	4	52	42	0.39
Unloaded			80	32	30.5	0.48	0.52	6.5	0.92			125			23			58	53	
Unloaded			84	29	28.3	0.47	0.50	6.0	0.94			124			24			55	52	
Unloaded		156/ 94	87	28	28.9	0.48	0.51	5.9	0.94	7.41	18	125	62	58	24	29	5	55	52	0.42
1.0	20		93	30	32.8	0.55	0.57	6.1	0.96			125			24			55	53	
2.0	40	162/ 94	96	32	37.4	0.62	0.62	6.5	1.00	7.40	17	125	59	63	24	28	4	56	56	0.42
3.0	60		104	40	50.8	0.80	0.76	7.3	1.05			126			24			59	62	
4.0	80	181/ 96	116	45	62.7	1.00	0.87	7.5	1.15	7.40	18	129	51	72	22	30	8	59	68	0.48
5.0	100		132	60	84.2	1.20	0.97	7.3	1.24			132			20			66	82	
5.5	120	187/100	144	57	78.6	1.19	0.99	6.9	1.20	7.39	17	133	54	72	20	28	8	62	75	0.47
Recovery			138	55	76.5	1.23	1.01	7.3	1.22			132			21			58	71	
Recovery			120	44	66.2	1.08	0.83	6.9	1.30			133			20			58	75	
Recovery		196/106								7.31	14		66			29				

FIGURE 29-A. *Pre-bullectomy Study*

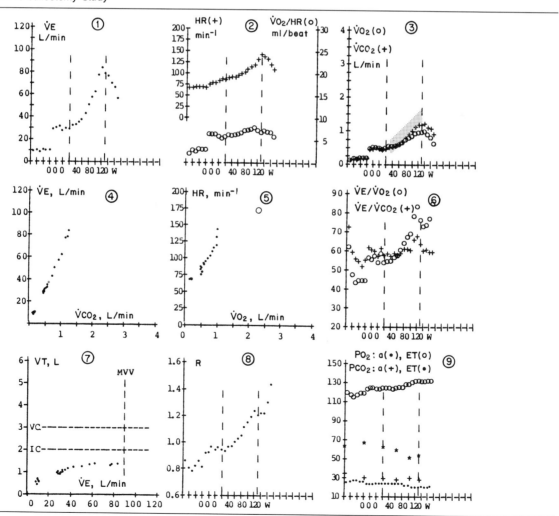

TABLE 29-4. *Post-bullectomy Study*

TIME min	WORK RATE W	BP mmHg	HR min⁻¹	f	V̇E BTPS	V̇CO₂	V̇O₂	O'₂ pulse	R	pH	HCO₃ mEq/L	PO₂ ET	PO₂ a	PO₂ A-a	PCO₂ ET	PCO₂ a	PCO₂ a-ET	V̇E/V̇CO₂	V̇E/V̇O₂	VD/VT
					—STPD— L/min			ml/beat				—mmHg—			—mmHg—					
Rest		150/ 94								7.44	21	76			32					
Rest		144/ 88	77	16	12.1	0.23	0.30	3.9	0.77	7.42	22	112	74	34	30	34	4	47	36	0.40
Unloaded			93	19	22.0	0.45	0.54	5.8	0.83			113			30			45	38	
Unloaded		163/ 88	92	19	22.2	0.47	0.49	5.3	0.96	7.42	22	113	68	48	31	33	2	44	42	0.37
1.0	20		95	20	24.3	0.51	0.61	6.4	0.84			114			30			44	37	
2.0	40	175/ 94	100	26	33.7	0.69	0.75	7.5	0.92	7.42	21	117	64	51	29	33	4	46	42	0.40
3.0	60		112	32	47.2	0.93	0.88	7.9	1.11			121			28			45	51	
4.0	80	225/ 94	130	42	62.4	1.25	1.03	7.9	1.21	7.39	20	123	66	55	28	34	6	47	57	0.43
5.0	100	238/ 94	138	48	75.7	1.48	1.06	7.7	1.40	7.35	17	126	74	52	28	31	3	48	69	0.40
5.5	120		144	57	79.5	1.52	1.06	7.4	1.43			128			26			49	70	
Recovery			144	45	74.5	1.49	1.00	6.9	1.49			129			26			47	71	
Recovery			114	36	63.5	1.26	0.85	7.5	1.43			130			26			48	71	
Recovery		231/100								7.31	14	88			29					

FIGURE 29-B. *Post-bullectomy Study*

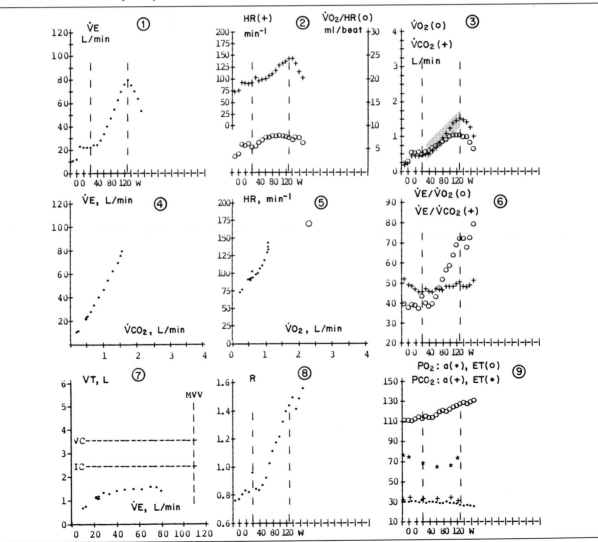

Interpretation

COMMENTS

Resting respiratory function studies show moderate obstructive lung disease with marked reduction in diffusing capacity (DL_{CO}). Following a bullectomy, the vital capacity increased, and the residual volume decreased with improvement in expiratory flow (Table 29-1). Although the diffusing capacity is slightly improved, it is still disproportionately reduced compared to the flow rate impairment. For example, postoperatively the MVV is 84% of predicted, while the diffusing capacity measurement is 50% of predicted. Exercise tolerance, surprisingly, is only slightly improved postoperatively.

ANALYSIS

Flow Chart 1: The maximum $\dot{V}O_2$ and anaerobic threshold are significantly reduced pre and postoperatively (Table 29-2). See *Flow Chart 4:* Preoperatively the exercise breathing reserve is low, but postoperatively the breathing reserve is normal *(branchpoint 4.1).* Taking the low breathing reserve branch directed by the preoperative study, VD/VT is high, consistent with lung disease with an O_2 flow problem *(branchpoint 4.2).* The confirmatory abnormalities noted in that diagnostic box are found in Table 29-3.

Taking the normal breathing reserve branch at *branchpoint 4.1,* consistent with the postbullectomy study, it is noted that the ventilatory equivalent for CO_2 is quite high and the indices of ventilation-perfusion mismatching are abnormal, supporting the diagnosis of an abnormal pulmonary circulation *(branchpoint 4.3).* The abnormality of the pulmonary circulation is also suggested by the low resting DL_{CO}. There is not an abrupt reduction in Pa_{O_2}, postoperatively, as might be expected with a right-to-left shunt. This is confirmed by a repeat exercise test with the patient breathing 100% oxygen (not shown). Referring to the diagnostic box under abnormal pulmonary circulation, confirmatory observations are: (1) A steep heart rate response to the increase in $\dot{V}O_2$, becoming more steep as the maximum $\dot{V}O_2$ is approached (Graph 5), (2) a low O_2 pulse with a flat contour as work rate is increased (Graph 2), and (3) a decreasing $\Delta\dot{V}O_2/\Delta WR$ as work rate is increased (Graph 3) for both the pre (Fig. 29-A) and postoperative (Fig. 29-B) studies. All of these findings are consistent with an oxygen flow problem of the type seen with functionally important pulmonary vascular disease. The latter is most likely related to this patient's lung disease. Although postoperatively, respiratory mechanics are improved, exercise performance did not improve significantly, and pulmonary vascular disease appears to be the predominant limiting factor. The ectopy noted during exercise, postbullectomy, might be secondary to the development of critically important pulmonary hypertension.

CONCLUSION

Bullous emphysema. Pulmonary vascular occlusive disease limited exercise performance, postbullectomy.

CASE 30 *Asbestosis*

CLINICAL FINDINGS

This 67-year-old woman was referred for exercise testing. She was exposed to asbestos for 3 years while working in a shipyard, approximately forty years ago. She never smoked. Three years prior to this evaluation she noted fatigability, clubbing of fingernails, and shortness of breath. She was unable to climb a flight of stairs or walk rapidly on the level. A transbronchial lung biopsy at that time was reported as showing "fibrosis." Her symptoms improved markedly on 80 mg of prednisone, but this medication was stopped after one year because of concern for its side effects. Five months prior to this evaluation she was started on oxygen therapy but corticosteroids were not reintroduced. Examination revealed a thin lady with fine inspiratory rales in the lateral and inferior lung fields that did not clear with coughing. There was dramatic digital clubbing. Chest roentgenograms showed extensive pulmonary infiltrates, compatible with interstitial pulmonary fibrosis. There was also a small patch of pleural calcification on the left. Resting ECG was normal.

EXERCISE FINDINGS

The patient performed exercise on a cycle ergometer. She pedalled at 60 rpm without added load for 3 minutes. The work rate was then increased 5 watts per minute to her symptom limited maximum. Blood was sampled every second minute and intra-arterial blood pressure was recorded from a percutaneously placed brachial artery catheter. The patient stopped exercising due to dyspnea. She developed some premature atrial contractions during exercise but ECG otherwise was not remarkable.

TABLE 30-1. *Selected Respiratory Function Data*

MEASUREMENT	PREDICTED	MEASURED
Age, yr		67
Sex		Female
Height, cm		163
Weight, kg	63	48
Hematocrit, %		38
VC, L	2.77	1.51
IC, L	1.85	0.70
TLC, L	4.82	2.65
FEV_1, L	2.19	1.24
FEV_1/VC, %	79	82
MVV, L/min	82	33
DL_{CO}, ml/mm Hg/min	22.3	6.4

TABLE 30-2. *Selected Exercise Data*

MEASUREMENT	PREDICTED	MEASURED
Maximum $\dot{V}O_2$, L/min	1.04	0.42
Maximum HR, beat/min	153	108
Maximum O_2 pulse, ml/beat	6.8	4.1
AT, L/min	> 0.42	indeterminate
Blood pressure, mm Hg (rest, max)		122/74,140/80
Maximum $\dot{V}E$, L/min		29
Exercise breathing reserve, L/min	> 15	4
Pa_{O_2}, mm Hg (rest, max ex)		58,46
$P(A-a)_{O_2}$, mm Hg (rest, max ex)		41,64
$P(a-ET)_{CO_2}$, mm Hg (rest, max ex)		8,10
VD/VT (rest, heavy ex)		0.56,0.55
HCO_3^-, mEq/L (rest, 2 min recov)		25,24

TABLE 30-3.

TIME min	WORK RATE W	BP mmHg	HR min⁻¹	f	V̇E BTPS	V̇CO₂ STPD	V̇O₂ STPD	O₂ pulse ml/beat	R	pH	HCO₃⁻ mEq/L	PO₂ ET	PO₂ a	PO₂ A-a	PCO₂ ET	PCO₂ a	PCO₂ a-ET	V̇E/V̇CO₂	V̇E/V̇O₂	VD/VT
Rest		122/ 74								7.44	25	48			37					
Rest			89	36	15.2	0.18	0.23	2.6	0.78			113			32			68	53	
Rest		119/ 71	90	36	15.0	0.17	0.22	2.4	0.77	7.40	25	109	58	41	33	41	8	70	54	0.56
Rest			92	37	15.1	0.16	0.20	2.2	0.80			113			32			74	60	
Unloaded			90	46	21.0	0.26	0.30	3.3	0.87			114			32			66	57	
Unloaded			92	49	24.0	0.32	0.36	3.9	0.89			114			33			62	55	
Unloaded			95	50	24.3	0.30	0.33	3.5	0.91			117			31			67	61	
1.0	10		97	51	25.0	0.32	0.36	3.7	0.89			114			33			65	58	
2.0	20	137/ 74	105	47	25.8	0.37	0.40	3.8	0.93	7.41	24	116	49	58	32	40	8	59	55	0.54
3.0	30		106	45	27.6	0.42	0.43	4.1	0.98			118			31			57	55	
3.5	40	140/ 80	108	45	29.1	0.44	0.42	3.9	1.05	7.39	24	120	46	64	31	41	10	57	60	0.55
Recovery			101	39	24.8	0.41	0.40	4.0	1.03			116			34			52	54	
Recovery			92	40	20.8	0.30	0.30	3.3	1.00			115			34			58	58	
Recovery			91	43	17.8	0.16	0.15	1.6	1.07			122			30			88	94	
Recovery		134/ 68								7.36	24			53			43			

FIGURE 30-A.

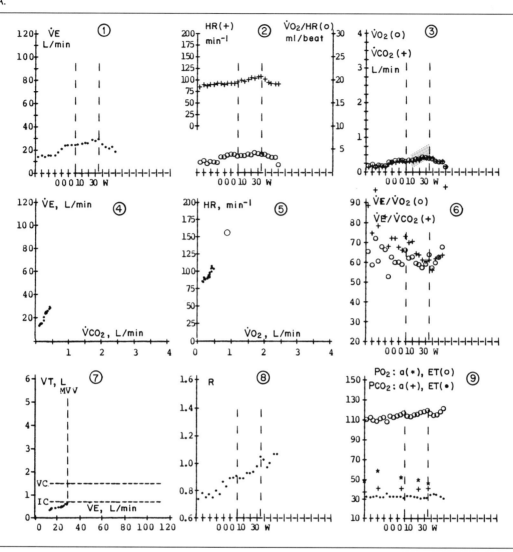

Interpretation

COMMENTS

Results of the respiratory function studies indicate that this patient has a moderately severe restrictive defect with a marked reduction in diffusing capacity (Table 30-1). The electrocardiogram is normal.

ANALYSIS

Flow Chart 1: The maximum $\dot{V}O_2$ is markedly reduced and the anaerobic threshold is indeterminate (Table 30-2). See *Flow Chart 5:* VD/VT, $P(a-ET)_{CO_2}$, and $P(A-a)_{O_2}$ during exercise are markedly abnormal *(branchpoint 5.1).* The breathing reserve is low *(branchpoint 5.3).* The breathing frequency is high at rest and is maintained at a high level of approxi-

mately 50 breaths/min through the incremental exercise period. The maximum ventilation achieved is approximately the patient's maximum ability to breathe *(branchpoint 5.7).* The above findings lead to the diagnosis of restrictive lung disease. Supporting this diagnosis is the progressive decrease in Pa_{O_2} and increase in $P(A-a)_{O_2}$ at each work rate performed (Table 30-3 and Graph 9, Figure 30-A). An additional measurement consistent with restrictive lung disease is the high tidal volume/inspiratory capacity ratio. An O_2 flow limitation is demonstrated by the small rise in $\dot{V}O_2$ and the failure of O_2 pulse to rise (Graphs 3 and 2, respectively, in Figure 30-A) as work rate is increased.

CONCLUSION

Exercise tolerance limited by restrictive lung disease.

CASE 31 *Intersitial pneumonitis: Pre- and post-corticosteroid therapy*

CLINICAL FINDINGS

This 37-year-old housewife developed progressive shortness of breath. She was found to have the pattern of interstitial lung disease on chest x-ray studies, and was referred for exercise testing.

EXERCISE FINDINGS

The patient performed exercise on a cycle ergometer. She pedalled at 60 rpm without added load for 3 minutes. The work rate was then increased 15 watts per minute to her symptom limited maximum. Blood was sampled every second minute and intra-arterial blood pressure was recorded from a percutaneously placed brachial artery catheter. Her resting and exercise ECG's were normal. In the initial study she stopped exercise because of shortness of breath.

After the first exercise test she was treated with prednisone. Her exercise test was repeated 6 months later, at which time she was taking 30 mgms of prednisone daily. She was asymptomatic at the time of the second test.

TABLE 31-1. *Selected Respiratory Function Data*

MEASUREMENT	PREDICTED	BEFORE TREATMENT	AFTER TREATMENT
Age, yr		37	
Sex		Female	
Height, cm		168	
Weight, kg	66	57	
Hematocrit, %		42	
VC, L	3.76	1.71	3.85
IC, L	2.50	1.31	2.25
FEV_1, L	3.08	1.52	3.10
FEV_1/VC, %	82	89	81
MVV, L/min	120	66	130
DL_{CO}, ml/mm Hg/min	28.5	16.2	

TABLE 31-2. *Selected Exercise Data*

MEASUREMENT	PREDICTED	BEFORE TREATMENT	AFTER TREATMENT
Maximum $\dot{V}O_2$, L/min	1.65	1.35	2.01
Maximum HR, beats/min	183	149	174
Maximum O_2 pulse, ml/beat	9.0	9.1	11.6
$\Delta\dot{V}O_2/\Delta WH$, ml/min/watt	10.3	9.5	9.8
$\dot{V}O_2$ difference, %	0.0	11.8	3.3
AT, L/min	> 0.66	0.6	1.0
Blood pressure, mm Hg (rest, max)		119/68,190/81	125/75,181/88
Maximum $\dot{V}E$, L/min		58	86
Exercise breathing reserve, L/min	> 15	8	44
Pa_{O_2}, mm Hg (rest, max ex)		65,51	117,98
$P(A-a)_{O_2}$, mm Hg (rest, max ex)		43,65	−1,26
$P(a-ET)_{CO_2}$, mm Hg (rest, max ex)		3,3	−3,−2
VD/VT (rest, heavy ex)		0.40,0.31	0.22,0.16
HCO_3^-, mEq/L (rest, 2 min recov)		25,21	23,16

TABLE 31-3. *Before Treatment*

TIME min	WORK RATE W	BP mmHg	HR min⁻¹	f	V̇E BTPS L/min	V̇CO₂ STPD L/min	V̇O₂ STPD L/min	O₂ pulse ml/beat	R	pH	HCO₃⁻ mEq/L	PO₂ ET mmHg	PO₂ a mmHg	PO₂ A-a mmHg	PCO₂ ET mmHg	PCO₂ a mmHg	PCO₂ a-ET mmHg	V̇E/V̇CO₂	V̇E/V̇O₂	VD/VT
Rest										7.47	25		74			35				
Rest			74	19	9.0	0.16	0.20	2.7	0.80			112			33			46	37	
Rest			74	22	9.5	0.14	0.18	2.4	0.78			112			33			55	42	
Rest		119/ 68	76	19	8.3	0.14	0.17	2.2	0.82	7.45	25	112	65	43	33	36	3	47	39	0.40
Unloaded			79	25	12.9	0.26	0.36	4.6	0.72			103			37			41	30	
Unloaded			78	23	11.3	0.23	0.29	3.7	0.79			107			35			41	32	
Unloaded		125/ 68	77	24	12.6	0.25	0.32	4.2	0.78	7.44	24	109	70	37	34	35	1	42	33	0.35
1.0	15		82	32	12.0	0.22	0.31	3.8	0.71			101			38			42	30	
2.0	30	131/ 68	95	23	17.1	0.42	0.56	5.9	0.75	7.44	25	104	68	35	37	37	0	36	27	0.31
3.0	45		102	23	17.6	0.46	0.58	5.7	0.79			103			38			34	27	
4.0	60	146/ 75	113	29	25.9	0.69	0.80	7.1	0.86	7.43	25	108	68	38	37	39	2	34	29	0.31
5.0	75		117	30	29.9	0.82	0.91	7.8	0.90			110			37			33	30	
6.0	90		127	37	37.8	1.03	1.05	8.3	0.98			112			36			34	33	
7.0	105	190/ 78	134	50	47.0	1.18	1.13	8.4	1.04	7.42	23	110	64	51	34	36	2	36	38	0.31
8.0	120	190/ 81	149	53	58.4	1.47	1.35	9.1	1.09	7.41	23	119	51	65	33	36	3	37	40	0.32
Recovery			104	41	37.6	0.95	0.83	8.0	1.14			117			36			36	41	
Recovery		190/ 81	83	34	23.1	0.51	0.48	5.8	1.06	7.36	21	116	80	35	35	37	2	40	42	0.36

FIGURE 31-A. *Before Treatment*

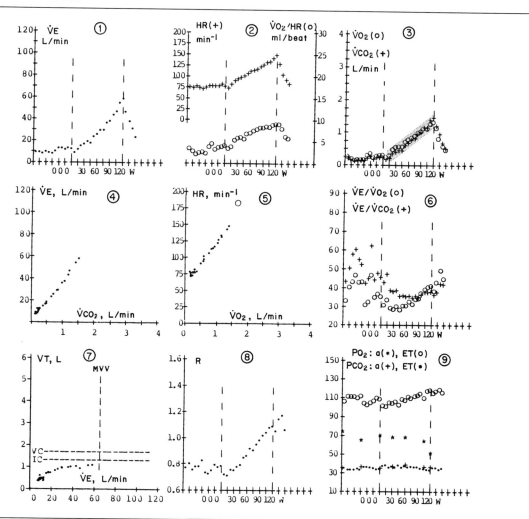

TABLE 31-4. *After Treatment*

TIME min	WORK RATE W	BP mmHg	HR min⁻¹	f	V̇E BTPS L/min	V̇CO2 STPD L/min	V̇O2 STPD L/min	O2 pulse ml/beat	R	pH	HCO3⁻ mEq/L	PO2 ET	PO2 a	PO2 A-a	PCO2 ET	PCO2 a	PCO2 a-ET	V̇E/V̇CO2	V̇E/V̇O2	VD/VT
Rest	125/ 75									7.45	23		94			34				
Rest			78	11	6.8	0.17	0.19	2.4	0.89			115			32			35	31	
Rest			83	24	8.2	0.13	0.15	1.8	0.87			115			31			47	41	
Rest	119/ 75		84	19	7.8	0.15	0.18	2.1	0.83	7.50	22	113	117	-1	32	29	-3	41	34	0.22
Unloaded			90	16	4.6	0.09	0.17	1.9	0.53			83			40			35	19	
Unloaded			88	15	12.8	0.37	0.51	5.8	0.73			100			38			31	23	
Unloaded	125/ 75		85	14	8.0	0.24	0.37	4.4	0.65	7.43	25	94	93	3	39	38	-1	28	18	0.17
1.0	15		89	23	7.5	0.21	0.33	3.7	0.64			90			41			26	17	
2.0	30	125/ 69	95	12	14.1	0.49	0.67	7.1	0.73	7.44	25	97	94	8	39	37	-2	27	20	0.12
3.0	45		109	17	19.2	0.66	0.84	7.7	0.79			99			40			27	21	
4.0	60	144/ 75	114	15	23.3	0.87	1.01	8.9	0.86	7.43	25	103	99	8	40	38	-2	25	22	0.10
5.0	75		126	16	25.3	0.93	1.03	8.2	0.90			103			41			26	23	
6.0	90	156/ 75	133	16	30.3	1.17	1.24	9.3	0.94	7.42	24	106	84	26	42	38	-4	25	23	0.08
7.0	105		145	20	41.4	1.50	1.47	10.1	1.02			106			42			26	27	
8.0	120	181/ 81	152	22	49.4	1.77	1.66	10.9	1.07	7.40	24	112	95	18	39	39	0	27	29	0.17
9.0	135		161	27	61.2	2.04	1.79	11.1	1.14			116			37			29	33	
10.0	150	181/ 88	174	38	85.6	2.49	2.01	11.6	1.24	7.40	19	122	98	26	33	31	-2	33	41	0.15
Recovery			146	22	46.9	1.42	0.96	6.6	1.48			123			35			32	47	
Recovery		181/ 81	126	26	31.4	0.85	0.64	5.1	1.33	7.36	16	124	101	25	32	30	-2	34	46	0.15
Recovery		175/ 75	113	23	22.2	0.58	0.48	4.2	1.21	7.36	17	123	93	30	31	31	0	35	42	0.19

FIGURE 31-B. *After Treatment*

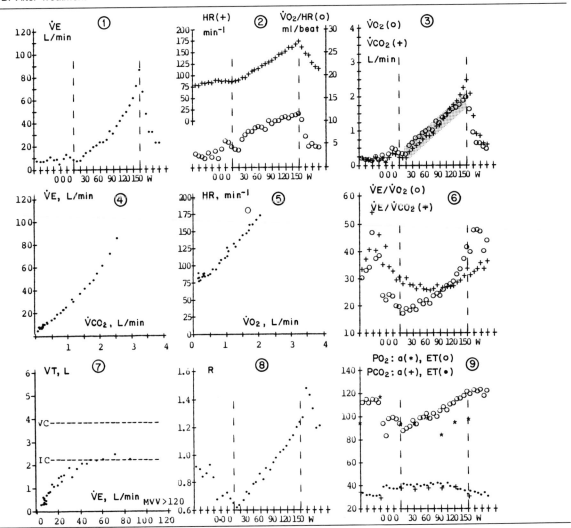

Interpretation

COMMENTS

The resting respiratory function studies indicate that this patient had severe restrictive lung disease, pretherapy, which improved markedly, post-therapy (Table 31-1). The resting electrocardiogram is normal. The "after-treatment" exercise test was performed 6 months after the first test.

ANALYSIS

Flow Chart 1: The maximum $\dot{V}O_2$ and the anaerobic threshold are abnormal (Table 31-2). See *Flow Chart 4:* The patient's breathing reserve is low *(branchpoint 4.1).* VD/VT is high *(branchpoint 4.2).* This leads to the diagnosis of lung disease with an O_2 flow problem. Characteristically, this is a restrictive lung disease. Confirming restrictive lung disease as the major pathophysiologic disorder are: A high $VT/$ IC ratio (Graph 7, Figure 31-A), breathing frequency exceeding 50 breaths/minute at the patient's maximum work rate (Table 31-3), $P(A-a)O_2$ increasing and PaO_2 decreasing systematically with work rate, and increased values of $P(a-ET)CO_2$ and VD/VT (Table 31-3).

After treatment, the maximum $\dot{V}O_2$ improved significantly and exceeded the predicted value. Arterial hypoxemia with exercise is no longer present and $P(a-ET)CO_2$ and VD/VT are normal, suggesting that the ventilation-perfusion abnormality observed before treatment was corrected. Also, the strikingly abnormal breathing pattern observed during pre-treatment exercise had resolved during post-treatment (compare Graphs 7 of Figures 31-A and 31-B).

CONCLUSION

Restrictive lung disease limited exercise performance. Reversal of abnormalities with therapy.

CASE 32 *Alveolar proteinosis: Pre- and post-whole lung lavage*

CLINICAL FINDINGS

This 25-year-old graduate student was found to have alveolar proteinosis, proven by transbronchial lung biopsy, several years previously. He had whole lung lavage twice previously, at yearly intervals, with improvement on both occasions. Despite the dyspnea associated with this illness, he was very physically active, running an average of 70 miles per week. He returned because of increasing dyspnea. Examination revealed a thin, muscular male who was not cyanotic. Chest roentgenograms showed bilateral infiltrates typical of alveolar proteinosis.

EXERCISE FINDINGS

The patient performed exercise on a cycle ergometer with similar protocols before and shortly after separate lavages of the right and left lungs. He pedalled at 60 rpm without added load for 3 minutes. The work rate was then increased 25 or 30 watts per minute to his symptom limited maximum. Blood was sampled every second minute and intra-arterial blood pressure was recorded from a percutaneously placed brachial artery catheter. Resting 12-lead and exercise single-lead ECG were normal. On both tests the patient stopped exercise because of leg fatigue.

TABLE 32-1. *Selected Respiratory Function Data*

MEASUREMENT	PREDICTED	PRE-LAVAGE	POST-LAVAGE
Age, yr		25	
Sex		Male	
Height, cm		165	
Weight, kg	70	52	
Hematocrit, %		48	47
VC, L	4.46	2.06	2.98
IC, L	2.98	1.36	1.60
TLC, L	5.93	3.28	4.10
FEV$_1$, L	3.63	1.67	2.44
FEV$_1$/VC, %	81	81	82
MVV, L/min	163	97	121
DL$_{CO}$, ml/mm Hg/min	29.5	20.0	28.7

TABLE 32-2. *Selected Exercise Data*

MEASUREMENT	PREDICTED	PRE-LAVAGE	POST-LAVAGE
Maximum $\dot{V}O_2$, L/min	2.15	2.70	3.07
Maximum HR, beats/min	195	165	175
Maximum O$_2$ pulse, ml/beat	11.0	16.4	17.5
$\Delta\dot{V}O_2/\Delta WR$, ml/min/watt	10.3	9.2	9.1
$\dot{V}O_2$ difference, %	0.0	8.8	10.1
AT, L/min	> 0.86	1.3	1.4
Maximum $\dot{V}E$, L/min		125	133
Exercise breathing reserve, L/min	> 15	−28	−12
Pa$_{O_2}$, mm Hg (rest, max ex)		82,53	93,64
P(A−a)$_{O_2}$, mm Hg (rest, max ex)		17,64	12,55
P(a−ET)$_{CO_2}$, mm Hg (rest, max ex)		−1,6	−2,−2
VD/VT (rest, heavy ex)		0.20,0.33	0.23,0.25
HCO$_3^-$, mEq/L (rest, 2 min recov)		26,20	24,15

TABLE 32-3. *Pre-whole Lung Lavage*

TIME min	WORK RATE W	BP mmHg	HR min⁻¹	f	V̇E BTPS L/min	V̇CO₂ STPD L/min	V̇O₂ STPD L/min	O₂ pulse ml/beat	R	pH	HCO₃⁻ mEq/L	PO₂ ET mmHg	PO₂ a	PO₂ A-a	PCO₂ ET mmHg	PCO₂ a	PCO₂ a-ET	V̇E/V̇CO₂	V̇E/V̇O₂	VD/VT
Rest										7.43	26		79		40					
Rest			74	15	6.3	0.15	0.21	2.8	0.71			101			39			33	24	
Rest			52	16	7.4	0.20	0.29	5.6	0.69	7.44	25	100	82	17	39	38	-1	30	21	0.20
Rest			67	21	6.4	0.12	0.18	2.7	0.67			104			38			38	25	
Unloaded			75	20	13.5	0.35	0.51	6.8	0.69			104			38			34	23	
Unloaded			71	25	16.8	0.42	0.58	8.2	0.72			105			38			35	25	
Unloaded			77	24	14.7	0.38	0.58	7.5	0.66	7.43	25	101	79	16	38	39	1	33	22	0.29
1.0	25		82	18	16.5	0.51	0.76	9.3	0.67			99			40			29	20	
2.0	50		90	30	23.9	0.63	0.98	10.9	0.64	7.43	24	101	70	27	39	37	-2	34	22	0.28
3.0	75		105	33	32.8	0.95	1.31	12.5	0.73			104			40			32	23	
4.0	100		108	44	40.7	1.21	1.56	14.4	0.78	7.44	25	106	66	39	41	37	-4	31	24	0.21
5.0	125		124	59	57.4	1.55	1.92	15.5	0.81			112			37			34	27	
6.0	150		137	61	65.6	1.84	2.11	15.4	0.87	7.43	24	118	58	51	34	37	3	33	29	0.27
7.0	175		146	63	70.2	2.03	2.33	16.0	0.87			116			36			32	28	
8.0	200		155	87	93.3	2.43	2.46	15.9	0.99	7.41	23	121	53	60	33	37	4	35	35	0.31
9.0	225		163	93	108.9	2.76	2.61	16.0	1.06			124			32			37	39	
10.0	250		165	96	124.9	3.07	2.70	16.4	1.14	7.36	20	125	53	64	31	37	6	38	43	0.36

FIGURE 32-A. *Pre-whole Lung Lavage*

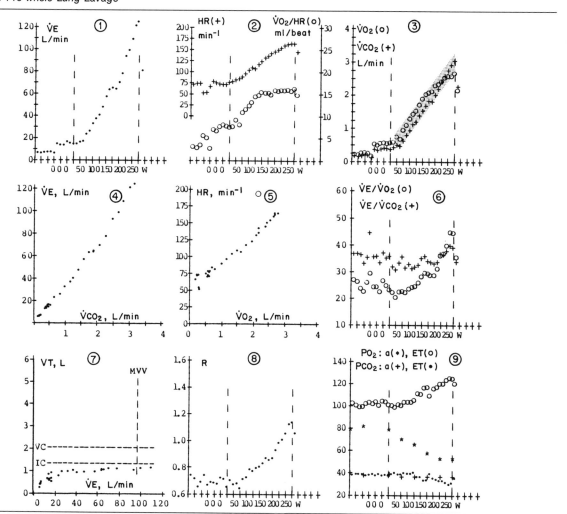

TABLE 32-4. *Post-whole Lung Lavage*

TIME min	WORK RATE W	BP mmHg	HR min⁻¹	f	V̇E BTPS L/min	V̇CO₂ STPD L/min	V̇O₂ STPD L/min	O₂ pulse ml/beat	R	pH	HCO₃⁻ mEq/L	PO₂ ET mmHg	PO₂ a	PO₂ A-a	PCO₂ ET mmHg	PCO₂ a	PCO₂ a-ET	V̇E/V̇CO₂	V̇E/V̇O₂	VD/VT
Rest										7.40	24		77			39				
Rest			52	17	8.9	0.22	0.29	5.6	0.76			107			36			34	26	
Rest			66	17	7.0	0.16	0.22	3.3	0.73	7.43	23	103	93	12	37	35	-2	35	25	0.23
Rest			55	15	9.7	0.25	0.30	5.5	0.83			108			37			34	28	
Unloaded			72	20	15.8	0.44	0.59	8.2	0.75			108			36			32	24	
Unloaded			75	12	11.5	0.34	0.55	7.3	0.62			97			38			31	19	
Unloaded			75	12	11.8	0.36	0.56	7.5	0.64	7.41	24	99	79	16	33	38	0	30	19	0.22
1.0	30		85	21	16.5	0.50	0.85	10.0	0.59			94			40			29	17	
2.0	60		92	24	20.8	0.64	0.95	10.3	0.67	7.41	23	99	79	20	40	37	-3	29	20	0.18
3.0	90		107	27	29.8	0.97	1.30	12.1	0.75			103			40			28	21	
4.0	120		117	31	40.0	1.30	1.59	13.6	0.82	7.40	23	104	75	31	41	37	-4	29	23	0.18
5.0	150		133	31	43.7	1.48	1.74	13.1	0.85			106			41			28	24	
6.0	180		140	41	56.8	1.81	2.05	14.6	0.88	7.40	22	109	71	38	40	37	-3	29	26	0.19
7.0	210		152	58	75.8	2.18	2.36	15.5	0.92			115			37			33	30	
8.0	240		158	57	81.3	2.36	2.56	16.2	0.92	7.40	20	109	65	49	40	34	-6	32	30	0.20
9.0	270		168	75	113.2	3.04	2.96	17.6	1.03			124			32			35	36	
10.0	300		172	96	132.8	3.17	3.06	17.8	1.04	7.30	15	125	64	55	31	32	1	39	41	0.30
Recovery			133	83	81.2	1.97	1.37	10.3	1.44			127			36			38	54	

FIGURE 32-B. *Post-whole Lung Lavage*

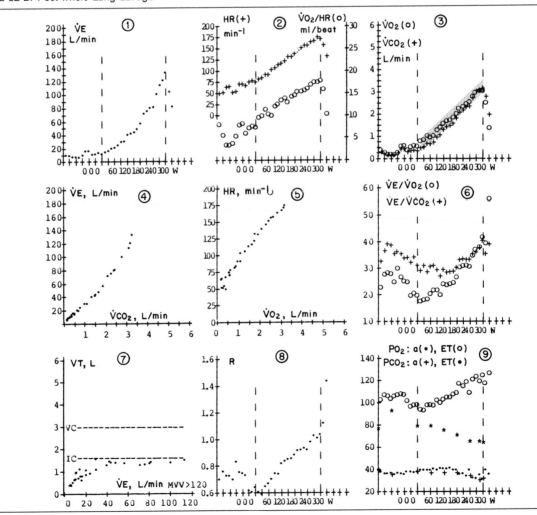

Interpretation

COMMENTS

Respiratory function studies indicate moderately severe restrictive lung disease that improves after lung lavage (Table 32-1). The resting electrocardiogram is normal. The postlavage exercise study was done 7 days after completion of whole-lung lavage and 11 days after the prelavage study.

ANALYSIS

Flow Chart 1: Because this patient is so exceptionally well trained, his maximum $\dot{V}O_2$ and anaerobic threshold are substantially greater than predicted. The maximum $\dot{V}O_2$, even pre-lavage, is significantly above predicted. His anaerobic threshold is normal (Table 32-2). See *Flow Chart 2:* The O_2 pulse is supra-normal and his electrocardiogram is normal at maximum $\dot{V}O_2$. However, his blood gases, while normal at rest, become abnormal during exercise, with PaO_2 progressively decreasing and $P(A-a)O_2$ progressively increasing with work rate (Table 32-3) *(branchpoint 2.1)*. The VD/VT is abnormal *(branchpoint 2.3)*. At the maximum work rate performed, the patient has a marked tachypnea (Table 32-3). The tidal volume remains constant at the level of the inspiratory capacity from a relatively light work rate to the maximum (Graph 7, Fig. 32-A), with the increase in minute ventilation being achieved, almost solely, by increasing breathing frequency. This exercise response is consistent with restrictive lung disease, despite a supra-normal maximum $\dot{V}O_2$.

Although the patient exceeds the predicted $\dot{V}O_2$ max value for sedentary males of his size, he clearly has physiological abnormalities that limit his exercise performance, as evidenced by his improved exercise performance following bilateral whole lung lavage (Table 32-2, and contrasting data in Tables 32-3 and 32-4). Because of the mechanical limitation to lung expansion imposed by the alveolar filling disorder, and perhaps some pulmonary fibrosis, the patient has to increase minute ventilation during exercise primarily by increasing breathing frequency. The minute ventilation at maximum exercise exceeds his MVV (negative breathing reserve), reflecting his high motivation and possibly some exercise bronchodilatation. In the second study the ventilatory pattern of restrictive disease persists but is more mild. The degree of arterial hypoxemia and increase in $P(A-a)O_2$ are also considerably reduced following whole lung lavage (compare Table 32-3 with Table 32-4).

CONCLUSION

Restrictive lung disease that improved following therapy.

CASE 33 *Interstitial pulmonary fibrosis: Air and oxygen breathing*

CLINICAL FINDINGS

This 47-year-old male developed dyspnea 12 years previously. A histological diagnosis of pulmonary alveolar proteinosis was then made by open lung biopsy. Following lung lavage he became asymptomatic until 10 months prior to evaluation when progressive dyspnea first became evident when skiing at higher altitudes. Although previously active in sports, he was unable to walk more than 30 yards on flat ground at a normal pace. He coughed with exercise and sometimes produced clear sputum. He denied smoking, wheezing, or edema. The results of his examination were normal except for digital clubbing and infrequent fine inspiratory rales at the lung bases. Chest roentgenogram showed increased interstitial markings with honeycombing.

EXERCISE FINDINGS

The patient performed exercise on a cycle ergometer breathing room air, and, after a 30 minute rest, breathing 100% oxygen. He pedalled at 60 rpm without added load for 3 minutes. The work rate was increased 15 watts every minute to his symptom limited maximum. Blood was sampled every second minute and intra-arterial blood pressure was recorded from a percutaneously placed brachial artery catheter. When breathing room air he stopped exercise due to fatigue and lightheadedness. When breathing oxygen he stopped due to leg pain and general fatigue. Resting and exercise ECG's were normal.

TABLE 33-1. *Selected Respiratory Function Data*

MEASUREMENT	PREDICTED	MEASURED
Age, yr		47
Sex		Male
Height, cm		174
Weight, kg	77	85
Hematocrit, %		41
VC, L	4.49	2.20
IC, L	2.99	1.14
TLC, L	6.48	3.17
FEV$_1$, L	3.58	2.01
FEV$_1$/VC, %	80	91
MVV, L/min	151	112
DL$_{CO}$, ml/mm Hg/min	30.7	13.9

TABLE 33-2. *Selected Exercise Data*

MEASUREMENT	PREDICTED	ROOM AIR	OXYGEN
Maximum V̇o$_2$, L/min	2.55	1.23	
Maximum HR, beats/min	173	150	154
Maximum O$_2$ pulse, ml/beat	14.7	8.2	
ΔV̇o$_2$/ΔWR, ml/min/watt	10.3	8.6	
V̇o$_2$ difference, %	0.0	8.4	
AT, L/min	> 1.02	0.8	
Blood pressure, mm Hg (rest, max)		120/75,175/84*	138/87,195/90*
Maximum V̇E, L/min		72	56
Exercise breathing reserve, L/min	> 15	40	56
Pa$_{O_2}$, mm Hg (rest, max ex)		62,37	568,284
P(A−a)$_{O_2}$, mm Hg (rest, max ex)		30,73	102,365
P(a−ET)$_{CO_2}$, mm Hg (rest, max ex)		6,10	4,12
VD/VT (rest, heavy ex)		0.54,0.54	0.51,0.56
HCO$_3^-$, mEq/L (rest, 2 min recov)		23,20	26,22

*systolic pulsus paradoxus of 70 mm Hg

TABLE 33-3. *Air Breathing*

TIME min	WORK RATE W	BP mmHg	HR min⁻¹	f	V̇E BTPS	V̇CO₂	V̇O₂	O₂ pulse	R	pH	HCO₃⁻ mEq/L	PO₂ ET	PO₂ a	PO₂ A-a	PCO₂ ET	PCO₂ a	PCO₂ a-ET	V̇E/V̇CO₂	V̇E/V̇O₂	VD/VT
					— L/min —	— L/min —		ml/beat				— mmHg —			— mmHg —					
Rest			79	20	14.6	0.22	0.34	4.3	0.65			102			33			58	38	
Rest		120/ 75	77	27	13.9	0.19	0.30	3.9	0.63	7.37	23	102	62	30	34	40	6	61	39	
Rest			79	20	14.1	0.21	0.31	3.9	0.68			103			33			59	40	0.54
Unloaded			98	25	23.0	0.40	0.57	5.8	0.70			104			35			52	37	
Unloaded			98	27	25.8	0.47	0.62	6.3	0.76			105			36			50	38	
Unloaded		153/ 81	101	31	31.0	0.58	0.70	6.9	0.83	7.35	23	108	49	51	35	43	8	49	40	0.54
1.0	15		105	35	34.8	0.66	0.80	7.6	0.83			104			38			48	40	
2.0	30	159/ 75	108	36	37.6	0.71	0.81	7.5	0.88	7.34	23	111	46	55	35	44	9	49	43	0.55
3.0	45		119	42	41.9	0.76	0.85	7.1	0.89			105			38			50	45	
4.0	60	156/ 90	126	46	54.3	1.03	1.02	8.1	1.01	7.33	23	116	40	66	34	44	10	49	49	0.56
5.0	75	162/ 90	145	52	62.1	1.18	1.08	7.4	1.09	7.33	22	110	38	73	38	42	4	49	53	0.54
6.0	90	168/ 93	150	52	67.5	1.38	1.21	8.1	1.14	7.31	22	119	37	73	34	44	10	46	52	0.53
Recovery			144	50	57.9	1.16	1.10	7.6	1.05			102			44			46	49	
Recovery		159/ 90	132	47	52.1	0.99	0.97	7.3	1.02	7.27	20	116	42	64	34	45	11	49	50	0.56

FIGURE 33-A. *Air Breathing*

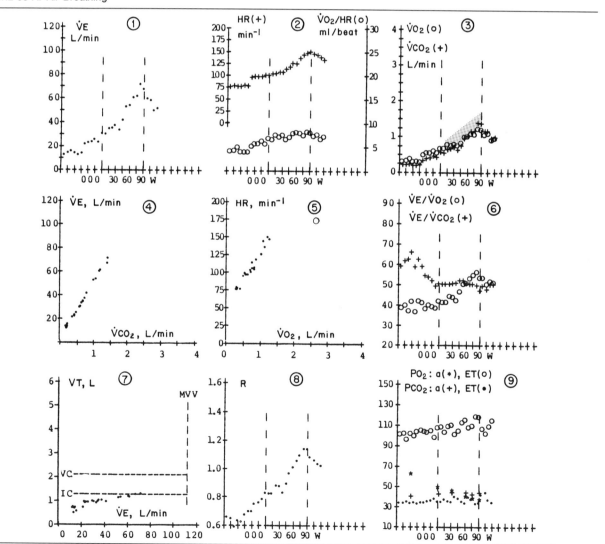

TABLE 33-4. *Oxygen Breathing*

TIME min	WORK RATE W	BP mmHg	HR min⁻¹	f	V̇E BTPS L/min	V̇CO2 —STPD— L/min	V̇O2 L/min	O2 pulse ml/beat	R	pH	HCO3 mEq/L	PO2 ET	PO2 a	PO2 A-a	PCO2 ET	PCO2 a	PCO2 a-ET	V̇E/V̇CO2	V̇E/V̇O2	VD/VT
Rest		132/ 84								7.44	24		66		36					
Rest			93	19	12.1	0.18									39				58	
Rest		138/ 87	91	29	14.5	0.23				7.39	26	568	102		39	43	4		52	0.51
Rest			96	25	14.0	0.18									36				66	
Rest			89	30	16.7	0.24									37				59	
Unloaded			100	26	20.1	0.34									39				53	
Unloaded			100	21	15.7	0.31									45				45	
Unloaded			114	24	17.2	0.42				7.33	26	540	122		46	51	5		36	0.47
1.0	15		120	28	20.1	0.59									49				30	
2.0	15		119	28	29.5	0.64									42				42	
3.0	30		117	28	27.1	0.58				7.31	26	505	156		44	52	8		43	0.56
4.0	45		120	32	32.0	0.74									44				40	
5.0	60		128	29	33.5	0.83				7.28	25	467	191		48	55	7		37	0.54
6.0	75		134	37	34.2	0.87									49				36	
7.0	90		132	35	37.5	0.99				7.25	25	409	245		54	59	5		35	0.53
8.0	105		145	37	41.3	1.10				7.23	25	350	302		54	61	7		35	0.55
9.0	120		152	40	48.3	1.39									52				32	
10.0	135		154	46	56.1	1.53				7.20	24	284	365		52	64	12		34	0.56
Recovery			144	43	51.7	1.38									52				35	
Recovery			133	39	44.1	1.03									47				40	
Recovery										7.22	22	475				55				

FIGURE 33-B. *Oxygen Breathing*

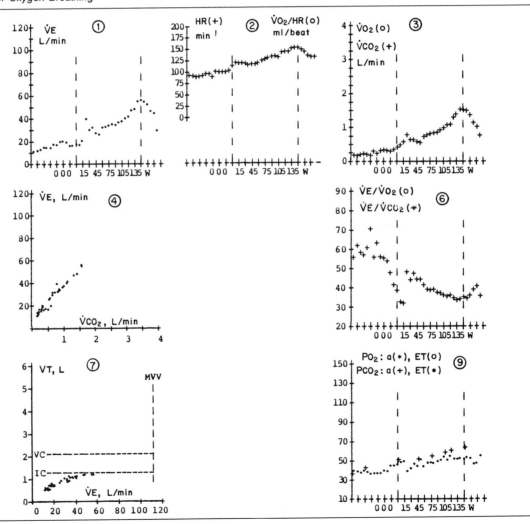

Interpretation

COMMENTS

This case of severe interstitial lung disease is presented to illustrate two major points: (1) The impaired peripheral oxygenation that may be caused by pulmonary fibrosis; and (2) the presence of a major increasing contribution of the carotid bodies to breathing, in association with arterial hypoxemia.

The results of the resting respiratory function studies indicate that this patient has a severe restrictive disorder, with no evidence of airflow obstruction (Table 33-1). The resting electrocardiogram is normal.

ANALYSIS

Flow Chart 1: The maximum $\dot{V}O_2$ and anaerobic threshold are reduced (Table 33-2). See *Flow Chart 4:* The breathing reserve is normal or high *(branchpoint 4.1).* The $\dot{V}E/\dot{V}CO_2$ at the anaerobic threshold is markedly elevated *(branchpoint 4.3).* This leads the interpreter to the diagnosis of "abnormal pulmonary circulation." However, *branchpoint 4.3* states that if the vital capacity is low, as it is in this patient, one should go to the low breathing reserve branch, i.e. go back to *branchpoint 4.1.* The reason for this is that patients with restrictive lung disease can have an unusually high MVV when measured directly. One can conclude, therefore, that the breathing reserve for the patient is high. However, if the MVV were calculated from the FEV_1 (2.01 × 40), the MVV would be 80.4 L/min in this patient, and the breathing reserve is then, in fact, low. Thus, this *branchpoint 4.3* instruction is designed to detect patients who have abnormal pulmonary circulation secondary to restrictive lung disease.

Following the low breathing reserve branch of *branchpoint 4.1,* we consider *branchpoint 4.2* and the high VD/VT. From this, we conclude that this patient has restrictive lung disease with an O_2 flow problem. Findings confirming this diagnosis are: (1) the high VT/IC ratio (Graph 7, Fig. 33-A), (2) the low and progressively decreasing PaO_2 as work rate is increased (Graph 9, Fig. 33-A), (3) a breathing frequency greater than 50 at the maximum $\dot{V}O_2$ (Table 33-3), (4) an increased $P(a-ET)CO_2$ (Graph 9, Fig. 33-A), (5) a steep heart rate response to the increasing oxygen uptake (Graph 5, Fig. 33-A), (6) a low O_2 pulse with a flat contour as the work rate is increased (Graph 2, Fig. 33-A), (7) a reduced $\Delta\dot{V}O_2/\Delta WR$ (Table 33-2 and Graph 3, Fig. 33-A), and (8) $P(A-a)O_2$ increasing with increasing work rate (Table 33-3). Note that all of these confirmatory findings, are characteristic of restrictive lung disease.

O_2 breathing allows the patient to increase his maximum work rate from 90 watts to 135 watts (Table 33-4 and Fig. 33-B). This was accomplished primarily by decreasing ventilatory drive. In contrast to regulating arterial PCO_2 around 40 as the patient did when breathing air, 100% O_2 breathing attenuated ventilatory drive (carotid body inhibition) causing $PaCO_2$ to increase to 64 at the maximum work rate achieved. At each work rate during O_2 breathing, the breathing frequency (f) is decreased (compare Table 33-3 with Table 33-4). O_2 breathing allows the patient to breathe less and to be less breathless. The breathing frequency is only 35 ($\dot{V}E=37.5$) at 90 watts when breathing O_2 as compared to 52 ($\dot{V}E=67.5$) during air breathing, at the same work rate. The heart rate is considerably more rapid during air breathing (150) than during O_2 breathing (132) at 90 watts.

CONCLUSION

Severe interstitial lung disease, with an important O_2 flow problem created largely by arterial hypoxemia. O_2 breathing attenuates ventilatory drive and provides relief of dyspnea.

CASE 34 *Ankylosing spondylitis*

CLINICAL FINDINGS

This 51-year-old airline employee first developed symptoms of ankylosing spondylitis, primarily involving the neck and thoracic spine, approximately 6 years prior to evaluation. He received some relief of pain with indomethacin. He stopped smoking over 10 years ago. On the basis of pleural changes at the apices, he was treated for tuberculosis several years ago although the tuberculin skin test was negative. To maintain fitness, he began running approximately three miles a day. In recent months he felt as if he "could not get enough air into his lungs" and found himself taking gasping breaths. Physical examination revealed reduced neck movement and thoracic expansion. Chest roentgenograms revealed apical pleural thickening. ECG was normal.

EXERCISE FINDINGS

The patient performed exercise on a cycle ergometer. He pedalled at 60 rpm without added load for 3 minutes. The work rate was then increased 20 watts per minute to his symptom limited maximum. He stopped exercise because of shortness of breath. Exercise ECGs were normal except for a single interpolated ventricular premature contraction.

TABLE 34-1. *Selected Respiratory Function Data*

MEASUREMENT	PREDICTED	MEASURED
Age, yr		51
Sex		Male
Height, cm		178
Weight, kg	80	79
Hematocrit, %		39
VC, L	4.62	3.61
IC, L	3.08	2.60
FEV_1, L	3.67	2.76
FEV_1/VC, %	79	76
MVV, L/min	151	132 at f = 80/min

TABLE 34-2. *Selected Exercise Data*

MEASUREMENT	PREDICTED	MEASURED
Maximum $\dot{V}O_2$, L/min	2.51	2.54
Maximum HR, beats/min	169	170
Maximum O_2 pulse, ml/beat	14.9	14.9
$\Delta\dot{V}O_2/\Delta WR$, ml/min/watt	10.3	9.4
$\dot{V}O_2$ difference, %	0.0	6.9
AT, L/min	> 1.0	1.1
Blood pressure, mm Hg (rest, max)		126/86,206/84
Maximum $\dot{V}E$, L/min		108
Exercise breathing reserve, L/min	> 15	24*

*Direct MVV was used for calculation. Based on indirect MVV ($FEV_1 \times 40$) the exercise breathing reserve is 2 L/ min (110 − 108 = 2).

TABLE 34-3.

TIME min	WORK RATE W	BP mmHg	HR min⁻¹	f	$\dot{V}E$ BTPS L/min	$\dot{V}CO_2$ STPD L/min	$\dot{V}O_2$ STPD L/min	O_2 pulse ml/beat	R	pH	HCO_3^- mEq/L	PO2 ET mmHg	PO2 a	PO2 A-a	PCO2 ET mmHg	PCO2 a	PCO2 a-ET	$\dot{V}E/\dot{V}CO_2$	$\dot{V}E/\dot{V}O_2$	VD/VT
Rest			72	17	11.5	0.30	0.38	5.3	0.79			102			37			34	27	
Rest			73	14	8.7	0.22	0.27	3.7	0.81			104			36			34	28	
Rest		126/ 86	71	16	7.2	0.16	0.22	3.1	0.73			104			36			37	27	
Rest			72	26	16.2	0.39	0.53	7.4	0.74			93			39			36	26	
Unloaded			77	18	7.8	0.20	0.29	3.8	0.69			84			44			32	22	
Unloaded			80	15	13.9	0.49	0.71	8.9	0.69			92			42			26	18	
Unloaded			77	16	14.3	0.46	0.62	8.1	0.74			94			42			28	21	
1.0	20	158/ 86	83	16	14.8	0.51	0.67	8.1	0.76			96			41			26	20	
2.0	40	174/ 84	86	17	20.7	0.70	0.97	11.3	0.72			89			44			28	20	
3.0	60		94	16	21.0	0.78	1.03	11.0	0.76			93			44			25	19	
4.0	80	178/ 78	105	20	33.6	1.23	1.48	14.1	0.83			86			47			26	22	
5.0	100		108	20	31.8	1.23	1.37	12.7	0.90			97			46			24	22	
6.0	120	190/ 86	125	18	37.5	1.51	1.59	12.7	0.95			96			48			24	23	
7.0	140		128	23	46.1	1.82	1.78	13.9	1.02			100			47			24	25	
8.0	160	206/ 84	144	25	52.7	2.08	1.94	13.5	1.07			102			48			24	26	
9.0	180		152	31	64.8	2.44	2.16	14.2	1.13			103			48			25	29	
10.0	200		163	37	77.2	2.80	2.29	14.0	1.22			108			45			26	32	
11.0	220		170	47	108.3	3.34	2.54	14.9	1.31			115			40			31	41	
Recovery			145	30	67.9	2.00	1.35	9.3	1.48			120			37			33	48	
Recovery			129	30	48.8	1.37	0.93	7.2	1.47			124			34			34	50	

FIGURE 34-A.

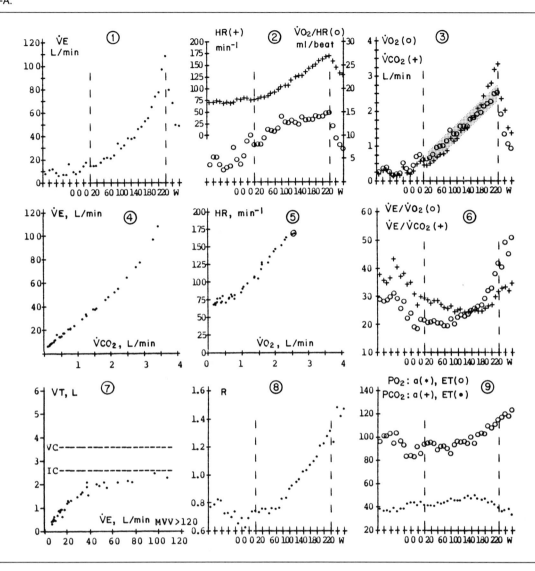

Interpretation

COMMENTS

The results of spirometry and total lung capacity measurement suggest that the patient has mild restrictive disease (Table 34-1) consequent to his ankylosing spondylitis. This is reflected in part by a reduction in the inspiratory capacity (loss of his ability to expand his chest wall). The resting electrocardiogram is normal.

ANALYSIS

Flow Chart 1: The maximum $\dot{V}O_2$ and the anaerobic threshold are normal (Table 34-2). See *Flow Chart 2:* The electrocardiogram and O_2 pulse at maximum

$\dot{V}O_2$ are normal *(branchpoint 2.1).* The subject is not obese *(branchpoint 2.2).* The normal ventilatory equivalent for CO_2 at the anaerobic threshold suggests that ventilation-perfusion matching is normal. The observation that tidal volume reaches the inspiratory capacity (Graph 7, Figure 34-A) reflects the changes that would be expected from restrictive pulmonary or chest wall disease. Note that the indirect MVV is very close to the maximum exercise ventilation resulting in virtually no breathing reserve. This is further evidence of ventilatory limitation.

CONCLUSION

Exertional dyspnea, developing secondary to restrictive changes in the chest wall, consequent to ankylosing spondylitis.

CASE 35 *Pulmonary vascular disease, thromboembolic*

CLINICAL FINDINGS

This 50-year-old shipyard worker felt well until one year prior to evaluation when he noted the insidious but progressive development of dyspnea and easy fatigability. Six months later he had the abrupt onset of severe substernal chest pain and dyspnea, which resulted in hospitalization and treatment for a suspected myocardial infarction. Following discharge from the hospital he lost 25 to 30 pounds by watching his diet but remained somewhat dyspneic. There was no personal or family history of hypertension or diabetes mellitus. He smoked 3 to 4 cigarettes daily until 2 years ago. Physical examination was normal. Chest roentgenograms showed minimal pleural thickening bilaterally. Resting ECG showed normal QRS complexes and negative T waves in V1 to V3, suggesting right ventricular strain.

EXERCISE FINDINGS

The patient performed exercise on a cycle ergometer. He pedalled at 60 rpm without added load for 3 minutes. The work rate was then increased 15 watts per minute. Blood was sampled every second minute and intra-arterial blood pressure was recorded from a percutaneously placed brachial artery catheter. At 105 watts work rate the pedal came off the cycle ergometer. After 30 minutes rest, the study was restarted with an increase of 20 watts every minute. The patient stopped exercise because of overall fatigue and exhaustion, denying chest pain or dyspnea. There was ½ mm ST segment depression in leads II,

V5 and V6 which disappeared at 3 minutes of recovery.

TABLE 35-1. *Selected Respiratory Function Data*

MEASUREMENT	PREDICTED	MEASURED
Age, yr		50
Sex		Male
Height, cm		185
Weight, kg	86	92
Hematocrit, %		46
VC, L	5.10	4.68
IC, L	3.40	2.94
TLC, L	7.45	5.94
FEV_1, L	4.06	3.62
FEV_1/VC, %	80	77
MVV, L/min	161	152
DL_{CO}, ml/mm Hg/min	32.3	21.2

TABLE 35-2. *Selected Exercise Data*

MEASUREMENT	PREDICTED	MEASURED
Maximum $\dot{V}O_2$, L/min	2.75	1.92
Maximum HR, beats/min	170	164
Maximum O_2 pulse, ml/beat	16.2	11.7
$\Delta\dot{V}O_2/\Delta WR$, ml/min/watt	10.3	8.9
$\dot{V}O_2$ difference, %	0.0	9.5
AT, L/min	> 1.1	0.9
Blood pressure, mm Hg (rest, max)		125/80,161/92
Maximum $\dot{V}E$, L/min		104
Exercise breathing reserve, L/min	> 15	48
PaO_2, mm Hg (rest, max ex)		83,56
$P(A-a)O_2$, mm Hg (rest, max ex)		28,63
$P(a-ET)O_2$, mm Hg (rest, max ex)		5,6
VD/VT (rest, heavy ex)		0.39,0.42
HCO_3^-, mEq/L (rest, 2 min recov)		22,19

TABLE 35-3.

TIME min	WORK RATE W	BP mmHg	HR min⁻¹	f	$\dot{V}E$ BTPS L/min	$\dot{V}CO_2$ STPD L/min	$\dot{V}O_2$ L/min	O_2 pulse ml/beat	R	pH	HCO_3 mEq/L	PO₂ ET mmHg	PO₂ a	PO₂ A-a	PCO₂ ET mmHg	PCO₂ a	PCO₂ a-ET	$\frac{\dot{V}E}{\dot{V}CO_2}$	$\frac{\dot{V}E}{\dot{V}O_2}$	$\frac{VD}{VT}$
Rest	125/ 80									7.41	21	73			34					
Rest			82	22	14.7	0.28	0.35	4.3	0.80			112			29			46	37	
Rest			81	16	12.0	0.23	0.29	3.6	0.79			112			29			46	37	
Unloaded	119/ 83		92	26	26.1	0.55	0.63	6.8	0.87	7.42	22	116	69	33	28	43	15	43	38	0.49
1.0	20		100	22	32.8	0.72	0.86	8.6	0.84			115			28			43	36	
2.0	40		108	22	37.1	0.84	0.99	9.2	0.85			115			28			42	36	
3.0	60		115	25	47.2	1.02	1.16	10.1	0.88			116			28			44	39	
4.0	80		125	29	56.5	1.21	1.31	10.5	0.92			120			25			45	41	
5.0	100	146/ 86	137	28	63.9	1.39	1.47	10.7	0.95	7.43	21	121	60	56	25	33	8	44	42	0.39
6.0	120		147	28	72.8	1.62	1.66	11.3	0.98			123			25			43	42	
7.0	140	161/ 92	156	31	89.7	1.88	1.79	11.5	1.05	7.41	21	124	58	60	24	33	9	46	49	0.42
8.0	160	155/ 86	164	37	104.5	2.07	1.92	11.7	1.08	7.40	20	126	56	63	24	33	9	49	53	0.45
Recovery			127	27	73.4	1.62	1.52	12.0	1.07			122			26			44	47	
Recovery		152/ 86	109	20	35.7	0.84	0.79	7.2	1.06	7.37	19	119	73	45	30	34	4	40	43	0.35

FIGURE 35-A.

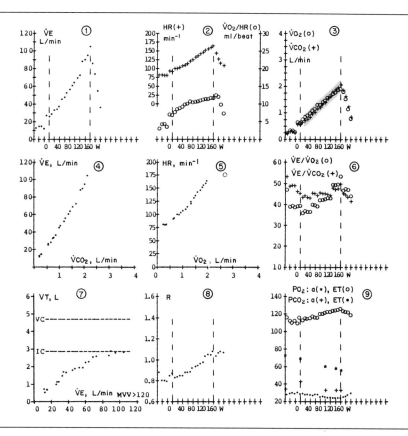

Interpretation

COMMENTS

This case is presented because it illustrates the use of exercise testing for detecting significant pulmonary vascular disease and correcting an erroneous diagnosis. The patient's physician assumed that symptoms of chest pain, dyspnea, and easy fatigability had been due to a myocardial infarction. That diagnosis could not be supported by myocardial enzyme concentrations or specific electrocardiographic changes. Radionuclide ventilation-perfusion scans confirmed the presence of many perfusion without ventilation defects, characteristic of pulmonary thromboembolic disease.

The results of the resting respiratory function studies indicate that this patient had normal lung mechanics. He had a significant reduction in diffusing capacity, however, (Table 35-1). The electrocardiogram was suggestive of right ventricular strain.

ANALYSIS

Flow Chart 1: The maximum $\dot{V}O_2$ and anaerobic threshold are reduced (Table 35-2). See *Flow Chart*

4: The breathing reserve is high *(branchpoint 4.1).* The ventilatory equivalent for CO_2 at the anaerobic threshold is increased *(branchpoint 4.3).* The finding of high VD/VT, $P(A-a)O_2$, $P(a-ET)CO_2$ values throughout exercise confirms that the defect is truly that of an abnormal pulmonary circulation (Table 35-3). Further measurements confirming the diagnosis of pulmonary vascular occlusive disease are the progressive decrease in PaO_2 (Graph 9, Figure 35-A) and the increase in $P(A-a)O_2$ as work rate is increased (Table 35-3). Hemodynamic effects of pulmonary vascular occlusion are reflected in the steep heart rate response as work rate is increased (Graph 5, Fig. 35-A), and the low O_2 pulse at maximum exercise (Table 35-2). The decrease in PaO_2 at the start of exercise was not unusually abrupt and thus did not suggest that a right-to-left shunt had developed in response to exercise *(branchpoint 4.5).*

CONCLUSION

Pulmonary vascular disease limited exercise performance, probably of thromboembolic etiology.

CASE 36 *Pulmonary vasculitis: Air and oxygen breathing*

CLINICAL FINDINGS

This 54-year-old executive was apparently in good health until 11 years ago when he had a documented acute myocardial infarction. Coronary arteriogram was normal one year later. Five years ago he developed fatigue, jaundice, Raynaud's phenomenon, renal failure, and peripheral neuropathy with a histologic diagnosis of membranoproliferative glomerulonephritis secondary to vasculitis. Diffuse cerebritis with panhypopituitarism followed; this responded well to corticosteroids, cyclophosphamide and endocrine-replacement therapy. Three years ago, progressive exertional dyspnea began without cough, pleurisy, or wheezing. A pulmonary nodule developed and was biopsied. Histological examination showed an organizing exudate, hemorrhage, and severe arteriolar wall thickening. The patient had never smoked nor abused drugs or alcohol. Physical examination revealed acrocyanosis without clubbing, clear lungs, and normal heart sounds. Exercise testing was performed to evaluate the possible efficacy of nifedipine. Subjectively, the patient had noted some benefit from its use.

EXERCISE FINDINGS

The patient performed repeated exercise tests on the cycle ergometer. On each occasion he pedalled at 60 rpm without added load for 3 minutes. The work rate was then increased 15 watts every minute.

The first three tests were performed 2 days after nifedipine was discontinued. The second test was 35 minutes after 20 mgms of oral nifedipine; the third test was 190 minutes after nifedipine while breathing 100% oxygen. Blood was sampled every second minute and intra-arterial blood pressure recorded from a percutaneously inserted brachial artery catheter. The fourth test was performed 3 weeks later after five 20 mgm doses of nifedipine over 24 hours, the last just 30 minutes prior to testing.

On all tests the patient stopped due to leg fatigue with complaints of shortness of breath on all but the oxygen test. Resting ECG showed a rightward axis, poor R wave progression in the precordial leads and T wave inversion in V4. There was no ectopy or abnormality of ST segments, although the T wave inversion increased during exercise.

TABLE 36-1. *Selected Respiratory Function Data*

MEASUREMENT	PREDICTED	MEASURED
Age, yr		54
Sex		Male
Height, cm		170
Weight, kg	74	64
Hematocrit, %		38
VC, L	4.03	4.07
IC, L	2.68	3.16
FEV$_1$, L	3.18	3.38
FEV$_1$/VC, %	79	83
MVV, L/min	137	143
DL$_{CO}$, ml/mm Hg/min	26.5	8.0

TABLE 36-2. *Selected Exercise Data*

MEASUREMENT	PREDICTED	TEST 1	TEST 2	TEST 3	TEST 4
Maximum work rate, watts	160	90	90	90	90
Maximum V̇O$_2$, L/min	1.95	0.96	0.99		1.06
Maximum HR, beats/min	166	132	137	131	137
Maximum O$_2$ pulse, ml/beat	11.7	7.3	7.5		8.0
ΔV̇O$_2$/ΔWR, ml/min/watt	10.3	8.8	8.6		8.2
V̇O$_2$ difference, %	0.0	6.7	8.3		9.4
AT, L/min	> 0.78	0.6	0.64		0.8
Blood pressure, mm Hg		129/69	126/72	126/75	118/54
(rest, max)		204/84	201/87	210/90	186/80
Maximum V̇E, L/min		117	131	89	123
Exercise breathing reserve, L/min	> 15	26	12	54	20
Pa$_{O_2}$, mm Hg (rest, max ex)		114,90	122,89	692,678	
P(A−a)$_{O_2}$, mm Hg (rest, max ex)		10,42	0,42		
P(a − ET)$_{CO_2}$, mm Hg (rest, max ex)		7,9	7,9	10,12	
VD/VT (rest, heavy ex)		0.44,0.50	0.43,0.51	0.52,0.56	
HCO$_3^-$, mEq/L (rest, 2 min recov)		18,12	17,12	17,15	

TABLE 36-3. *Air Breathing*

TIME min	WORK RATE W	BP mmHg	HR min⁻¹	f	V̇E BTPS L/min	V̇CO₂ STPD L/min	V̇O₂ STPD L/min	O₂ pulse ml/beat	R	pH	HCO₃⁻ mEq/L	PO₂ ET mmHg	PO₂ a mmHg	PO₂ A-a mmHg	PCO₂ ET mmHg	PCO₂ a mmHg	PCO₂ a-ET mmHg	V̇E/V̇CO₂	V̇E/V̇O₂	VD/VT
Rest		129/ 69								7.38	18		99		31					
Rest			70	13	20.1	0.32	0.29	4.1	1.10			131			19			59	66	
Rest			72	12	22.3	0.34	0.32	4.4	1.06			129			20			63	67	
Rest		126/ 69	71	13	17.3	0.26	0.26	3.7	1.00	7.44	17	130	114	10	19	26	7	62	62	0.44
Rest			73	13	16.1	0.25	0.27	3.7	0.93			129			19			60	55	
Rest			72	13	16.3	0.25	0.26	3.6	0.96			130			20			61	58	
Unloaded			82	22	23.5	0.34	0.34	4.1	1.00			124			22			64	64	
Unloaded			83	16	27.6	0.46	0.53	6.4	0.87			125			21			57	50	
Unloaded		147/ 75	83	19	29.4	0.49	0.54	6.5	0.91	7.41	18	125	96	24	21	28	7	57	51	0.43
1.0	15		88	21	25.8	0.47	0.59	6.7	0.80			119			25			51	41	
2.0	30	156/ 78	98	16	34.9	0.67	0.71	7.2	0.94	7.39	18	124	85	35	23	29	6	50	47	0.39
3.0	45		107	20	48.1	0.86	0.80	7.5	1.08			127			22			54	58	
4.0	60	183/ 84	115	26	68.3	1.10	0.88	7.7	1.25	7.38	17	130	85	41	21	29	8	60	75	0.49
5.0	75		124	29	87.6	1.30	0.95	7.7	1.37			134			19			65	90	
5.5	90	204/ 84	131	40	109.1	1.43	0.96	7.3	1.49	7.39	14	137	90	42	16	25	9	74	110	0.52
Recovery			132	42	116.9	1.47	0.84	6.4	1.75			138			16			77	135	
Recovery		198/ 87	126	32	93.1	1.22	0.78	6.2	1.56	7.33	12	137	86	46	16	25	9	74	116	0.52
Recovery			118	34	70.6	0.87	0.63	5.3	1.38			136			16			78	107	

FIGURE 36-A. *Air Breathing*

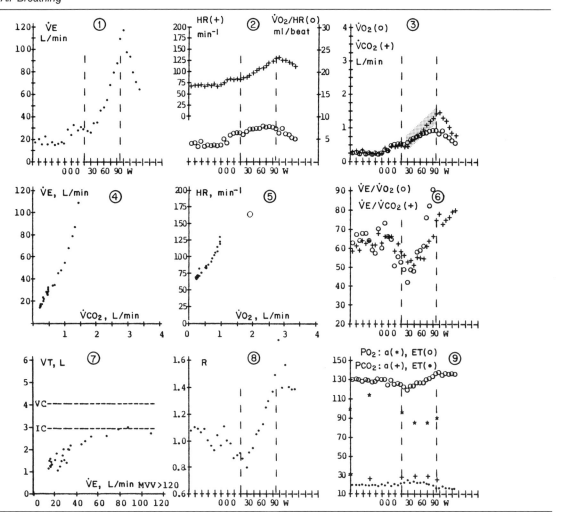

TABLE 36-4. *Oxygen Breathing*

TIME min	WORK RATE W	BP mmHg	HR min⁻¹	f	V̇E BTPS L/min	V̇CO₂ STPD L/min	V̇O₂ STPD L/min	O₂ pulse ml/beat	R	pH	HCO₃⁻ mEq/L	PO₂ ET mmHg	PO₂ a mmHg	PO₂ A-a mmHg	PCO₂ ET mmHg	PCO₂ a mmHg	PCO₂ a-ET mmHg	V̇E/V̇CO₂	V̇E/V̇O₂	VD/VT
Rest			83	12	16.1	0.23									20			66		
Rest			86	12	16.2	0.23									19			66		
Rest		120/ 72	84	12	16.9	0.24				7.40	17		692	-8	19	29	10	66		0.52
Rest			86	12	23.5	0.31									17			73		
Unloaded			91	22	30.2	0.40									19			71		
Unloaded			90	25	21.4	0.35									23			55		
Unloaded		132/ 72	91	19	22.3	0.39				7.36	18		678	1	24	34	10	53		0.48
1.0	15		96	16	30.4	0.55									23			53		
2.0	30	156/ 75	100	19	38.4	0.65				7.35	18		645	34	24	34	10	57		0.53
3.0	45		107	21	43.3	0.73									22			57		
4.0	60	189/ 81	117	27	60.1	0.93				7.35	18		683	-3	20	33	13	62		0.56
5.0	75		124	32	72.0	1.08									20			64		
6.0	90	201/ 81	131	43	89.4	1.26				7.34	17		678	4	19	31	12	68		0.57
6.5	105		127	29	71.7	1.11									21			62		
Recovery			123	32	76.5	1.12									20			66		
Recovery		186/ 78	118	30	62.9	0.78				7.31	15		682	0	19	31	12	77		0.61

Figure 36-B. *Oxygen Breathing*

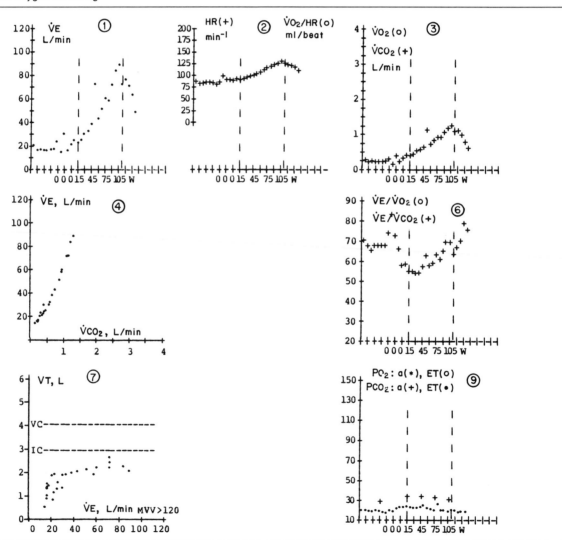

Interpretation

COMMENTS

Except for the very low diffusing capacity, the results of this patient's respiratory function studies are normal (Table 36-1). The patient had four exercise tests to his symptom limited maximum to determine the effect of nifedipine and O_2. Test 1 was performed during air breathing without drugs. Tests 2 and 4 were done to determine the acute and chronic effects, respectively, of nifedipine on this patient's exercise performance. Test 3 was performed to determine the effect of hyperoxia on exercise performance. The graphs and tables containing the detailed data at submaximal work rates are shown for only tests 1 and 3, because the data for tests 2 and 4 are similar to test 1. The summary data are given for all four tests in Table 36-2.

ANALYSIS

Flow Chart 1: The maximum $\dot{V}O_2$ and the anaerobic threshold are significantly reduced (Test 1, Table 36-2). See *Flow Chart 4:* The breathing reserve is normal *(branchpoint 4.1).* The ventilatory equivalent is significantly increased but part of this increase is due to chronic and acute hyperventilation (Table 36-3) *(branchpoint 4.3).* However, the patient has a very high V_D/V_T and abnormal $P(a\text{-}ET)_{CO_2}$ and $P(A\text{-}a)_{O_2}$ at the maximum work rate performed, providing confirmatory evidence of marked ventilation-perfusion mismatching. In view of the patient's normal respiratory mechanics, the ventilation-perfusion abnormality is probably due to pulmonary vascular disease. Further support that pulmonary vascular disease is limiting the cardiac output increase is provided by the confirmatory findings listed in the abnormal pulmonary circulation diagnostic box in *Flow Chart 4:* (1) a steep and steepening heart rate increase with increasing $\dot{V}O_2$ (Graph 5, Fig. 36-A), (2) a low O_2 pulse that fails to increase as work rate is increased (Graph 2, Fig. 36-A), and (3) a low $\Delta\dot{V}O_2/\Delta WR$ that decreases with increasing work rate (Graph 3, Fig. 36-A).

Pa_{O_2} decreases during exercise but remains within the normal range (Graph 9, Fig. 36-A). Test 3, in which Pa_{O_2} was measured during exercise with the patient breathing 100% O_2, confirms the absence of the development of a right-to-left shunt (usually through the foramen ovale). This might be contrasted with Case 37, a patient with pulmonary vascular disease in whom a right-to-left shunt through the foramen ovale did develop during exercise.

Acutely, nifedipine has very little effect (Test 2, Table 36-2). Chronically, the major effect noted is a slightly increased maximum $\dot{V}O_2$, O_2 pulse, and anaerobic threshold (Test 4, Table 36-2). These changes suggest a slight improvement in cardiovascular status. The resting and exercise blood pressure is mildly reduced with the chronically administered nifedipine.

100% O_2 breathing has no effect on this patient's exercise performance. This suggests that this patient has very little vasodilatation in response to high O_2 breathing. Ventilation, however, is considerably reduced with O_2 breathing demonstrating a suppression of ventilatory drive during exercise. Despite this reduction, there is no improvement in exercise performance. This suggests that the patient is not ventilatory limited.

It should be noted that resting arterial bicarbonate is low in all four studies demonstrating a compensated metabolic acidosis at rest. The metabolic acidosis worsens with exercise (Table 36-2).

CONCLUSION

Severe pulmonary vascular disease limited exercise performance.

CASE 37 *Pulmonary hypertension with patent foramen ovale*

CLINICAL FINDINGS

This 61-year-old lady first noted mild exertional dyspnea 3 years prior to evaluation. Four months prior to evaluation she "caught the flu" and soon thereafter developed recurring episodes of depression, confusion, and urinary incontinence. Medical evaluation revealed hypoxemia. With oxygen therapy her mental status returned to normal. She also experienced squeezing substernal chest pain, usually associated with exercise. There was no history of cigarette smoking, exposure to environmental toxins, pulmonary emboli, or thrombophlebitis. She was given alprazolam for her mental symptoms and propranolol for systemic hypertension. On referral, examination revealed mild obesity, hypertension, and a prominent S4. Chest roentgenogram showed enlarged pulmonary arteries. Resting ECG revealed right axis deviation, an R much greater than S in V1, and negative T waves in leads V1 to V4.

EXERCISE FINDINGS

The patient performed exercise on a cycle ergometer. She pedalled at 60 rpm without added load for 3 minutes. The work rate was then increased 5 watts per minute to her symptom limited maximum. Blood was sampled every second minute and intra-arterial blood pressure was recorded from a percutaneously placed brachial artery catheter. She stopped exercise because of shortness of breath. There were no arrhythmias, ST segment, or T wave changes with exercise. Following a rest period of 30 minutes, the exercise study was repeated breathing 100% oxygen.

TABLE 37-1. *Selected Respiratory Function Data*

MEASUREMENT	PREDICTED	MEASURED
Age, yr		61
Sex		Female
Height, cm		147
Weight, kg	53	61
Hematocrit, %		37
VC, L	2.33	2.31
IC, L	1.56	1.59
TLC, L	3.66	4.53
FEV_1, L	1.90	1.59
FEV_1/VC, %	81	69
MVV, L/min	73	59
DL_{CO}, ml/mm Hg/min	17.6	17.3

TABLE 37-2. *Selected Exercise Data*

MEASUREMENT	PREDICTED	ROOM AIR	OXYGEN
Maximum work rate, watts		20	25
Maximum $\dot{V}O_2$, L/min	1.15	0.62	
Maximum HR, beats/min	159	87	85
Maximum O_2 pulse, ml/beat	7.2	7.1	
AT, L/min	>0.46	0.3	
Blood pressure, mm Hg (rest, max)		186/90,204/90	172/84,210/102
Maximum $\dot{V}E$, L/min		38	42
Exercise breathing reserve, L/min	>15	21	17
Pa_{O_2}, mm Hg (rest, max ex)		71,40	550,70
$P(A-a)_{O_2}$, mm Hg (rest, max ex)		42,79	138,612
$P(a-ET)_{CO_2}$, mm Hg (rest, max ex)		5,12	4,9
VD/VT (rest, heavy ex)		0.31,0.47	0.34,0.47
HCO_3^-, mEq/L (rest, 2 min recov)		23,20	22,18

TABLE 37-3. *Air Breathing*

TIME min	WORK RATE W	BP mmHg	HR min⁻¹	f	V̇E BTPS L/min	V̇CO2 STPD L/min	V̇O2 STPD L/min	O2 pulse ml/beat	R	pH	HCO3⁻ mEq/L	PO2 ET mmHg	PO2 a mmHg	PO2 A-a mmHg	PCO2 ET mmHg	PCO2 a mmHg	PCO2 a-ET mmHg	V̇E/V̇CO2	V̇E/V̇O2	VD/VT
Rest		186/ 90								7.56	22		77			24				
Rest			60	11	6.7	0.12	0.16	2.7	0.75			120			23			48	36	
Rest		206/114	61	14	8.4	0.15	0.21	3.4	0.71	7.52	23	120	71	42	23	28	5	48	34	0.31
Unloaded			67	17	11.2	0.20	0.27	4.0	0.74			121			23			49	36	
Unloaded		191/ 94	73	23	14.9	0.27	0.35	4.8	0.77	7.50	23	121	58	55	23	30	7	48	37	0.35
1.0	5		76	23	15.3	0.30	0.39	5.1	0.77			119			25			45	34	
2.0	10	202/ 96	81	27	25.3	0.46	0.52	6.4	0.88	7.47	23	125	43	72	22	32	10	50	44	0.42
3.0	15		84	32	26.6	0.47	0.54	6.4	0.87			124			23			51	44	
4.0	20	204/ 90	87	35	37.7	0.61	0.62	7.1	0.98	7.45	22	130	40	79	19	31	12	57	56	0.47
Recovery			80	28	29.1	0.51	0.55	6.9	0.93			127			21			52	49	
Recovery		198/ 87	79	27	24.8	0.43	0.48	6.1	0.90	7.45	20	126	50	67	22	30	8	52	47	0.41

FIGURE 37-A. *Air Breathing*

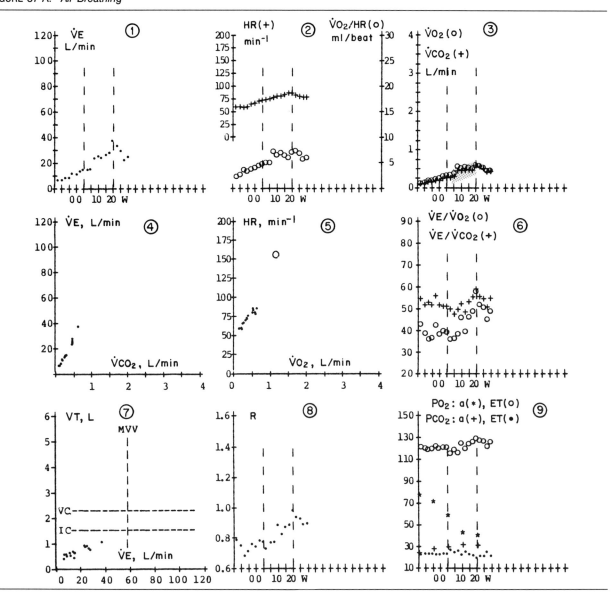

TABLE 37-4. *Oxygen Breathing*

TIME min	WORK RATE W	BP mmHg	HR min⁻¹	f	V̇E BTPS L/min	V̇CO₂ STPD L/min	V̇O₂ STPD L/min	O₂ pulse ml/beat	R	pH	HCO₃⁻ mEq/L	PO₂ ET mmHg	PO₂ a	PO₂ A-a	PCO₂ ET mmHg	PCO₂ a	PCO₂ a-ET	V̇E/V̇CO₂	V̇E/V̇O₂	VD/VT
Rest		171/ 78								7.50	21	67			28					
Rest			58	16	9.9	0.14									20			61		
Rest		172/ 84	58	15	9.3	0.14				7.53	20	550	138		21	25	4	57		0.34
Unloaded			68	27	14.5	0.20									21			61		
Unloaded		180/ 87	67	29	16.5	0.26				7.43	22	386	297		22	30	8	54		0.40
Unloaded			70	23	17.5	0.31									23			50		
1.0	5		73	26	18.3	0.32									25			50		
2.0	10	180/ 84	77	26	24.2	0.42				7.44	22	100	580		23	33	10	52		0.45
3.0	15		81	34	29.9	0.48									22			56		
4.0	20	210/102	84	32	34.5	0.56				7.45	21	70	612		22	31	9	57		0.47
4.5	25		85	36	42.3	0.64									19			61		
Recovery			80	31	38.4	0.62									20			58		
Recovery			76	24	28.2	0.49									21			53		

FIGURE 37-B. *Oxygen Breathing*

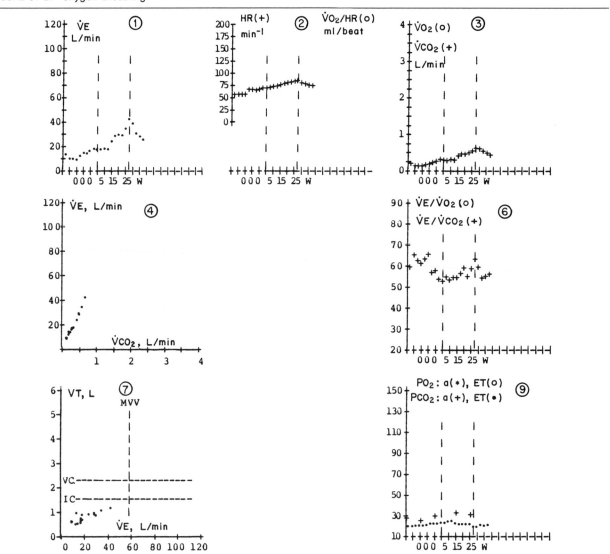

Interpretation

COMMENTS

The results of this patient's resting respiratory function tests show mild airway obstruction (Table 37-1). The electrocardiogram is compatible with right ventricular hypertrophy. The exercise test was repeated with the subject breathing 100% oxygen in order to evaluate the possible development of a right-to-left shunt through a foramen ovale when exercise-induced right atrial pressure exceeds left atrial pressure — a possible cause of activity-induced hypoxemia, which might contribute to this patient's symptoms.

ANALYSIS

Flow Chart 1: The maximum oxygen uptake and the anaerobic threshold are significantly reduced (Table 37-2). See *Flow Chart 4:* The breathing reserve is normal *(branchpoint 4.1).* The $\dot{V}_E/\dot{V}_{CO_2}$ at the anaerobic threshold is high *(branchpoint 4.3).* The patient is hyperventilating, however, and the arterial CO_2 must be taken into account (Fig. 3-13), or the indices of ventilation-perfusion mismatching $(V_D/V_T, P(A-a)_{O_2}$ and $P(a-ET)_{CO_2})$ must be directly measured. Since they were measured and, in fact, are quite high (Table 37-3), the diagnosis of an abnormal pulmonary circulation is made. The abnormal measurements listed under this diagnosis provides confirmation.

At the lowest work rate, Pa_{O_2} abruptly decreases and continues to decrease as the work rate is increased. Also, $P(a-ET)_{CO_2}$ continues to increase as work rate is increased and the abnormalities in V_D/V_T become progressively more severe (Table 37-3). The changes in Pa_{O_2}, P_{CO_2} and V_D/V_T suggest the development of a right-to-left shunt during exercise. Clearly, the patient is also oxygen-flow limited in that $\dot{V}_{O_2}$ and oxygen pulse fail to increase with increasing work rate (Graphs 3 and 2, respectively, Fig. 37-A).

To document that a right-to-left shunt develops with exercise, Pa_{O_2} was measured at rest and during exercise while breathing 100% oxygen. At rest, Pa_{O_2} is normal (550 mm Hg); with mild exercise, it drops to 70 mm Hg. This can be explained only by the development of a right-to-left shunt with exercise (in contrast with Case 36).

Subsequently, the patient had a right heart catheterization. Pulmonary artery pressures were confirmed to be at systemic pressure levels; the catheter slipped easily through the foramen ovale into the left atrium.

CONCLUSION

Pulmonary hypertension with an exercise-induced right-to-left shunt through a foramen ovale.

CASE 38 *Pulmonary vascular disease, primary or secondary*

CLINICAL FINDINGS

This 61-year-old shipyard worker noted occasional chest pain with effort following a myocardial infarction 15 years prior to evaluation. He also noted slight shortness of breath when walking rapidly about 3 blocks. He had a 45 pack year history of smoking. He had a frequent cough, scant sputum, and occasional wheezing. He took no medication. A physical examination revealed fine end-inspiratory rales at both lung bases. Chest roentgenogram revealed bilateral minimal pleural and parenchymal scarring. There was slight improvement in flow rates after inhalation of isoproterenol. ECG showed an old inferior wall infarction.

EXERCISE FINDINGS

The patient performed exercise on a cycle ergometer. He pedalled at 60 rpm without added load for 3 minutes. The work rate was then increased 15 watts per minute to his symptom limited maximum. Blood was sampled every second minute and intra-arterial blood pressure was recorded from a percutaneously placed brachial artery catheter. The patient stopped exercise due to general fatigue. There were no abnormal ST segments or arrhythmia.

TABLE 38-1. *Selected Respiratory Function Data*

MEASUREMENT	PREDICTED	MEASURED
Age, yr		61
Sex		Male
Height, cm		173
Weight, kg	76	82
Hematocrit, %		42
VC, L	4.00	3.46
IC, L	2.67	2.69
TLC, L	6.15	6.74
FEV_1, L	3.13	2.17
FEV_1, VC, %	78	63
MVV, L/min	131	101
DL_{CO}, ml/mm Hg/min	27.1	17.8

TABLE 38-2. *Selected Exercise Data*

MEASUREMENT	PREDICTED	MEASURED
Maximum $\dot{V}O_2$, L/min	2.13	1.43
Maximum HR, beats/min	159	130
Maximum O_2 pulse, ml/beat	13.4	11.0
$\Delta\dot{V}O_2/\Delta WR$, ml/min/watt	10.3	9.0
$\dot{V}O_2$ difference, %	0.0	8.0
AT, L/min	>0.85	0.7
Blood pressure, mm Hg (rest, max)		156/87,213/93
Maximum $\dot{V}E$, L/min		64
Exercise breathing reserve, L/min	>15	37
Pa_{O_2}, mm Hg (rest, max ex)		81,96
$P(A-a)_{O_2}$, mm Hg (rest, max ex)		29,22
$P(a-ET)_{CO_2}$, mm Hg (rest, max ex)		7,2
VD/VT (rest, heavy ex)		0.48,0.37
HCO_3^-, mEq/L (rest, 2 min recov)		22,18

TABLE 38-3.

TIME min	WORK RATE W	BP mmHg	HR min⁻¹	f	$\dot{V}E$ BTPS	$\dot{V}CO_2$	$\dot{V}O_2$	O_2 pulse	R	pH	HCO_3^- mEq/L	PO2 ET	PO2 a	PO2 A-a	PCO2 ET	PCO2 a	PCO2 a-ET	$\dot{V}E$/$\dot{V}CO_2$	$\dot{V}E$/$\dot{V}O_2$	VD/VT
Rest		156/ 87								7.41	22	80			36					
Rest			80	20	14.5	0.24	0.28	3.5	0.86			117			28			53	46	
Rest		162/ 87	80	19	13.2	0.22	0.25	3.1	0.88	7.41	22	117	81	29	29	36	7	52	46	0.48
Rest			80	22	15.1	0.24	0.28	3.5	0.86			118			28			55	47	
Unloaded			93	19	21.1	0.43	0.50	5.4	0.86			113			31			45	39	
Unloaded			95	19	22.6	0.48	0.56	5.9	0.86			112			32			44	38	
Unloaded		183/ 84	95	20	24.7	0.53	0.59	6.2	0.90	7.40	22	113	92	19	31	36	5	43	39	0.42
1.0	15		96	19	26.9	0.62	0.69	7.2	0.90			112			32			41	37	
2.0	30	186/ 87	100	23	28.6	0.57	0.65	6.5	0.88	7.39	22	112	88	21	32	37	5	47	41	0.47
3.0	45		109	21	33.6	0.76	0.82	7.5	0.93			112			33			42	39	
4.0	60	204/ 90	114	24	40.2	0.91	0.91	8.0	1.00	7.39	22	115	93	20	33	37	4	42	42	0.42
5.0	75		119	27	47.3	1.09	1.06	8.9	1.03			116			32			41	42	
6.0	90	216/ 93	123	29	52.7	1.25	1.18	9.6	1.06	7.37	20	117	94	23	32	35	3	40	43	0.37
7.0	105	213/ 93	130	31	64.4	1.53	1.43	11.0	1.07	7.37	19	118	96	22	32	34	2	40	43	0.36
Recovery			116	34	51.5	1.24	1.07	9.2	1.16			118			33			39	45	
Recovery		204/ 90	112	38	32.4	0.70	0.59	5.3	1.19	7.35	18	116	107	14	35	33	-2	42	49	0.33

FIGURE 38-A.

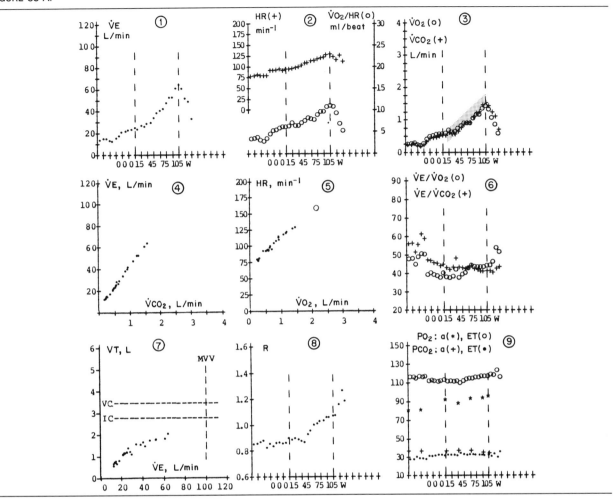

Interpretation

COMMENTS

This patient has mild airflow obstruction and a moderate reduction in diffusing capacity (Table 38-1). The resting electrocardiogram shows evidence of an old inferior wall infarction.

ANALYSIS

Flow Chart 1: The maximum $\dot{V}O_2$ and anaerobic threshold are significantly reduced (Table 38-2). See *Flow Chart 4:* The breathing reserve is normal *(branchpoint 4.1).* The ventilatory equivalent for CO_2 at the anaerobic threshold is significantly elevated. While the Pa_{CO_2} is slightly reduced *(branchpoint 4.3),* hyperventilation does not account for the high ventilatory equivalent. Ventilation-perfusion mismatching is confirmed by the high V_D/V_T and positive $P(a-_{ET})_{CO_2}$ during exercise. $P(A-a)_{O_2}$ and Pa_{O_2} are normal at rest and remain normal during exercise, suggesting that the ventilation-perfusion abnormality does not consist of many low $\dot{V}A/\dot{Q}$ lung units (as with airway disease) but rather a reduction of perfusion relative to ventilation (as with pulmonary vascular disease). Supporting the diagnosis of pulmonary vascular disease is the moderate reduction in diffusing capacity. Some of the other supporting data that one might expect to find with hemodynamically important pulmonary vascular disease, e.g., a steep heart rate response, a low O_2 pulse, and decreasing $\Delta\dot{V}O_2/\Delta WR$ with increasing work rate, are not evident. The patient did not hyperventilate in response to the metabolic acidosis (see $\dot{V}E/\dot{V}CO_2$, Graph 6, Fig. 38-A). The pulmonary vascular abnormalities may be secondary to interstitial or obstructive airway disease.

CONCLUSION

Pulmonary vascular defect, primary or secondary to lung disease, at an early stage of development.

CASE 39 *Pulmonary vascular disease of unknown etiology*

CLINICAL FINDINGS

This 64-year-old gentleman was evaluated because of increasing dyspnea on exertion. He was a retired shipyard worker who had hypertension for many years that was being treated with a beta-adrenergic blocking drug. He never smoked cigarettes but did smoke a pipe and 3 cigars daily. Physical examination was unremarkable except for bilaterally absent dorsalis pedis and posterior tibial pulsations. Chest roentgenograms were normal except for fullness in the right hilum, which was considered to be vascular on tomography.

EXERCISE FINDINGS

The patient performed exercise on a cycle ergometer. He pedalled at 60 rpm without added load for 3 minutes. The work rate was then increased 15 watts per minute to his symptom limited maximum. Blood was sampled every second minute and intra-arterial blood pressure was recorded from a percutaneously placed brachial artery catheter. Resting and exercise ECG recordings were normal. Patient stopped exercising because of general fatigue.

TABLE 39-1. *Selected Respiratory Function Data*

MEASUREMENT	PREDICTED	MEASURED
Age, yr		64
Sex		Male
Height, cm		178
Weight, kg	79	87
Hematocrit, %		46
VC, L	3.82	4.38
IC, L	2.55	3.43
TLC, L	5.93	6.19
FEV_1, L	2.98	3.14
FEV_1/VC, %	78	72
MVV, L/min	121	129
DL_{CO}, ml/min Hg/min	22.0	21.5

TABLE 39-2. *Selected Exercise Data*

MEASUREMENT	PREDICTED	MEASURED
Maximum $\dot{V}O_2$, L/min	2.15	1.78
Maximum HR, beats/min	156	135
Maximum O_2 pulse, ml/beat	13.8	14.0
$\Delta\dot{V}O_2/\Delta WR$, ml/min/watt	10.3	8.9
$\dot{V}O_2$ difference, %	0.0	8.5
AT, L/min	>0.90	1.1
Blood pressure, mm Hg (rest, max)		152/98,212/110
Maximum $\dot{V}E$, L/min		89
Exercise breathing reserve, L/min	>15	40
Pa_{O_2}, mm Hg (rest, max ex)		81,77
$P(A-a)_{O_2}$, mm Hg (rest, max ex)		30,44
$P(a-ET)_{CO_2}$, mm Hg (rest, max ex)		4,2
VD/VT (rest, heavy ex)		0.37,0.34
HCO_3^-, mEq/L (rest, 2 min recov)		25,19

TABLE 39-3.

TIME min	WORK RATE W	BP mmHg	HR min⁻¹	f	V̇E BTPS L/min	V̇CO2 STPD L/min	V̇O2 STPD L/min	O2 pulse ml/beat	R	pH	HCO3 mEq/L	PO2 ET mmHg	PO2 a mmHg	PO2 A-a mmHg	PCO2 ET mmHg	PCO2 a mmHg	PCO2 a-ET mmHg	V̇E/V̇CO2	V̇E/V̇O2	VD/VT
Rest	152/ 98									7.43	25	85			38					
Rest			66	19	13.4	0.30	0.33	5.0	0.91			111			33			39	36	
Rest			66	17	11.7	0.27	0.28	4.2	0.96			113			33			38	37	
Rest	152/ 98		66	17	11.5	0.25	0.27	4.1	0.93	7.42	24	113	81	30	33	37	4	40	37	0.37
Unloaded			81	21	21.8	0.57	0.65	8.0	0.88			107			35			35	31	
Unloaded			82	26	26.5	0.68	0.74	9.0	0.92			108			36			36	33	
Unloaded		191/110	83	28	26.7	0.69	0.75	9.0	0.92	7.41	24	110	80	28	35	39	4	35	32	0.34
1.0	15		84	30	29.5	0.74	0.79	9.4	0.94			111			34			36	34	
2.0	30	191/104	91	30	31.0	0.81	0.90	9.9	0.90	7.42	24	109	74	35	35	38	3	35	32	0.32
3.0	45		99	30	37.3	0.99	1.07	10.8	0.93			110			35			35	32	
4.0	60	209/110	106	31	41.1	1.10	1.17	11.0	0.94	7.41	24	111	69	40	35	39	4	35	33	0.34
5.0	75		110	39	52.6	1.38	1.38	12.5	1.00			112			35			36	36	
6.0	90	212/107	118	34	57.0	1.56	1.50	12.7	1.04	7.40	23	114	72	41	34	38	4	35	36	0.33
7.0	105		121	41	68.5	1.79	1.65	13.6	1.08			117			33			36	39	
8.0	120	212/110	126	53	89.3	2.04	1.77	14.0	1.15	7.40	21	121	73	47	29	34	5	42	48	0.37
8.5	135	188/ 95	135	52	88.2	2.02	1.78	13.2	1.13	7.41	20	120	77	44	30	32	2	41	47	0.33
Recovery			118	38	67.4	1.79	1.66	14.1	1.08			117			33			36	39	
Recovery			95	39	58.9	1.34	0.95	10.0	1.41			125			29			41	59	
Recovery		188/104								7.38	19	110			32					

FIGURE 39-A.

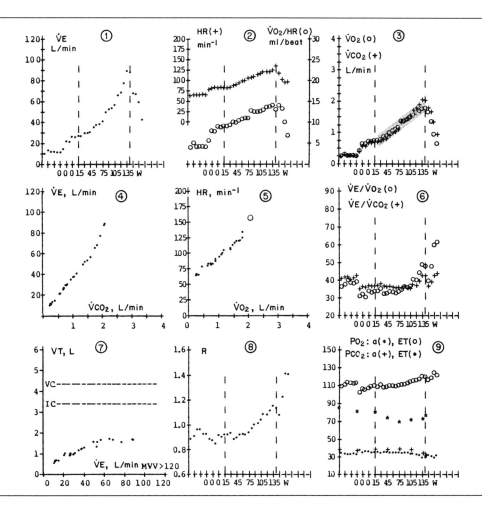

Interpretation

COMMENTS

This patient's lung mechanics and resting diffusing capacity are normal (Table 39-1). The resting electrocardiogram is normal. The patient is slightly overweight and has hypertension that is being treated with a beta-adrenergic blocking drug.

ANALYSIS

Flow Chart 1: Maximum $\dot{V}O_2$ is slightly reduced but the anaerobic threshold is normal (Table 39-2). See *Flow Chart 3:* The breathing reserve is normal *(branchpoint 3.1)*. The ECG is normal *(branchpoint 3.3)*. This leads to the diagnosis of poor effort or limitation because of musculoskeletal disorder. This is obviously an incorrect diagnosis, however, because a $\dot{V}O_2$ max is reached, i.e. a plateau in $\dot{V}O_2$ in response to increasing work rate (Graph 3, Fig. 39-A). Also, the HCO_3^- decrease of 6 mEq/L at the two minute

recovery period and increase in R at maximum exercise reflect good effort. Despite the observation that the measurements of respiratory function are normal at rest, hypoxemia develops during exercise and the $P(A-a)O_2$ increases as work rate is increased. Also, $P(a-ET)CO_2$ and VD/VT at maximum exercise are abnormally elevated. Therefore, we must conclude that this patient has ventilation-perfusion mismatching during exercise, consistent with pulmonary vascular disease. The severity is such that the diffusing capacity measurement is not abnormal at rest, although it might not have increased normally if measured during exercise.

CONCLUSION

Ventilation-perfusion mismatching probably secondary to pulmonary vascular disease of unknown etiology. Contributing factors to the patient's symptoms of dyspnea might be his systemic hypertension and obesity.

CASE 40 *Pulmonary vascular disease and mild chronic bronchitis*

CLINICAL FINDINGS

A 55-year-old former shipyard worker first noted exertional dyspnea and a morning cough with small amounts of sputum approximately five years ago. He retired three years ago because of an injury to the left foot. The patient had a sixty pack year smoking history but stopped one year ago. Hypertension, diagnosed one year previously, was being treated with hydrochlorothiazide and propranolol. There is no history of angina or congestive heart failure. Examination revealed normal breath sounds, cardiovascular examination, and peripheral pulses. Chest roentgenograms showed minimal pleural plaques without evidence of parenchymal lung disease.

EXERCISE FINDINGS

The patient performed exercise on a cycle ergometer. He pedalled at 60 rpm without added load for 3 minutes. The work rate was then increased 20 watts per minute to his symptom limited maximum. Blood was sampled every second minute and intra-arterial blood pressure was recorded from a percutaneously placed brachial artery catheter. Resting and exercise ECGs were normal except for relative bradycardia. The patient stopped exercise complaining of general fatigue and shortness of breath.

TABLE 40-1. *Selected Respiratory Function Data*

MEASUREMENT	PREDICTED	MEASURED
Age, yr		55
Sex		Male
Height, cm		173
Weight, kg	76	85
Hematocrit, %		48
VC, L	4.20	4.54
IC, L	2.80	3.66
TLC, L	6.26	6.88
FEV_1, L	3.32	3.16
FEV_1/VC, %	79	70
MVV, L/min	140	121
DL_{CO}, ml/mm Hg/min	28.1	16.6

TABLE 40-2. *Selected Exercise Data*

MEASUREMENT	PREDICTED	MEASURED
Maximum $\dot{V}O_2$, L/min	2.30	1.59
Maximum HR, beats/min	165	113
Maximum O_2 pulse, ml/beat	13.9	14.4
$\Delta\dot{V}O_2/\Delta WR$, ml/min/watt	10.3	9.8
$\dot{V}O_2$ difference, %	0.0	2.9
AT, L/min	>0.92	0.7
Blood pressure, mm Hg (rest, max)		182/107,206/113
Maximum $\dot{V}E$, L/min		72
Exercise breathing reserve, L/min	>15	49
Pa_{O_2}, mm Hg (rest, max ex)		73,71
$P(A-a)_{O_2}$, mm Hg (rest, max ex)		31,46
$P(a-ET)_{CO_2}$, mm Hg (rest, max ex)		3,4
VD/VT (rest, heavy ex)		0.33,0.35
HCO_3^-, mEq/L (rest, 2 min recov)		24,18

TABLE 40-3.

TIME min	WORK RATE W	BP mmHg	HR min⁻¹	f	$\dot{V}E$ BTPS L/min	$\dot{V}CO_2$ STPD L/min	$\dot{V}O_2$ STPD L/min	O_2 pulse ml/beat	R	pH	HCO_3^- mEq/L	PO₂ ET mmHg	PO₂ a mmHg	PO₂ A-a mmHg	PCO₂ ET mmHg	PCO₂ a mmHg	PCO₂ a-ET mmHg	$\dot{V}E/\dot{V}CO_2$	$\dot{V}E/\dot{V}O_2$	VD/VT
Rest										7.47	24	59			33					
Rest			57	17	11.0	0.21	0.29	5.1	0.72			109			31			46	33	
Rest		182/107	57	14	12.1	0.25	0.32	5.6	0.78			113			29			44	34	
Rest			57	12	8.9	0.20	0.28	4.9	0.71	7.45	24	108	73	31	32	35	3	40	28	0.33
Unloaded		193/107	69	19	18.5	0.40	0.53	7.7	0.75			107			33			42	32	
Unloaded			69	17	19.5	0.50	0.64	9.3	0.78			106			34			36	28	
Unloaded			70	19	21.4	0.54	0.66	9.4	0.82	7.44	24	110	73	36	33	35	2	37	30	0.30
1.0	20	194/107	73	17	21.6	0.57	0.67	9.2	0.85			109			34			35	30	
2.0	40		79	20	32.2	0.85	0.94	11.9	0.90	7.44	24	111	72	40	33	35	2	36	32	0.30
3.0	60	197/110	83	21	35.4	0.95	1.01	11.5	0.94			112			34			35	33	
4.0	80		97	22	44.0	1.21	1.21	12.5	1.00	7.42	25	113	70	41	34	39	5	35	35	0.35
5.0	100	206/113	104	28	61.0	1.52	1.45	13.9	1.05			117			32			39	40	
6.0	120		113	31	66.4	1.65	1.56	13.8	1.06	7.42	23	118	71	46	31	35	4	39	41	0.35
Recovery		213/107	89	29	58.6	1.37	1.22	13.7	1.12			120			30			41	46	
Recovery			77	25	39.0	0.87	0.73	9.5	1.19	7.40	18	123	86	39	29	29	0	42	50	0.28

FIGURE 40-A.

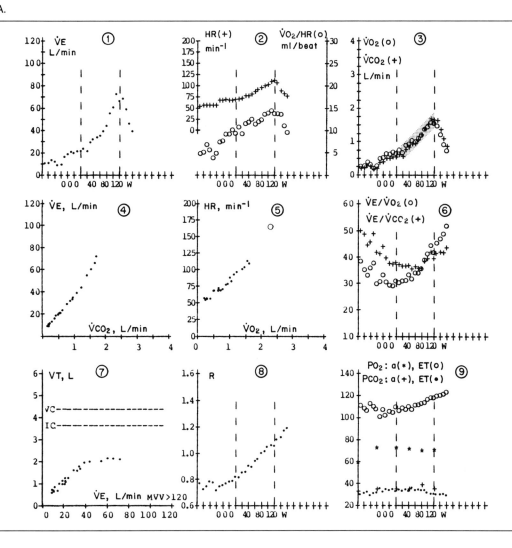

Interpretation

COMMENTS

The mechanics of breathing are normal but the diffusing capacity is significantly reduced (Table 40-1). The resting electrocardiogram is normal.

ANALYSIS

Flow Chart 1: Maximum $\dot{V}_{O_2}$ and the anaerobic threshold are reduced (Table 40-2). See *Flow Chart 4:* The breathing reserve is high *(branchpoint 4.1)*. The ventilatory equivalent for CO_2 at the anaerobic threshold is high *(branchpoint 4.3)*. This suggests that the patient has an abnormal pulmonary circulation. Confirmation of this is demonstrated by high V_D/V_T, $P(A-a)_{O_2}$, and $P(a-ET)_{CO_2}$ values (indices of ventilation-perfusion mismatching). Since there is no associated disturbance in respiratory mechanics, we must conclude that these findings are on the basis of primary pulmonary vascular disease. The significant reduction in diffusing capacity (DL_{CO}) is compatible with this conclusion. There is no abrupt decrease in Pa_{O_2} or O_2 saturation at the start of exercise *(branchpoint 4.5)*, indicating that a right-to-left shunt does not accompany the pulmonary vascular disease. Because the patient is being treated with propranolol, the heart rate response is unusually low for this kind of abnormality. The systemic hypertension and beta-adrenergic blockade might be contributing factors to the low maximum $\dot{V}_{O_2}$ and anaerobic threshold.

CONCLUSION

Exercise limitation caused by pulmonary vascular disease. Systemic hypertension might be contributory. Beta-adrenergic blockade prevents a normal heart rate response.

CASE 41 *Pulmonary vascular disease, probably secondary to asbestosis*

CLINICAL FINDINGS

This 66-year-old shipyard worker stated that he was in excellent health. Two weeks prior to evaluation he had an episode of severe shortness of breath, awakening him from his sleep at a Colorado camp site at 11,000 feet of altitude. He had driven there from Los Angeles in the previous 24 hours. He had no relief until he was driven down to an altitude of 7,000 feet. He had a 40 pack year history of cigarette smoking with a nonproductive cough. He denied other symptoms. The physical examination was normal except for mild obesity. Chest roentgenograms revealed moderate nodular pleural plaques with evidence of minimal pulmonary fibrosis. Resting ECG showed left anterior superior hemiblock.

EXERCISE FINDINGS

The patient performed exercise on a cycle ergometer. He pedalled at 60 rpm without added load for 3 minutes. The work rate was then increased 20 watts per minute to his symptom limited maximum. Blood was sampled every second minute and intra-arterial blood pressure was recorded from a percutaneously placed brachial artery catheter. The patient stopped exercising because of leg fatigue and shortness of breath. Exercise ECGs were normal except for the appearance of infrequent premature ventricular contractions during the last two work rates.

TABLE 41-1. *Selected Respiratory Function Data*

MEASUREMENT	PREDICTED	MEASURED
Age, yr		66
Sex		Male
Height, cm		178
Weight, kg	80	84
Hematocrit, %		41
VC, L	4.18	3.48
IC, L	2.79	2.96
TLC, L	6.56	5.95
FEV_1, L	3.26	2.76
FEV_1/VC, %	78	79
MVV, L/min	132	93
DL_{CO}, ml/mm Hg/min	25.6	22.7

TABLE 41-2. *Selected Exercise Data*

MEASUREMENT	PREDICTED	MEASURED
Maximum $\dot{V}O_2$, L/min	2.06	1.58
Maximum HR, beats/min	154	141
Maximum O_2 pulse, ml/beat	13.4	11.6
$\Delta\dot{V}O_2/\Delta WR$, ml/min/watt	10.3	7.7
$\dot{V}O_2$ difference, %	0.0	15.7
AT, L/min	>0.82	indeterminate
Blood pressure, mm Hg (rest, max)		167/86,241/104
Maximum $\dot{V}E$, L/min		70
Exercise breathing reserve, L/min	>15	23
PaO_2, mm Hg (rest, max ex)		87,90
$P(A-a)O_2$, mm Hg (rest, max ex)		19,23
$P(a-ET)CO_2$, mm Hg (rest, max ex)		−2,3
VD/VT (rest, heavy ex)		0.38,0.33
HCO_3^-, mEq/L (rest, 2 min recov)		24,16

TABLE 41-3.

TIME min	WORK RATE W	BP mmHg	HR min⁻¹	f	$\dot{V}E$ BTPS L/min	$\dot{V}CO_2$ STPD L/min	$\dot{V}O_2$ STPD L/min	O_2 pulse ml/beat	R	pH	HCO_3^- mEq/L	PO2 ET mmHg	PO2 a mmHg	PO2 A-a mmHg	PCO2 ET mmHg	PCO2 a mmHg	PCO2 a-ET mmHg	$\dot{V}E/\dot{V}CO_2$	$\dot{V}E/\dot{V}O_2$	VD/VT
Rest		167/ 86								7.42	24	78			37					
Rest			89	18	17.8	0.41	0.53	6.0	0.77			102			35			40	31	
Rest		161/ 89	87	20	13.6	0.28	0.36	4.1	0.78	7.41	23	102	87	19	38	36	−2	42	33	0.38
Rest			91	15	16.3	0.38	0.45	4.9	0.84			105			36			39	33	
Unloaded			102	20	21.4	0.50	0.62	6.1	0.81			107			34			39	32	
Unloaded			103	20	21.5	0.53	0.64	6.2	0.83			103			38			37	31	
Unloaded		191/ 95	105	20	23.0	0.59	0.69	6.6	0.86	7.39	23	106	85	21	37	39	2	36	31	0.36
1.0	20		107	20	25.8	0.66	0.74	6.9	0.89			109			35			37	33	
2.0	40	194/ 92	109	21	30.5	0.84	0.99	9.1	0.85	7.39	23	107	81	25	36	39	3	34	29	0.33
3.0	60		116	20	29.0	0.84	0.98	8.4	0.86			101			42			33	28	
4.0	80	218/ 98	122	23	39.1	1.11	1.14	9.3	0.97	7.37	22	109	84	26	38	39	1	33	33	0.32
5.0	100		126	26	48.3	1.41	1.37	10.9	1.03			110			38			33	34	
6.0	120	239/ 98	133	29	57.8	1.68	1.50	11.3	1.12	7.34	21	113	90	23	37	40	3	33	37	0.33
7.0	140	241/104	141	35	65.0	1.82	1.53	10.9	1.19			116			37			34	41	
Recovery			131	27	62.4	1.70	1.23	9.4	1.38			121			36			35	49	
Recovery		200/ 80	120	26	43.3	1.04	0.65	5.4	1.60	7.29	16	126	120	5	32	35	3	40	63	0.36

FIGURE 41-A.

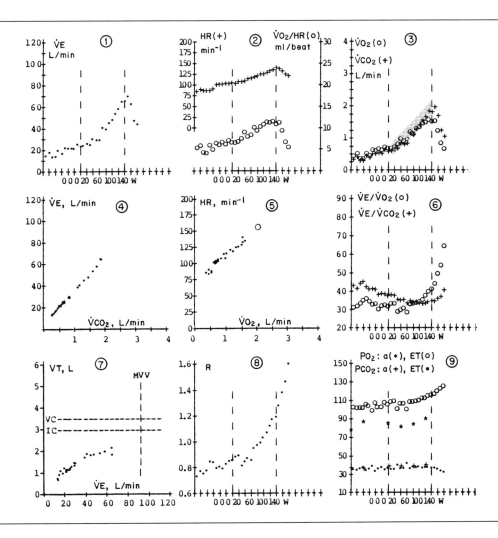

Interpretation

COMMENTS

Results of the resting respiratory function studies show the vital capacity to be at the low end of the normal range (Table 41-1). The resting ECG is slightly abnormal as noted in "Clinical Findings."

ANALYSIS

Flow Chart 1: The maximum $\dot{V}O_2$ is reduced and the anaerobic threshold is indeterminate (Table 41-2). See *Flow Chart 5:* The VD/VT and $P(a–ET)_{CO_2}$ are elevated, although $P(A–a)_{O_2}$ is within normal limits *(branchpoint 5.1)*. Taking the abnormal branch, the breathing reserve is found to be normal *(branchpoint 5.3)*. Pa_{O_2} does not decrease with increasing work rate *(branchpoint 5.6)*. The results of these findings are compatible with a circulatory limi-

tation. The ECG is normal except for infrequent premature ventricular contractions. The patient does not have a chronic metabolic acidosis but does develop an acute metabolic acidosis at the highest work rate performed (Table 41-3). $\Delta\dot{V}O_2/\Delta WR$ is low (Table 41-2) and $\dot{V}O_2$ and O_2 pulse fail to increase as the subject approaches his symptom limited maximum work rate, confirmatory evidence of a circulatory limitation. The abnormalities in gas exchange at the lung are compatible with pulmonary vascular disease. However, systemic hypertension and peripheral vascular disease might also be contributory to the impaired O_2 utilization.

CONCLUSION

Circulatory limitation. Pulmonary vascular disease possibly secondary to fibrosing alveolitis.

CASE 42 *Pulmonary vascular disease, secondary to interstitial and obstructive lung disease*

CLINICAL FINDINGS

This 70-year-old retired shipyard worker complained of shortness of breath after climbing one flight of stairs. He had a 50 pack year smoking history but stopped 3 months prior to the evaluation. He took triamterene, hydrochlorothiazide, and methyldopa for hypertension but denied any history of heart or lung disease. The physical examination was not remarkable. Resting ECG showed left axis deviation, left atrial enlargement, and left ventricular hypertrophy. Chest roentgenograms showed moderate pleural thickening with some calcification plus moderate interstitial fibrosis.

EXERCISE FINDINGS

The patient performed exercise on a cycle ergometer. He pedalled at 60 rpm without added load for 3 minutes. The work rate was then increased 15 watts per minute to his symptom limited maximum. Blood was sampled every second minute and intra-arterial blood pressure was recorded from a percutaneously placed brachial artery catheter. Except for an increase in rate, the ECG pattern remained unchanged during exercise. The patient stopped exercise because of shortness of breath and a dry mouth.

TABLE 42-1. *Selected Respiratory Function Data*

MEASUREMENT	PREDICTED	MEASURED
Age, yr		70
Sex		Male
Height, cm		187
Weight, kg	87	76
Hematocrit, %		47
VC, L	4.69	3.64
IC, L	3.13	2.28
TLC, L	7.39	6.02
FEV_1, L	3.65	2.19
FEV_1/VC, %	78	60
MVV, L/min	140	90
DL_{CO}, ml/mm Hg/min	29.4	10.8

TABLE 42-2. *Selected Exercise Data*

MEASUREMENT	PREDICTED	MEASURED
Maximum $\dot{V}O_2$, L/min	1.85	1.32
Maximum HR, beats/min	150	152
Maximum O_2 pulse, ml/beat	12.3	8.7
$\Delta\dot{V}O_2/\Delta WR$, ml/min/watt	10.3	7.4
$\dot{V}O_2$ difference, %	0.0	17.3
AT, L/min	>0.74	<0.6
Blood pressure, mm Hg (rest, max)		176/86,227/89
Maximum $\dot{V}E$, L/min		88
Exercise breathing reserve, L/min	>15	2
PaO_2, mm Hg (rest, max ex)		62,52
$P(A-a)O_2$, mm Hg (rest, max ex)		48,68
$P(a-ET)CO_2$, mm Hg (rest, max ex)		9,4
VD/VT (rest, heavy ex)		0.49,0.48
HCO_3^-, mEq/L (rest, 2 min recov)		27,19

TABLE 42-3.

TIME min	WORK RATE W	BP mmHg	HR min⁻¹	f	$\dot{V}E$ BTPS L/min	$\dot{V}CO_2$ STPD L/min	$\dot{V}O_2$ STPD L/min	O_2 pulse ml/beat	R	pH	HCO_3^- mEq L	ET PO₂ mmHg	a PO₂	A-a PO₂	ET PCO₂ mmHg	a PCO₂	a-ET PCO₂	$\dfrac{\dot{V}E}{\dot{V}CO_2}$	$\dfrac{\dot{V}E}{\dot{V}O_2}$	$\dfrac{VD}{VT}$
Rest		176/ 86								7.45	27	59			39					
Rest			89	22	18.8	0.34	0.37	4.2	0.92			116			30			50	46	
Rest			89	20	16.0	0.30	0.33	3.7	0.91			114			31			48	43	
Rest			88	19	15.2	0.30	0.32	3.6	0.94			115			31			45	43	
Rest			89	22	17.8	0.33	0.35	3.9	0.94			116			30			48	46	
Unloaded			95	28	23.1	0.42	0.45	4.7	0.93			115			31			49	46	
Unloaded			98	34	31.2	0.57	0.59	6.0	0.97			117			30			50	48	
Unloaded		197/ 89	101	31	32.4	0.65	0.65	6.4	1.00	7.43	26	116	62	48	31	40	9	46	46	0.49
1.0	15		102	33	37.6	0.76	0.74	7.3	1.03			119			30			46	47	
2.0	30	206/ 86	107	36	41.8	0.85	0.82	7.7	1.04	7.42	25	117	60	53	31	38	7	46	47	0.47
3.0	45		113	53	53.3	0.96	0.92	8.1	1.04			121			28			51	53	
4.0	60	209/ 86	120	55	66.6	1.24	1.11	9.3	1.12	7.42	25	123	57	57	27	39	12	50	56	0.52
5.0	75		124	53	72.1	1.40	1.21	9.8	1.16			123			28			48	56	
6.0	90	221/ 92	134	54	72.4	1.45	1.22	9.1	1.19	7.40	23	121	53	65	30	37	7	47	56	0.47
7.0	105	227/ 89	152	60	87.5	1.68	1.32	8.7	1.27	7.38	21	125	52	68	32	36	4	49	62	0.48
Recovery			131	39	64.1	1.39	1.08	8.2	1.29			123			30			44	56	
Recovery		233/ 98	122	34	48.1	1.03	0.76	6.2	1.36	7.34	19	121	74	47	34	36	2	44	59	0.43

FIGURE 42-A.

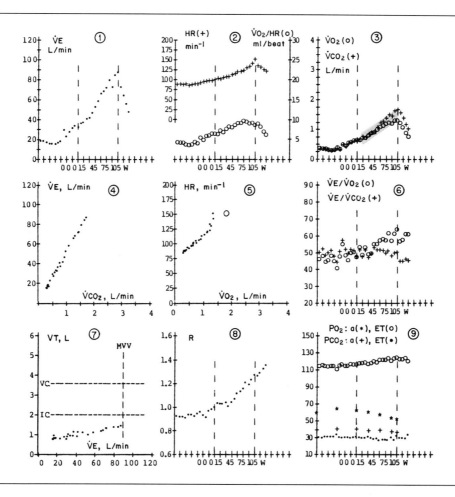

Interpretation

COMMENTS

This case is presented because of its mixed pathophysiology. Despite the patient's denial of a history of lung disease, the results of his respiratory function studies indicate that he has mild to moderate obstructive as well as mild restrictive lung disease as evidenced by the reduced FEV_1/VC, total lung capacity, and vital capacity. Accompanying these changes is a marked reduction in diffusing capacity (Table 42-1). The resting electrocardiogram reflects changes associated with long standing systemic hypertension, for which he is being treated.

ANALYSIS

Flow Chart 1: The maximum $\dot{V}O_2$ and the anaerobic threshold are reduced (Table 42-2). See *Flow Chart 4:* The breathing reserve is low *(branchpoint 4.1).* The V_D/V_T at rest and throughout exercise is

increased *(branchpoint 4.2).* This supports the diagnosis of lung disease with an O_2 flow problem (usually interstitial lung disease). Sufficient disease of the pulmonary circulation is present to limit the cardiac output increase in response to exercise (items 1, 2 and 3 under the diagnosis of pulmonary vascular disease without right-to-left shunt in *Flow Chart 4*). The arterial hypoxemia and increase in $P(A-a)_{O_2}$ that become progressively more marked at each work rate (Table 42-3), are characteristic of pulmonary vascular and interstitial lung disease. The increased $P(a-ET)_{CO_2}$ is expected due to ventilation-perfusion mismatching. The high breathing frequency (f = 60) at the maximum work rate achieved suggests that interstitial or restrictive lung disease is the cause of the pulmonary vascular disorder limiting exercise performance.

CONCLUSION

Pulmonary vascular disease limited exercise performance probably secondary to interstitial lung disease.

CASE 43 *Asbestosis and chronic bronchitis*

CLINICAL FINDINGS

This 48-year-old shipyard worker denied having breathing difficulties and could climb 3 to 4 flights of stairs before noting shortness of breath. He was treated for pneumonia 14 years ago and for a pleural effusion 12 years ago. Two years ago a benign "calcified mass" attached to a left lower rib was removed. He smoked a pack of cigarettes daily for 25 years and had a morning cough with small amounts of yellow sputum. There was no deformity, rhonchi, rales, or clubbing on physical examination. Chest roentgenograms, including computerized tomographic views, showed bilateral pleural plaques and marked coarse parenchymal scarring at both bases.

EXERCISE FINDINGS

The patient performed exercise on a cycle ergometer. He pedalled at 60 rpm without added load for 3 minutes. The work rate was then increased 20 watts per minute to his symptom limited maximum. Blood was sampled every second minute and intra-arterial blood pressure was recorded from a percutaneously placed brachial artery catheter. The patient stopped exercise because of chest discomfort. Resting and exercise ECG were normal. Carboxyhemoglobin was 8.3%.

TABLE 43-1. *Selected Respiratory Function Data*

MEASUREMENT	PREDICTED	MEASURED
Age, yr		48
Sex		Male
Height, cm		180
Weight, kg	82	97
Hematocrit, %		49
VC, L	4.87	4.84 (5.04*)
IC, L	3.25	3.12
TLC, L	7.06	7.12
FEV$_1$, L	3.88	3.23 (3.59*)
FEV$_1$/VC, %	80	67
MVV, L/min	158	183 (172*)
DL$_{CO}$, ml/mm Hg/min	31.8	20.0

*after 4 breaths of aerosolized isoproterenol

TABLE 43-2. *Selected Exercise Data*

MEASUREMENT	PREDICTED	MEASURED
Maximum V̇O$_2$, L/min	2.68	2.37
Maximum HR, beats/min	172	149
Maximum O$_2$ pulse, ml/beat	15.6	15.9
ΔV̇O$_2$/ΔWR, ml/min/watt	10.3	10.3
V̇O$_2$ difference, %	0.0	0.0
AT, L/min	>1.07	1.1
Blood pressure, mm Hg (rest, max)		120/81,213/84
Maximum V̇E, L/min		98
Exercise breathing reserve, L/min	>15	85
Pa$_{O_2}$, mm Hg (rest, max ex)		96,72
P(A−a)$_{O_2}$, mm Hg (rest, max ex)		17,47
P(a−ET)$_{CO_2}$, mm Hg (rest, max ex)		3,2
VD/VT (rest, heavy ex)		0.41,0.28
HCO$_3^-$, mEq/L (rest, 2 min recov)		25,17

TABLE 43-3.

TIME min	WORK RATE W	BP mmHg	HR min⁻¹	f	V̇E BTPS L/min	V̇CO₂ STPD L/min	V̇O₂ STPD L/min	O₂ pulse ml/beat	R	pH	HCO₃⁻ mEq/L	PO₂ ET mmHg	PO₂ a mmHg	PO₂ A-a mmHg	PCO₂ ET mmHg	PCO₂ a mmHg	PCO₂ a-ET mmHg	V̇E/V̇CO₂	V̇E/V̇O₂	VD/VT
Rest	120/ 81									7.43	25	90			38					
Rest			62	14	22.6	0.54	0.64	10.3	0.84			104			36			40	33	
Rest	120/ 78		60	18	17.3	0.35	0.38	6.3	0.92	7.45	24	114	96	17	32	35	3	45	42	0.41
Rest			58	17	16.8	0.34	0.39	6.7	0.87			108			35			45	39	
Unloaded			69	14	20.7	0.52	0.63	9.1	0.83			106			34			37	31	
Unloaded			65	17	21.5	0.58	0.77	11.8	0.75			101			37			35	26	
Unloaded	120/ 72		67	17	16.3	0.43	0.57	8.5	0.75	7.43	25	103	85	17	37	38	1	35	26	0.31
1.0	20		76	14	20.4	0.59	0.78	10.3	0.76			103			37			33	25	
2.0	40	129/ 72	84	20	22.1	0.65	0.88	10.5	0.74	7.42	25	97	81	18	41	40	−1	31	23	0.29
3.0	60		91	13	23.3	0.74	0.95	10.4	0.78			91			44			30	23	
4.0	80	150/ 75	98	21	37.7	1.16	1.34	13.7	0.87	7.39	24	101	77	27	41	41	0	31	27	0.31
5.0	100		105	21	47.8	1.48	1.55	14.8	0.95			107			39			31	30	
6.0	120	174/ 75	114	25	47.9	1.56	1.61	14.1	0.97	7.38	24	104	73	35	42	41	−1	29	28	0.27
7.0	140		126	29	70.1	2.18	2.04	16.2	1.07			109			41			31	33	
8.0	160	204/ 78	138	34	83.6	2.48	2.14	15.5	1.16	7.37	22	116	74	42	36	38	2	33	38	0.29
9.0	180	213/ 84	149	40	97.6	2.86	2.37	15.9	1.21	7.36	20	119	72	47	34	36	2	33	40	0.26
Recovery			122	35	84.5	2.26	1.59	13.0	1.42			124			33			36	51	
Recovery		213/ 72	106	23	51.2	1.32	0.96	9.1	1.38	7.33	17	123	99	24	32	34	2	37	51	0.31

FIGURE 43-A.

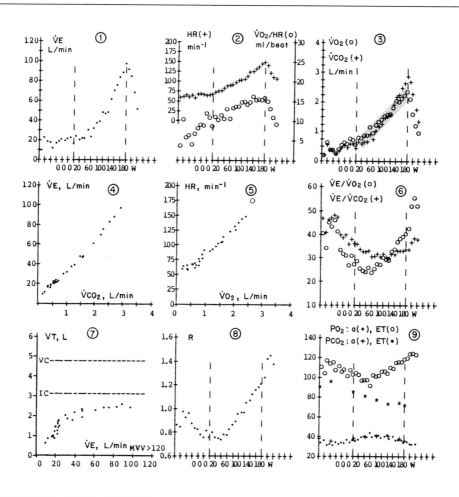

Interpretation

COMMENTS

The results of the resting respiratory function studies indicate that this patient has mild, reversible airflow obstruction and a moderate reduction in diffusing capacity (Table 43-1). His resting and exercise electrocardiograms are normal. It should be noted that the man is a cigarette smoker with a high carboxyhemoglobin level in his blood.

ANALYSIS

Flow Chart 1: The maximum $\dot{V}O_2$ and anaerobic threshold are at the lower limits of normal (Table 43-2). *(See Flow Chart 2.)* Despite these values being within the normal range and the electrocardiogram at the maximum work rate being normal, certain measurements become abnormal during exercise, indicating that the patient has ventilation-perfu-

sion mismatching *(branchpoint 2.3).* These include mild arterial hypoxemia and a significant progressive increase in $P(A-a)O_2$ as work rate is increased. Also, $P(a-ET)_{CO_2}$ is increased at the maximum $\dot{V}O_2$ and VD/VT is borderline normal.

CONCLUSION

Ventilation-perfusion mismatching during exercise in an asymptomatic, 48-year-old man, with maximum exercise performance at the lower limit of normal. Putting this together with the history of a pleural effusion 12 years previously, pleural plaques, and pulmonary fibrosis evident on chest x-ray studies, the strong possibility exists that this patient is evidencing early features of pulmonary asbestosis. The persistent cigarette smoking (high level of blood carboxyhemoglobin) in this asbestos exposed worker provides a major neoplastic threat. It also makes him a high risk candidate for heart disease and emphysema.

CASE 44 *Obesity*

CLINICAL FINDINGS

This 53-year-old former mechanic retired because of medical disability 3 years previously with symptoms of vertigo, nausea, and ataxia, and a diagnosis of vestibular neuronitis. He had no other complaints except for some shortness of breath when bicycling uphill. He had 30 pack years of cigarette smoking and claimed to be smoking one-half pack per day. Hypertension, diagnosed 14 years ago, was being treated with methyldopa. Chest roentgenograms were normal except for symmetrical pleural thickening considered to represent extrapleural fat.

EXERCISE FINDINGS

The patient performed exercise on a cycle ergometer. He pedalled at 60 rpm without added load for 3 minutes. The work rate was then increased 15 watts per minute to his symptom limited maximum. Blood was sampled every second minute and intra-arterial blood pressure was recorded from a percutaneously placed brachial artery catheter. Resting and exercise ECGs were normal. Resting carboxyhemoglobin was 7.4%. The patient stopped exercise complaining of leg fatigue.

TABLE 44-1. *Selected Respiratory Function Data*

MEASUREMENT	PREDICTED	MEASURED
Age, yr		53
Sex		Male
Height, cm		171
Weight, kg	74	104
Hematocrit, %		51
VC, L	4.15	4.00
IC, L	2.77	3.64
TLC, L	6.15	5.69
FEV$_1$, L	3.28	3.25
FEV$_1$/VC, %	79	81
MVV, L/min	140	126
DL$_{CO}$, ml/mm Hg/min	28.8	29.8

TABLE 44-2. *Selected Exercise Data*

MEASUREMENT	PREDICTED	MEASURED
Maximum V̇O$_2$, L/min	2.31	2.45
Maximum HR, beats/min	167	168
Maximum O$_2$ pulse, ml/beat	13.8	15.6
ΔV̇O$_2$/ΔWR, ml/min/watt	10.3	10.4
V̇O$_2$ difference, %	0.0	−0.6
AT, L/min	>0.92	1.1
Blood pressure, mm Hg (rest, max)		
Maximum V̇E, L/min		116
Exercise breathing reserve, L/min	>15	10
Pa$_{O_2}$, mm Hg (rest, max ex)		81,85
P(A−a)$_{O_2}$, mm Hg (rest, max ex)		26,37
P(a−ET)$_{CO_2}$, mm Hg (rest, max ex)		1,−7
VD/VT (rest, heavy ex)		0.31,0.21
HCO$_3^-$, mEq/L (rest, 2 min recov)		24,14

TABLE 44-3.

TIME min	WORK RATE W	BP mmHg	HR min⁻¹	f	V̇E BTPS L/min	V̇CO$_2$ STPD L/min	V̇O$_2$ STPD L/min	O$_2$ pulse ml/beat	R	pH	HCO$_3^-$ mEq/L	PO$_2$ ET mmHg	PO$_2$ a mmHg	PO$_2$ A-a mmHg	PCO$_2$ ET mmHg	PCO$_2$ a mmHg	PCO$_2$ a-ET mmHg	V̇E/V̇CO$_2$	V̇E/V̇O$_2$	VD/VT
Rest										7.44	24		72			36				
Rest			84	17	11.9	0.30	0.37	4.4	0.81			106			36			35	28	
Rest			84	14	12.6	0.32	0.39	4.6	0.82	7.43	24	108	81	26	36	37	1	36	29	0.31
Unloaded			101	23	26.9	0.75	0.89	8.8	0.84			105			37			33	28	
Unloaded			98	23	27.3	0.75	0.83	8.5	0.90			109			36			34	30	
Unloaded			100	24	27.4	0.76	0.82	8.2	0.93	7.43	23	105	90	23	39	35	−4	33	31	0.24
1.0	15		102	26	26.3	0.75	0.82	8.0	0.91			103			40			32	29	
2.0	30		107	22	30.6	0.90	1.00	9.3	0.90	7.43	24	106	93	18	39	36	−3	32	29	0.23
3.0	45		109	19	34.6	1.09	1.17	10.7	0.93			104			40			30	28	
4.0	60		111	20	41.2	1.30	1.29	11.6	1.01	7.42	23	108	89	25	39	36	−3	30	31	0.20
5.0	75		118	23	45.2	1.46	1.43	12.1	1.02			108			40			30	30	
6.0	90		123	24	51.4	1.68	1.61	13.1	1.04	7.39	22	108	87	27	40	37	−3	29	31	0.20
7.0	105		130	26	62.6	1.99	1.77	13.6	1.12			111			40			30	34	
8.0	120		139	32	73.3	2.32	2.03	14.6	1.14	7.38	21	104	82	36	45	36	−9	30	35	0.20
9.0	135		144	34	84.5	2.61	2.19	15.2	1.19			107			44			31	37	
10.0	150		156	41	108.4	3.13	2.43	15.6	1.29	7.37	19	111	85	37	41	34	−7	34	43	0.23
10.5	165		168	41	115.8	3.30	2.45	14.6	1.35			121			34			34	46	
Recovery			156	33	102.3	3.08	2.05	13.1	1.50			123			37			32	49	
Recovery			138	25	68.7	1.76	1.04	7.5	1.69			124			34			38	64	
Recovery			129	26	54.4	1.24	0.71	5.5	1.75			130			28			42	74	
Recovery										7.32	14		112			27				

FIGURE 44-A.

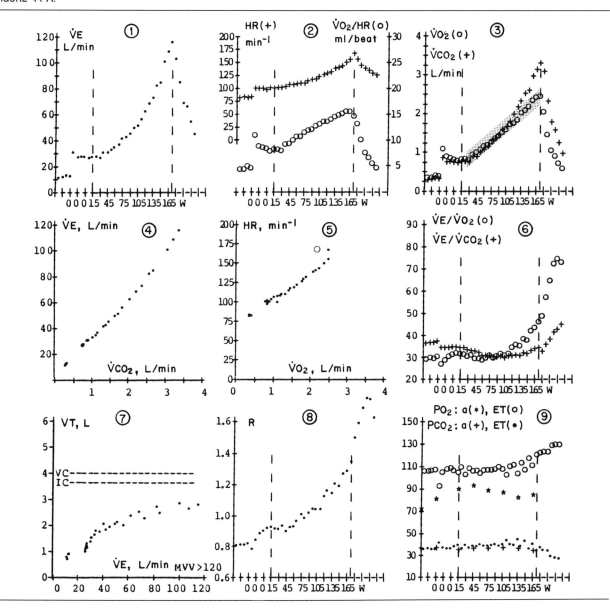

Interpretation

COMMENTS

Results of this patient's resting respiratory function studies are normal except for a low ERV/IC ratio consistent with obesity (Table 44-1). The resting electrocardiogram is normal. The patient is 30 kg overweight (Table 44-1); his resting carboxyhemoglobin of 7.4% suggests recent cigarette smoking.

ANALYSIS

Flow Chart 1: Maximum $\dot{V}O_2$ and anaerobic threshold are within normal limits (Table 44-2). See *Flow*

Chart 2: The electrocardiogram, arterial blood gases, and O_2 pulse at maximum $\dot{V}O_2$ are normal *(branchpoint 2.1)*. The patient is 30 kg overweight *(branchpoint 2.2)*. Supporting the diagnosis of obesity as the cause of this patient's shortness of breath is his high oxygen cost for unloaded cycling ($\dot{V}O_2$ = 0.9 L/min.), and low breathing reserve at the maximum work rate (Table 44-2).

CONCLUSION

Obesity contributed to dyspnea in an otherwise normal patient.

CASE 45 *Skeletal disease limiting exercise*

CLINICAL FINDINGS

This 60-year-old former shipyard worker had enjoyed apparent good health except for arthritis of the right hip of many years duration and hypertension, which had not been treated. He smoked cigarettes for a short period of time 3 decades previously. Chest roentgenograms showed fibrotic changes at both bases but no rales were heard on physical examination.

EXERCISE FINDINGS

The patient felt more comfortable walking on the treadmill than pedalling the cycle ergometer. After insertion of a brachial artery catheter he walked at 1.6 mph on the level followed by increments in grade of 2% per minute. He stopped exercise after 11 minutes because of pain in the right hip. He had no shortness of breath or palpitations. The ECG remained normal.

TABLE 45-1. *Selected Respiratory Function Data*

MEASUREMENT	PREDICTED	MEASURED
Age, yr		60
Sex		Male
Height, cm		175
Weight, kg	78	97
Hematocrit, %		44
VC, L	3.77	4.09
IC, L	2.52	3.01
TLC, L	5.77	5.72
FEV_1, L	2.96	3.21
FEV_1/VC, %	78	78
MVV, L/min	122	94
DL_{CO}, ml/min Hg/min	25.0	23.9

TABLE 45-2. *Selected Exercise Data*

MEASUREMENT	PREDICTED	MEASURED
Maximum $\dot{V}O_2$, L/min	2.44	1.62
Maximum HR, beats/min	160	123
Maximum O_2 pulse, ml/beat	15.3	14.0
AT, L/min	>0.98	1.3
Blood pressure, mm Hg (rest, max)		186/117,213/123
Maximum $\dot{V}E$, L/min		52
Exercise breathing reserve, L/min	>15	42
Pa_{O_2}, mm Hg (rest, max ex)		90,80
$P(A-a)_{O_2}$, mm Hg (rest, max ex)		10,32
$P(a-ET)_{CO_2}$, mm Hg (rest, max ex)		1,−3
VD/VT (rest, heavy ex)		0.39,0.28
HCO_3^-, mEq/L (rest, 2 min recov)		24,23

TABLE 45-3.

TIME min	WORK RATE %	BP mmHg	HR min⁻¹	f	$\dot{V}E$ BTPS L/min	$\dot{V}CO_2$ STPD L/min	$\dot{V}O_2$ STPD L/min	O_2 pulse ml/beat	R	pH	HCO_3^- mEq/L	PO₂ ET mmHg	PO₂ a mmHg	PO₂ A-a mmHg	PCO₂ ET mmHg	PCO₂ a mmHg	PCO₂ a-ET mmHg	$\dot{V}E/\dot{V}CO_2$	$\dot{V}E/\dot{V}O_2$	VD/VT
Rest		186/117								7.44	23	100			34					
Rest			85	20	13.7	0.30	0.37	4.4	0.81			110			35			40	32	
Rest		192/126	84	20	11.1	0.23	0.31	3.7	0.74	7.41	24	102	90	10	38	39	1	41	30	0.39
Rest			90	20	13.4	0.29	0.34	3.8	0.85			111			35			40	34	
	0		95	24	27.7	0.70	0.76	3.0	0.92			110			36			37	34	
	0	216/129	103	29	22.4	0.64	0.91	8.8	0.70	7.41	23	93	74	28	41	36	−5	31	22	0.20
	0		111	22	28.6	0.84	1.17	10.5	0.72			90			41			32	23	
1.0	2		105	26	33.0	0.90	1.18	11.2	0.76			100			39			34	26	
2.0	4	216/126	106	33	31.9	0.88	1.06	10.0	0.83	7.41	23	103	80	27	39	37	−2	33	27	0.27
3.0	6		107	38	29.4	0.80	1.06	9.9	0.75			97			40			33	25	
4.0	8	210/123	109	25	35.8	1.02	1.20	11.0	0.85	7.41	23	106	81	27	38	37	−1	33	28	0.28
5.0	10		111	28	36.8	1.07	1.31	11.8	0.82			102			40			33	26	
6.0	12	216/123	114	33	44.3	1.23	1.42	12.5	0.87	7.40	23	106	81	26	39	38	−1	34	29	0.31
7.0	14		119	30	48.3	1.41	1.55	13.0	0.91			106			40			32	30	
8.0	16	213/123	123	32	49.9	1.44	1.56	12.7	0.92	7.40	22	107	80	32	39	36	−3	33	30	0.25
Recovery			112	27	40.4	1.21	1.34	12.0	0.90			107			40			32	28	
Recovery		192/126	97	38	21.7	0.50	0.61	6.3	0.82	7.39	23	100	90	14	42	39	−3	37	30	0.34

FIGURE 45-A.

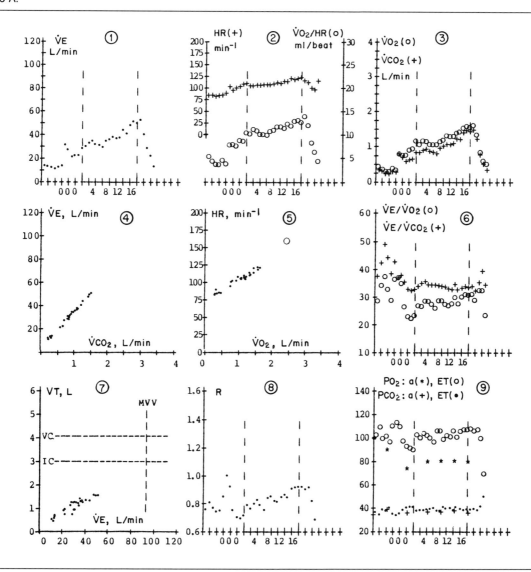

Interpretation

COMMENTS

The results of the respiratory function studies are within normal limits (Table 45-1). The patient had significant systemic hypertension at the time of the study (Table 45-3). Because of arthritis of the right hip, treadmill walking was used for exercise testing. The rate of walking was slow (1.6 mph) to avoid discomfort to the patient and also so that the arterial pressure could be closely monitored.

ANALYSIS

Flow Chart 1: The maximum $\dot{V}O_2$ is significantly reduced but the anaerobic threshold is normal (Table 45-2). See *Flow Chart 3:* The breathing reserve at maximum exercise is high *(branchpoint 3.1).* The electrocardiogram is normal *(branchpoint 3.3).* The diagnosis at this point reveals either poor effort or that the patient has a musculoskeletal disorder. The normal V_D/V_T, borderline $P(A-a)_{O_2}$, normal $P(a-ET)_{CO_2}$, high heart rate reserve, and only 1 mEq/L decrease in bicarbonate two minutes after the start of recovery support either of these diagnoses. From the history, musculoskeletal disorder seems most likely.

CONCLUSION

Musculoskeletal disorder limited exercise performance.

CASE 46 *Myasthenia gravis*

CLINICAL FINDINGS

This 62-year-old retired shipyard worker was found to have myasthenia gravis 21 years ago. He took 30 mgm of pyridostigmine bromide with benefit for many years. He had a 20 pack year history of smoking cigarettes but stopped 21 years ago. He had a daily minimally productive cough. He took digoxin for an arrhythmia and reserpine for hypertension. He complained of gradually increasing shortness of breath in the last 3 years, evident when walking 2 to 3 blocks slowly or climbing one flight of stairs. There was no evidence of pulmonary or cardiovascular disease on physical examination. Chest roentgenogram was normal except for old granulomatous disease. Resting ECG showed sinus bradycardia and ST segment depression in V5 and V6 consistent with digitalis effect.

EXERCISE FINDINGS

The patient performed exercise on a cycle ergometer. He pedalled at 60 rpm without added load for 3 minutes. The work rate was then increased 15 watts per minute to his symptom limited maximum. Blood was sampled every second minute and intra-arterial blood pressure was recorded from a percutaneously placed brachial artery catheter. He stopped exercise complaining of leg pain and generalized fatigue. A single premature ventricular contraction occurred at 60 watts.

TABLE 46-1. *Selected Respiratory Function Data*

MEASUREMENT	PREDICTED	MEASURED
Age, yr		62
Sex		Male
Height, cm		178
Weight, kg	80	80
Hematocrit, %		39
VC, L	3.87	2.96
IC, L	2.58	2.08
TLC, L	5.95	4.64
FEV_1, L	3.03	2.42
FEV_1/VC, %	78	82
MVV, L/min	123	56
DL_{CO}, ml/min Hg/min	24.7	25.6

TABLE 46-2. *Selected Exercise Data*

MEASUREMENT	PREDICTED	MEASURED
Maximum $\dot{V}O_2$, L/min	2.21	1.09
Maximum HR, beats/min	158	102
Maximum O_2 pulse, ml/beat	14.0	10.8
$\Delta\dot{V}O_2/\Delta WR$, ml/min/watt	10.3	10.5
$\dot{V}O_2$ difference, %	0.0	−1.0
AT, L/min	>0.88	>1.1
Blood pressure, mm Hg (rest, max)		153/84,210/84
Maximum $\dot{V}E$, L/min		37
Exercise breathing reserve, L/min	>15	19
Pa_{O_2}, mm Hg (rest, max ex)		95,86
$P(A-a)_{O_2}$, mm Hg (rest, max ex)		8,21
$P(a-ET)_{CO_2}$, mm Hg (rest, max ex)		3,0
VD/VT (rest, heavy ex)		0.39,0.32
HCO_3^-, mEq/L (rest, 2 min recov)		25,23

TABLE 46-3.

TIME min	WORK RATE W	BP mmHg	HR min⁻¹	f	$\dot{V}E$ BTPS	$\dot{V}CO_2$ STPD	$\dot{V}O_2$ L/min	O_2 pulse ml/beat	R	pH	HCO_3^- mEq/L	PO_2 ET	PO_2 a	PO_2 A-a	PCO_2 ET	PCO_2 a	PCO_2 a-ET	$\dot{V}E/\dot{V}CO_2$	$\dot{V}E/\dot{V}O_2$	VD/VT
Rest		153/ 84								7.42	24	97			38					
Rest			74	32	13.6	0.27	0.30	4.1	0.90			112			34			40	36	
Rest		138/ 78	77	23	10.6	0.20	0.26	3.4	0.77	7.43	25	107	95	8	35	38	3	43	33	0.39
Unloaded			80	25	15.2	0.39	0.55	6.9	0.71			96			39			34	24	
Unloaded			80	24	14.8	0.37	0.47	5.9	0.79			99			41			35	27	
Unloaded		165/ 81	80	27	15.8	0.42	0.53	6.6	0.79	7.41	26	101	86	15	40	41	1	32	25	0.30
1.0	15		82	26	28.1	0.76	0.78	9.5	0.97			103			39			34	33	
2.0	30	162/ 78	90	27	24.2	0.69	0.84	9.3	0.82			101			39			32	26	
3.0	45		93	39	28.0	0.77	0.84	9.0	0.92			106			40			32	29	
4.0	60	192/ 81	101	32	35.3	1.06	1.09	10.8	0.97	7.38	24	104	86	21	41	42	1	31	30	0.31
4.5	75		102	35	32.8	1.00	1.06	10.4	0.94			107			40			30	28	
Recovery		210/ 84	93	36	37.4	1.05	0.93	9.9	1.07	7.33	24	108	92	19	41	41	0	33	35	0.33
Recovery			84	33	22.3	0.61	0.59	7.0	1.03			109			40			32	33	
Recovery		174/ 84	82	30	21.8	0.54	0.46	5.6	1.17	7.38	23	117	94	22	36	39	3	36	42	0.33

FIGURE 46-A.

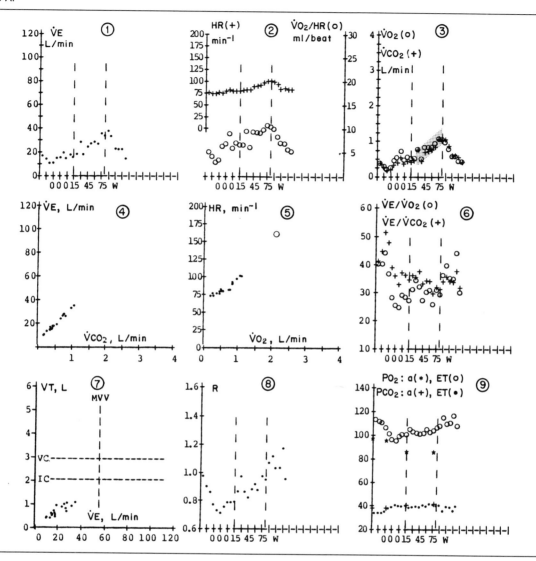

Interpretation

COMMENTS

This patient appears to have mild restrictive lung or chest wall disease (Table 46-1). Because the diffusing capacity is within normal limits and the MVV is significantly reduced, the latter is more likely. The resting electrocardiogram is normal except for the digitalis effect.

ANALYSIS

Flow Chart 1: The maximum oxygen uptake is reduced but the anaerobic threshold is normal (Table 46-2). See *Flow Chart 3:* The breathing reserve at the maximum work rate is normal *(branchpoint 3.1).* The electrocardiogram remained normal except for

the digitalis effect *(branchpoint 3.3).* This suggests that the patient either made poor effort or had a musculoskeletal disorder. The indices of ventilation-perfusion mismatching are normal, supporting the concept that this patient does not have significant pulmonary disease (Note V_D/V_T of 0.31 to 0.33 is considered to be normal in view of the low level of exercise performed.) The high heart rate reserve and small decrease in bicarbonate support the observation that the cardiovascular system was not highly stressed. The reduced maximum $\dot{V}O_2$, with the strikingly reduced MVV, suggests that this patient is limited by a musculoskeletal defect.

CONCLUSION

Exercise limitation secondary to myasthenia gravis.

CASE 47 *Coronary artery disease and chronic bronchitis*

CLINICAL FINDINGS

This 65-year-old man sustained an acute myocardial infarction 6 years ago. Since then he requires one to two nitroglycerin tablets per day and propranolol for "stable angina." He had 30 years of asbestos exposure in the shipyards and smoked 23 pack years of cigarettes. He can walk 2 to 3 miles before becoming dyspneic and admitted to a scantily-productive morning cough. Resting ECG was normal. An exercise study was performed to evaluate the relative contributions of his pulmonary and cardiac illnesses.

EXERCISE FINDINGS

The patient performed exercise on a cycle ergometer. He pedalled at 60 rpm without added load for 3 minutes. The work rate was then increased 10 watts per minute. Blood was sampled every second minute and intra-arterial blood pressure was recorded from a percutaneously placed brachial artery catheter. The incremental cycle exercise test was terminated at 70 watts due to moderate substernal chest pain and the development of 3 mm of ST segment depression in leads 2, 3, and AVF, and occasional premature ventricular beats. These abnormalities resolved promptly after termination of exercise.

TABLE 47-1. *Selected Respiratory Function Data*

MEASUREMENT	PREDICTED	MEASURED
Age, yr		65
Sex		Male
Height, cm		167
Weight, kg	71	55
Hematocrit, %		41
VC, L	3.54	3.42
IC, L	2.36	1.81
TLC, L	5.57	6.16
FEV_1, L	2.75	2.33
FEV_1/VC, %	78	68
MVV, L/min	120	101
DL_{CO}, ml/mm Hg/min	22.6	26.4

TABLE 47-2. *Selected Exercise Data*

MEASUREMENT	PREDICTED	MEASURED
Maximum $\dot{V}O_2$, L/min	1.46	1.01
Maximum HR, beats/min	155	152
Maximum O_2 pulse, ml/beat	9.4	7.3
$\Delta\dot{V}O_2/\Delta WR$, ml/min/watt	10.3	5.7
$\dot{V}O_2$ difference, %	0.0	20.6
AT, L/min	>0.58	indeterminate
Blood pressure, mm Hg (rest, max)		165/87,159/84
Maximum $\dot{V}E$, L/min		39
Exercise breathing reserve, L/min	>15	62
PaO_2, mm Hg (rest, max ex)		94,95
$P(A-a)O_2$, mm Hg (rest, max ex)		13,18
$P(a-ET)CO_2$, mm Hg (rest, max ex)		4,2
VD/VT (rest, heavy ex)		0.39,0.27
HCO_3^-, mEq/L (rest, 2 min recov)		27,24

TABLE 47-3.

TIME min	WORK RATE W	BP mmHg	HR min⁻¹	f	VE BTPS	VCO₂ —STPD—	VO₂ —L/min—	O₂ pulse ml/beat	R	pH	HCO₃⁻ mEq L	PO₂ ET	PO₂ a	PO₂ A-a	PCO₂ ET	PCO₂ a	PCO₂ a-ET	VE VCO₂	VE VO₂	VD VT
Rest	165/ 87									7.43	27	86			41					
Rest			85	16	14.1	0.34	0.36	4.2	0.94			113			34			37	35	
Rest		156/ 84	82	15	9.8	0.21	0.24	2.9	0.88	7.44	27	111	94	13	35	39	4	40	35	0.39
Rest			86	15	9.2	0.17	0.20	2.3	0.85			112			34			47	40	
Rest			84	17	12.8	0.28	0.31	3.7	0.90			114			33			41	37	
Unloaded			105	22	20.3	0.52	0.73	7.0	0.71			92			39			35	25	
Unloaded			105	23	20.6	0.55	0.65	6.2	0.85			105			37			34	29	
Unloaded		162/ 84	103	23	21.1	0.58	0.68	6.6	0.85	7.44	26	107	92	14	37	39	2	33	28	0.30
1.0	10		105	27	20.8	0.55	0.61	5.8	0.90			110			36			34	30	
2.0	20	165/ 87	111	20	19.9	0.56	0.61	5.5	0.92	7.45	26	107	98	12	39	37	-2	32	30	0.26
3.0	30		115	20	23.3	0.67	0.70	6.1	0.96			112			36			32	31	
4.0	40	156/ 84	121	23	27.9	0.81	0.88	7.3	0.92	7.44	26	110	94	15	36	38	2	32	30	0.27
5.0	50		135	30	25.7	0.73	0.80	5.9	0.91			101			44			32	29	
6.0	60		152	28	36.2	0.96	0.92	6.1	1.04			116			34			35	37	
6.5	70	159/ 84	138	30	38.9	1.03	1.01	7.3	1.02			116			34			35	36	
Recovery			134	30	36.3	1.00	1.02	7.6	0.98			112			36			34	33	
Recovery		162/ 84	113	27	31.7	0.86	0.82	7.3	1.05	7.43	24	114	101	14	36	36	0	34	36	0.28

FIGURE 47-A.

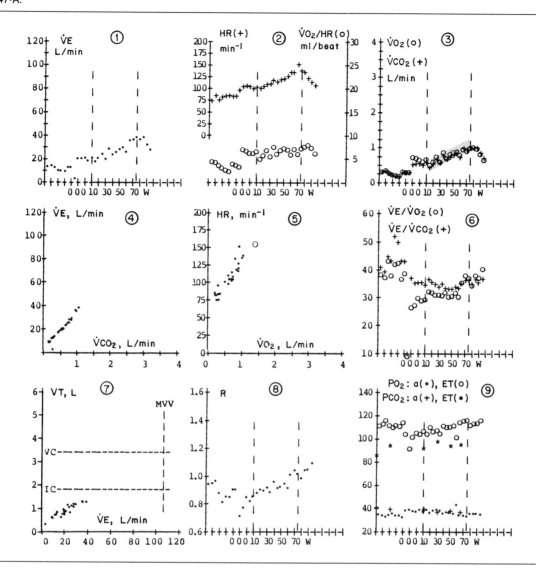

Interpretation

COMMENTS

The resting respiratory function studies indicate that the patient has mild airflow obstruction (Table 47-1). The resting ECG is normal.

ANALYSIS

Flow Chart 1: The maximum $\dot{V}O_2$ is low but the anaerobic threshold is indeterminate from the data provided (Table 47-2 and Fig. 47-A). See *Flow Chart 5.* The indices of ventilation-perfusion matching are normal *(branchpoint 5.1).* The heart rate reserve is normal *(branchpoint 5.2).* The hematocrit is normal *(branchpoint 5.4).* This leads to the diagnosis of heart disease. Confirmatory evidence of ischemic heart disease is provided by the electrocardiogram that develops characteristic changes of myocardial ischemia during exercise. Chest pain was described as only moderate. The shallow $\Delta\dot{V}O_2/\Delta WR$, increased $\dot{V}O_2$ difference, and the low O_2 pulse throughout exercise that fails to rise as work rate is increased all provide support for the cardiac diagnosis. The high breathing reserve and normal indices of ventilation-perfusion matching clearly suggest that the lungs and pulmonary circulation are functioning normally. In contrast, the cardiovascular response to exercise is quite abnormal.

CONCLUSION

Coronary artery disease limited exercise performance in a patient with mild airflow obstruction.

CASE 48 *Myocardial ischemia, systemic hypertension, and mild interstitial lung disease*

CLINICAL FINDINGS

This 65-year-old man was referred for evaluation. He had retired from work in the shipyard 5 years previously. He noted slight dyspnea on exertion beginning 6 years prior to evaluation but could still climb 2 flights of stairs without shortness of breath. He smoked one half of a pack of cigarettes a day between the ages 24 and 40. He denied cough, sputum production, or wheezing. He recently became very short of breath on a fishing trip at high altitude. At age 25 he was discharged from the Army because of a "cardiac murmur," but this was not noted on later examinations. There was no history of rheumatic fever or congestive heart failure. He took no medications. Physical examination was normal except for bilateral arcus senilis. Chest roentgenograms revealed bilateral pleural plaques and possible bibasilar interstitial disease.

EXERCISE FINDINGS

The patient performed exercise on a cycle ergometer. He pedalled at 60 rpm without added load for 3 minutes. The work rate was then increased 20 watts per minute. Blood was sampled every second minute and intra-arterial blood pressure was recorded from a percutaneously placed brachial artery catheter. Resting ECG showed deep Q waves in leads 2, 3, and AVF compatible with an old inferior infarction. During exercise, occasional single ventricular premature contractions were noted. At 120 watts the ST segments were depressed 2 mm in V4 through V6 and then 4 mm before exercise was stopped at 160 watts. The ST segments became isoelectric within 5 minutes of recovery. Patient experienced leg fatigue but denied any chest pain or discomfort.

TABLE 48-1. *Selected Respiratory Function Data*

MEASUREMENT	PREDICTED	MEASURED
Age, yr		65
Sex		Male
Height, cm		174
Weight, kg	77	65
Hematocrit, %		45
VC, L	3.97	3.58
IC, L	2.64	2.24
TLC, L	6.21	6.68
FEV_1, L	3.09	2.60
FEV_1/VC, %	78	73
MVV, L/min	128	117
DL_{CO}, ml/mm Hg/min	25.6	21.7

TABLE 48-2. *Selected Exercise Data*

MEASUREMENT	PREDICTED	MEASURED
Maximum $\dot{V}O_2$, L/min	1.71	1.41
Maximum HR, beats/min	155	176
Maximum O_2 pulse, ml/beat	11.0	8.0
$\Delta \dot{V}O_2 / \Delta WR$, ml/min/watt	10.3	7.3
$\dot{V}O_2$ difference, %	0.0	21.1
AT, L/min	>0.68	0.9
Blood pressure, mm Hg (rest, max)		189/108,234/126
Maximum $\dot{V}E$, L/min		74
Exercise breathing reserve, L/min	>15	43
PaO_2, mm Hg (rest, max ex)		89,89
$P(A-a)O_2$, mm Hg (rest, max ex)		16,27
$P(a-ET)CO_2$, mm Hg (rest, max ex)		1,1
VD/VT (rest, heavy ex)		0.34,0.32

TABLE 48-3.

TIME min	WORK RATE W	BP mmHg	HR min⁻¹	f	$\dot{V}E$ BTPS L/min	$\dot{V}CO_2$ STPD L/min	$\dot{V}O_2$ STPD L/min	O_2 pulse ml/beat	R	pH	HCO_3^- mEq/L	PO_2 ET	PO_2 a	PO_2 A-a	PCO_2 ET	PCO_2 a	PCO_2 a-ET	$\dot{V}E/\dot{V}CO_2$	$\dot{V}E/\dot{V}O_2$	VD/VT
Rest		189/108								7.44	26	86			39					
Rest			85	13	11.5	0.30	0.37	4.4	0.81			105			37			35	28	
Rest			84	16	12.4	0.31	0.38	4.5	0.82			104			39			36	29	
Rest			84	12	11.2	0.27	0.29	3.5	0.93			111			35			38	35	
Unloaded			101	17	19.2	0.49	0.66	6.5	0.74			100			38			36	27	
Unloaded			96	18	16.8	0.41	0.48	5.0	0.85			106			37			37	32	
Unloaded		213/120	97	17	16.2	0.42	0.50	5.2	0.84	7.43	26	105	89	16	38	39	1	35	29	0.34
1.0	20		100	18	23.6	0.56	0.58	5.8	0.97			107			37			39	38	
2.0	30	210/114	103	20	20.9	0.51	0.59	5.7	0.86	7.50	28	106	90	20	38	36	-2	38	33	0.33
3.0	60		115	21	29.0	0.76	0.91	7.9	0.84			103			39			36	30	
4.0	80	219/117	137	24	38.3	1.10	1.15	8.4	0.96	7.36	22	108	102	7	39	40	1	33	32	0.33
5.0	100		154	28	50.1	1.44	1.28	8.3	1.13			113			38			33	37	
6.0	120	234/126	167	32	56.6	1.65	1.33	8.0	1.24	7.35	22	115	89	27	39	40	1	33	41	0.32
7.0	140		176	41	69.8	1.96	1.41	8.0	1.39			117			39			34	47	
7.5	160	234/126	175	44	73.9	2.00	1.13	6.5	1.77			120			36			35	62	
Recovery			174	36	61.1	1.95	1.36	7.8	1.43			116			42			30	43	
Recovery			158	31	53.3	1.58	0.89	5.6	1.78			124			38			32	57	
Recovery			138	27	44.0	1.20	0.63	4.6	1.90			126			36			35	66	

FIGURE 48-A.

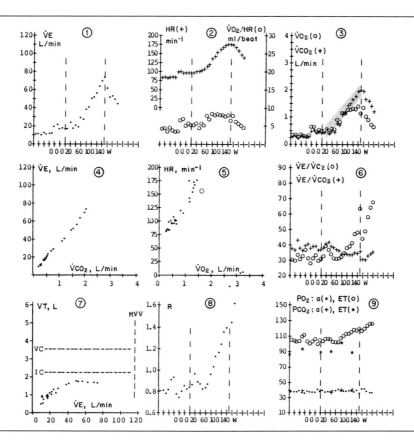

Interpretation

COMMENTS

Results of the resting respiratory function studies are within normal limits (Table 48-1). The resting electrocardiogram is abnormal and suggests that the patient had an inferior wall myocardial infarction in the past.

ANALYSIS

Flow Chart 1: The maximum $\dot{V}O_2$ is reduced but the anaerobic threshold is within normal limits (Table 48-2). See *Flow Chart 3:* The breathing reserve is high *(branchpoint 3.1).* The electrocardiogram became abnormal as the maximum work rate was approached *(branchpoint 3.3).* While the patient did not experience chest pain, the diagnosis of myocardial ischemia is supported by the marked change in slope in $\dot{V}O_2$ in response to increasing work rate (Graph 3, Fig. 48-A), a reduced $\Delta\dot{V}O_2/\Delta WR$, and a large difference between the predicted and observed $\dot{V}O_2$ at maximum work rate ($\dot{V}O_2$ difference in Table 48-2). The very marked increase in R at 80 watts (Table 48-3 and Graph 8, Fig. 48-A) reflects the de-

velopment of a significant metabolic acidosis as the anaerobic threshold is exceeded. The steepening heart rate response with increasing oxygen uptake (Graph 5, Fig. 48-A) and the failure of O_2 pulse to increase at a low work rate (Graph 2, Fig. 48-A) reflect a low stroke volume and a maximal $C(a - \bar{v})O_2$ being reached at a relatively low work rate.

It should be noted that this patient has significant systemic hypertension. We cannot, therefore, exclude the possibility that the myocardial ischemia and impaired cardiac function demonstrated here is due, in part, to abnormally increased myocardial work as well as coronary artery disease.

There is evidence of ventilation-perfusion mismatching (high V_D/V_T and positive $P(a - ET)_{CO_2}$). These abnormalities, despite normal resting respiratory function, give support to the diagnosis of interstitial lung disease, consistent with the radiological finding.

CONCLUSION

Myocardial ischemia limited exercise performance, secondary to coronary artery disease and/or systemic hypertension. Interstitial lung disease.

CASE 49 *Cardiac disease and mild obstructive airways disease: Cycle and treadmill*

CLINICAL FINDINGS

This 64-year-old shipyard worker was referred for evaluation. He stated that he was not limited in any of his activities; he had no shortness of breath walking on the level and only mild dyspnea after climbing 25 steps. He smoked a half a pack of cigarettes daily until one year prior to this evaluation. Physical examination revealed no abnormality of the cardiovascular or respiratory systems except for a resting blood pressure of 160/84. Questionable pleural thickening was noted on chest x-ray studies. There was a small but consistent improvement in expiratory flow rates and MVV following inhalation of aerosolized isoproterenol.

EXERCISE FINDINGS

The patient performed exercise on a cycle ergometer and, one month later, on a treadmill. He first pedalled at 60 rpm, without added load, for 3 minutes. The work rate was then increased 20 watts per minute to his symptom limited maximum. Blood was sampled every second minute and intra-arterial blood pressure was recorded from a percutaneously placed brachial artery catheter. The resting ECG was normal. He stopped exercising because of leg fatigue. Near the end of cycle exercise 1 mm horizontal ST depression was noted in leads 2, 3, and AVF. On repeat testing one month later on the treadmill the patient stopped exercising because he "could not get a good deep breath" and felt tired. There were no abnormal ECG findings on that test.

TABLE 49-1. *Selected Respiratory Function Data*

MEASUREMENT	PREDICTED	MEASURED
Age, yr		64
Sex		Male
Height, cm		182
Weight, kg	83	80
Hematocrit, %		47
VC, L	4.49	4.25
IC, L	2.99	3.95
TLC, L	6.94	7.61
FEV_1, L	3.51	2.96
FEV_1/VC, %	78	70
MVV, L/min	140	121
DL_{CO}, ml/mm Hg/min	28.8	28.1

TABLE 49-2. *Selected Exercise Data*

MEASUREMENT	PREDICTED		MEASURED	
	CYCLE	TREADMILL	CYCLE	TREADMILL
Maximum $\dot{V}O_2$, L/min	2.16	2.40	1.56	1.65
Maximum HR, beats/min	156	156	143	157
Maximum O_2 pulse, ml/beat	13.8	15.4	10.9	10.5
$\Delta\dot{V}O_2/\Delta WR$, ml/min/watt	10.3		9.7	
$\dot{V}O_2$ difference, %	0.0		3.7	
AT, L/min	>0.86	>0.96	0.83	indeterminate
Blood pressure, mm Hg (rest, max)			194/98,230/98	
Maximum $\dot{V}E$, L/min			68	77
Exercise breathing reserve, L/min			53	44
Pa_{O_2}, mm Hg (rest, max ex)			98,104	
$P(A-a)_{O_2}$, mm Hg (rest, max ex)			22,18	
$P(a-ET)_{CO_2}$, mm Hg (rest, max ex)			2,-3	
VD/VT (rest, heavy ex)			0.30,0.23	
HCO_3^-, mEq/L (rest, 2 min recov)			24,17	

TABLE 49-3. *Cycle Ergometry*

TIME min	WORK RATE W	BP mmHg	HR min⁻¹	f	V̇E BTPS L/min	V̇CO₂ STPD L/min	V̇O₂ STPD L/min	O₂ pulse ml/beat	R	pH	HCO₃⁻ mEq/L	PO₂ ET mmHg	PO₂ a mmHg	PO₂ A-a mmHg	PCO₂ ET mmHg	PCO₂ a mmHg	PCO₂ a-ET mmHg	V̇E/V̇CO₂	V̇E/V̇O₂	VD/VT
Rest		194/ 98								7.42	24	77			38					
Rest			72	17	17.9	0.38	0.38	5.3	1.00			118			29			43	43	
Rest		176/ 95	82	14	13.7	0.29	0.30	3.7	0.97			118			30			43	42	
Rest			80	20	14.3	0.30	0.29	3.6	1.03	7.48	23	119	98	22	29	31	2	42	44	0.30
Unloaded			92	12	26.5	0.58	0.48	5.2	1.21			124			27			44	53	
Unloaded		194/ 95	85	15	23.2	0.52	0.52	6.1	1.00			116			31			42	42	
Unloaded			92	16	24.0	0.56	0.56	6.1	1.00	7.47	22	117	100	19	30	31	1	40	40	0.29
1.0	20	209/ 92	99	17	27.7	0.65	0.68	6.9	0.96			114			32			40	39	
2.0	40		105	21	27.6	0.72	0.83	7.9	0.87			104			36			36	31	
3.0	60	212/ 92	112	26	40.0	0.93	0.96	8.6	0.97			113			33			41	39	
4.0	80		119	31	29.8	0.87	1.02	8.6	0.85	7.40	22	97	92	16	42	37	-5	31	27	0.23
5.0	100	230/ 98	131	25	60.3	1.53	1.36	10.4	1.13			116			34			38	43	
6.0	120		143	27	68.2	1.77	1.56	10.9	1.13	7.40	19	117	104	18	34	31	-3	37	42	0.24
Recovery		221/ 95	134	23	53.4	1.32	0.95	7.1	1.39			121			34			39	54	
Recovery			120	18	38.2	0.89	0.61	5.1	1.46	7.38	17	126	114	14	30	29	-1	41	60	0.27

FIGURE 49-A. *Cycle Ergometry*

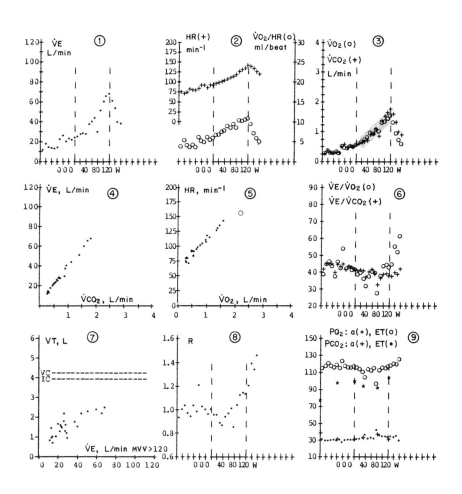

TABLE 49-4. *Treadmill Ergometry*

TIME min	WORK RATE %	BP mmHg	HR min⁻¹	f	$\dot{V}E$ BTPS	$\dot{V}CO_2$ STPD L/min	$\dot{V}O_2$ STPD L/min	O_2 pulse ml/beat	R	pH	HCO₃⁻ mEq/L	PO₂ ET mmHg	PO₂ a	PO₂ A-a	PCO₂ ET mmHg	PCO₂ a	PCO₂ a-ET	$\dot{V}E/\dot{V}CO_2$	$\dot{V}E/\dot{V}O_2$	VD/VT
Rest			102	15	15.4	0.34	0.37	3.6	0.92			112			33			45	42	
Rest			105	11	13.5	0.33	0.35	3.3	0.94			116			31			41	39	
Rest			109	21	14.9	0.28	0.28	2.6	1.00			118			30			53	53	
	0		113	13	19.3	0.51	0.66	5.8	0.77			104			34			38	29	
	0		112	19	15.6	0.38	0.52	4.6	0.73			99			37			41	30	
1.0	2		116	18	24.9	0.70	0.93	8.0	0.75			101			36			36	27	
2.0	4		117	20	29.7	0.85	1.07	9.1	0.79			98			39			35	28	
3.0	6		124	18	27.2	0.76	0.92	7.4	0.83			99			40			36	30	
4.0	8		131	20	32.0	0.96	1.13	8.6	0.85			102			40			33	28	
5.0	10		139	21	41.8	1.25	1.35	9.7	0.93			106			38			33	31	
6.0	12		146	20	54.7	1.61	1.50	10.3	1.07			111			38			34	36	
7.0	14		153	25	61.9	1.82	1.56	10.2	1.17			114			38			34	40	
7.5	16		157	31	76.8	2.06	1.65	10.5	1.25			119			34			37	47	
Recovery			153	29	69.2	1.82	1.46	9.5	1.25			116			37			38	47	
Recovery			148	23	58.1	1.42	1.07	7.2	1.33			121			33			41	54	

FIGURE 49-B. *Treadmill Ergometry*

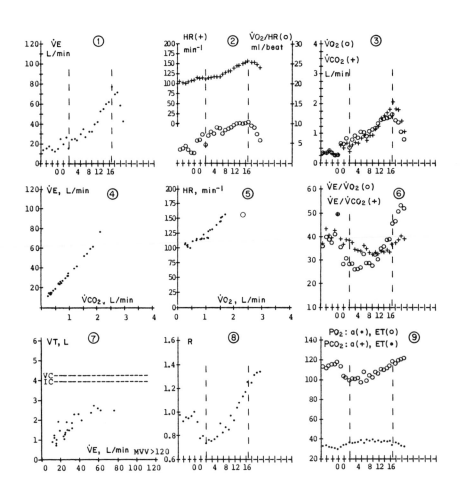

Interpretation

COMMENTS

This case is presented to contrast cycle with treadmill incremental exercise testing. Respiratory function measurements at rest suggest that this patient has mild obstructive lung disease (Table 49-1). Also, note that the patient hyperventilated at rest (Pa_{CO_2} and R values in Table 49-3) when first starting to breathe on the mouthpiece.

ANALYSIS

Flow Chart 1: The maximum $\dot{V}O_2$ is significantly reduced in both the cycle and treadmill exercise studies, and the anaerobic threshold is borderline in the former and indeterminate in the latter (Table 49-2). See *Flow Chart 4:* The breathing reserve at maximum exercise (Table 49-2) is high *(branchpoint 4.1)* and the indices of ventilation-perfusion matching are normal *(branchpoint 4.3)*, although the subject did evidence hyperventilation. The hematocrit is normal *(branchpoint 4.4)*. The O_2 pulse at the highest work rate for both the cycle and treadmill tests is low (Table 49-2). The heart rate-$\dot{V}O_2$ relationship is abnormally steep in both forms of ergometry (Graph 5 in Figures 49-A and B). This suggests that the patient's primary diagnosis is heart disease rather than peripheral vascular disease. $\dot{V}O_2$ also reaches a plateau at a low value as the patient's highest work rate is approached in the treadmill study. Although the patient has mild obstructive airway disease, his breathing reserve is high at his maximum work rate suggesting that he is not ventilatory limited. Also, indices of ventilation-perfusion matching are normal. In contrast, the patient reaches his predicted maximal heart rate during both the cycle and treadmill exercise studies.

CONCLUSION

Cardiac disease limited exercise performance. This is confirmed by the absence of a cardiac reserve at the reduced maximum work rate, failure for $\dot{V}O_2$ to rise normally with increasing work rate (treadmill exercise study), as well as the reduced maximal O_2 pulse.

CASE 50 *Pulmonary vascular disease, chronic bronchitis, asbestosis, and myocardial ischemia*

CLINICAL FINDINGS

This 51-year-old shipyard worker noted increased dyspnea on exertion for 2 years, until he was unable to finish cleaning his one bedroom apartment. For several years he had a morning cough productive of small amounts of yellow sputum. He had over 40 pack years of cigarette smoking and continued to smoke. He denied chest pain, tightness, or pressure. Chest x-ray studies showed a streaky infiltrate in the lower lung fields with nodular scarring in the upper lung zones. Physical examination of the chest was normal. There was equivocal clubbing of the digits. Peripheral pulses were normal. ECG showed left axis deviation.

EXERCISE FINDINGS

The patient performed exercise on a cycle ergometer. He first pedalled at 60 rpm, without added load, for 3 minutes. The work rate was then increased 15 watts per minute to his symptom limited maximum. Blood was sampled every second minute and intra-arterial blood pressure was recorded from a percutaneously placed brachial artery catheter. The patient stopped exercising because of severe knee cramps. During incremental exercise he developed premature atrial and ventricular contractions, and 3 to 4 mm ST segment depression in leads V4 and V5. He denied any chest pain or discomfort, dizziness or light headedness. The ST segments returned to normal within 1 minute of recovery.

TABLE 50-1. *Selected Respiratory Function Data*

MEASUREMENT	PREDICTED	MEASURED
Age, yr		51
Sex		Male
Height, cm		166
Weight, kg	70	55
Hematocrit, %		49
VC, L	3.88	3.83
IC, L	2.59	2.37
TLC, L	5.71	6.81
FEV_1, L	3.07	2.41
FEV_1/VC, %	79	63
MVV, L/min	136	120
DL_{CO}, ml/mm Hg/min	26.9	21.5

TABLE 50-2. *Selected Exercise Data*

MEASUREMENT	PREDICTED	MEASURED
Maximum $\dot{V}O_2$, L/min	1.75	1.77
Maximum HR, beats/min	169	150
Maximum O_2 pulse, ml/beat	10.4	11.8
$\Delta\dot{V}O_2/\Delta WR$, ml/min/watt	10.3	9.7
$\dot{V}O_2$ difference, %	0.0	4.0
AT, L/min	>0.70	indeterminate
Blood pressure, mm Hg (rest, max)		132/72,189/99
Maximum $\dot{V}E$, L/min		79
Exercise breathing reserve, L/min	>15	41
PaO_2, mm Hg (rest, max ex)		69,63
$P(A-a)O_2$, mm Hg (rest, max ex)		30,44
$P(a-ET)CO_2$, mm Hg (rest, max ex)		10,6
VD/VT (rest, heavy ex)		0.53,0.44
HCO_3^-, mEq/L (rest, 2 min recov)		25,16

TABLE 50-3.

TIME min	WORK RATE W	BP mmHg	HR min⁻¹	f	$\dot{V}E$ BTPS L/min	$\dot{V}CO_2$ STPD L/min	$\dot{V}O_2$ STPD L/min	O_2 pulse ml/beat	R	pH	HCO_3^- mEq/L	PO2 ET mmHg	PO2 a mmHg	PO2 A-a mmHg	PCO2 ET mmHg	PCO2 a mmHg	PCO2 a-ET mmHg	$\dot{V}E$/$\dot{V}CO_2$	$\dot{V}E$/$\dot{V}O_2$	VD/VT
Rest	132/ 72									7.42	25	76			40					
Rest	159/ 81	66	21	11.4	0.19	0.26	3.9	0.73				107			33			51	37	
Rest		66	22	14.1	0.24	0.32	4.8	0.75				106			33			51	38	
Rest		65	19	11.8	0.19	0.24	3.7	0.79	7.39	25	110	69	30	32	42	10	54	42	0.53	
Unloaded		88	21	15.0	0.32	0.40	4.5	0.80				101			38			41	33	
Unloaded	165/ 90	87	16	20.1	0.49	0.57	6.6	0.86				99			40			38	33	
Unloaded		81	16	19.9	0.49	0.56	6.9	0.88	7.38	25	103	69	33	39	43	4	38	33	0.44	
1.0	15	180/ 93	88	18	20.6	0.52	0.59	6.7	0.88			99			41			37	32	
2.0	30		90	21	22.5	0.56	0.63	7.0	0.89	7.37	25	102	70	32	40	44	4	37	33	0.43
3.0	45	186/ 93	105	26	32.3	0.82	0.93	8.9	0.88			102			40			37	32	
4.0	60		108	24	36.4	1.01	1.09	10.1	0.93	7.35	25	99	66	35	44	46	2	34	31	0.42
5.0	75	189/ 93	119	24	38.1	1.13	1.17	9.8	0.97			101			44			32	31	
6.0	90		124	26	43.0	1.28	1.28	10.3	1.00	7.31	24	101	61	41	45	48	3	32	32	0.41
7.0	105	191/ 99	138	32	54.2	1.59	1.48	10.7	1.07			105			44			32	35	
8.0	120		148	48	72.8	1.91	1.64	11.1	1.16	7.28	22	109	63	44	42	48	6	36	42	0.47
9.0	135	189/ 99	150	42	78.7	2.19	1.77	11.8	1.24			110			44			34	42	
Recovery	184/ 84	124	34	62.6	1.57	0.97	7.8	1.62				121			39			38	62	
Recovery		115	27	45.8	1.06	0.67	5.8	1.58	7.24	16	123	97	25	35	40	5	41	65	0.45	

FIGURE 50-A.

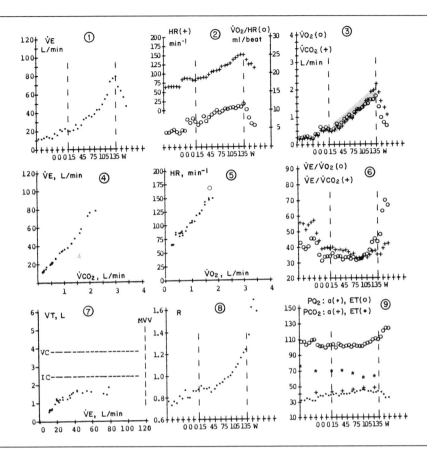

Interpretation

COMMENTS

Resting respiratory function tests are compatible with mild airflow obstruction (Table 50-1). The diffusing capacity is at the lower limits of normal. The resting electrocardiogram is essentially normal.

ANALYSIS

Flow Chart 1: The maximum $\dot{V}O_2$ is normal but the anaerobic threshold is indeterminate (Table 50-2). (Note that the predicted values are based on the patient's actual weight as this patient is 15 kg underweight. Thus, the predicted $\dot{V}O_2$ may be spuriously low). See *Flow Chart 2:* The electrocardiogram at maximum exercise is abnormal suggesting ischemic changes. The arterial blood gases are also significantly abnormal during exercise *(branchpoint 2.1).* The indices of ventilation-perfusion matching (V_D/V_T, $P(a - ET)_{CO_2}$ and $P(A-a)_{O_2}$) *(branchpoint 2.3)* are clearly abnormal suggesting that this patient has lung disease and/or pulmonary vascular disease. Since the results of the resting respiratory function tests are not consistent with a diagnosis of restrictive lung disease and suggest that the patient's airflow obstruction is only mild, it is likely that the major abnormalities in ventilation-perfusion mismatching observed in this patient are attributable to pulmonary vascular disease. The electrocardiographic abnormalities that this patient developed as he approached his maximum work rate, despite the absence of chest pain, suggest that the patient also develops myocardial ischemia under exercise stress.

CONCLUSION

Normal maximum exercise capacity in a patient with pulmonary vascular disease and myocardial ischemia. There is clear evidence of significant ventilation-perfusion mismatching of the type seen with pulmonary vascular disease. However, his pulmonary mechanics are only mildly abnormal. Presumably, this is an instance of changes in the pulmonary circulation disproportionate to airway or parenchymal disease. Additionally, the exercise induced ST segment depression and arrhythmia, typical of myocardial ischemia, suggest coronary artery disease. The pulmonary vascular disease and exercise hypoxemia possibly contribute to this cardiac abnormality.

CASE 51 *Peripheral vascular, pulmonary vascular and obstructive airway diseases*

CLINICAL FINDINGS

This 69-year-old retired shipyard worker was a heavy cigarette smoker until 5 years ago. For more than a decade he noted excessive shortness of breath on climbing one flight of stairs. For the last several years his activity was limited by cramps in the calves after walking approximately 100 yards; they were relieved by rest. He took no medication. Examination revealed a left cataract and reduced arterial pulsations in the legs, but no rales, wheezing, or edema. Chest x-ray studies showed pleural thickening on the right, an elevated left diaphragm, and normal heart size.

EXERCISE FINDINGS

The patient performed exercise on a cycle ergometer. He pedalled at 60 rpm without added load for 3 minutes. The work rate was then increased 10 watts per minute to his symptom limited maximum. Blood was sampled every second minute and intra-arterial blood pressure was recorded from a percutaneously placed brachial artery catheter. The patient stopped exercise because of pain in both calves. He developed frequent premature ventricular contractions and hypertension during exercise that resolved during recovery. Resting, exercise, and recovery ECG tracings were otherwise normal.

TABLE 51-1. *Selected Respiratory Function Data*

MEASUREMENT	PREDICTED	MEASURED
Age, yr		69
Sex		Male
Height, cm		165
Weight, kg	70	76
Hematocrit, %		40
VC, L	3.68	3.25
IC, L	2.45	2.69
TLC, L	6.11	6.05
FEV_1, L	2.87	1.92
FEV_1/VC, %	78	59
MVV, L/min	113	87
DL_{CO}, ml/mm Hg/min	21.8	17.5

TABLE 51-2. *Selected Exercise Data*

MEASUREMENT	PREDICTED	MEASURED
Maximum $\dot{V}O_2$, L/min	1.75	0.83
Maximum HR, beats/min	151	155
Maximum O_2 pulse, ml/beat	11.6	7.2
$\Delta\dot{V}O_2/\Delta WR$, ml/min/watt	10.3	5.2
$\dot{V}O_2$ difference, %	0.0	16.5
AT, L/min	>0.70	not reached
Blood pressure, mm Hg (rest, max)		198/84,264/120
Maximum $\dot{V}E$, L/min		30
Exercise breathing reserve, L/min	>15	57
Pa_{O_2}, mm Hg (rest, max ex)		87,80
$P(A-a)_{O_2}$, mm Hg (rest, max ex)		11,28
$P(a-ET)_{CO_2}$, mm Hg (rest, max ex)		5,1
VD/VT (rest, heavy ex)		0.46,0.38
HCO_3^-, mEq/L (rest, 2 min recov)		24,23

TABLE 51-3.

TIME min	WORK RATE W	BP mmHg	HR min⁻¹	f	$\dot{V}E$ BTPS L/min	$\dot{V}CO_2$ STPD L/min	$\dot{V}O_2$ STPD L/min	O_2 pulse ml/beat	R	pH	HCO_3^- mEq L	PO2 ET mmHg	PO2 a mmHg	PO2 A-a mmHg	PCO2 ET mmHg	PCO2 a mmHg	PCO2 a-ET mmHg	$\frac{\dot{V}E}{\dot{V}CO_2}$	$\frac{\dot{V}E}{\dot{V}O_2}$	$\frac{VD}{VT}$
Rest		210/ 84								7.43	24	80			36					
Rest			75	22	11.6	0.20	0.28	3.7	0.71			110			33			48	35	
Rest			71	22	10.3	0.16	0.23	3.2	0.70			110			33			53	37	
Rest		198/ 84	72	20	10.4	0.17	0.25	3.5	0.68	7.41	24	111	87	11	33	38	5	51	35	0.46
Unloaded			94	21	18.3	0.40	0.49	5.2	0.82			112			34			41	34	
Unloaded			103	22	20.7	0.47	0.64	6.2	0.73			109			35			40	29	
Unloaded		246/ 93	102	24	22.4	0.51	0.66	6.5	0.77	7.40	25	111	76	25	35	40	5	40	31	0.42
1.0	10		104	23	20.7	0.47	0.58	5.6	0.81			110			36			40	32	
2.0	20	252/114	105	24	18.5	0.42	0.51	4.9	0.82	7.40	23	110	77	27	36	39	3	39	32	0.39
3.0	30		112	25	20.7	0.46	0.54	4.8	0.85			114			34			40	34	
4.0	40	264/120	115	26	30.3	0.71	0.83	7.2	0.86	7.40	23	111	80	28	36	37	1	39	34	0.38
Recovery			103	21	24.8	0.61	0.71	6.9	0.86			108			38			38	32	
Recovery		210/ 96	96	21	18.9	0.42	0.42	4.4	1.00	7.37	23	117	96	13	35	41	6	41	41	0.44

FIGURE 51-A.

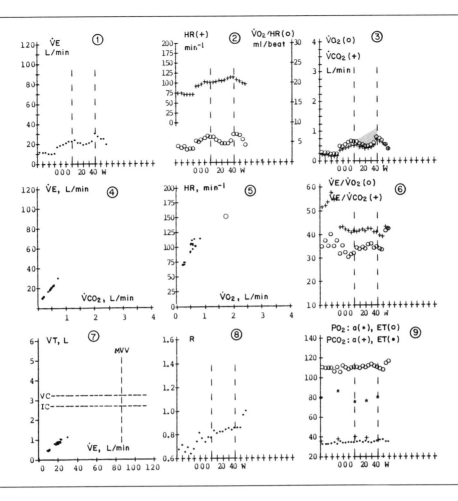

Interpretation

COMMENTS

Resting respiratory function studies show the patient to have moderate airflow obstruction (Table 51-1). The resting electrocardiogram is normal.

ANALYSIS

Flow Chart 1: The maximum $\dot{V}O_2$ is low; the anaerobic threshold, however, is indeterminate (Table 51-2). See *Flow Chart 5.* While the maximum word rate performed is quite low, the maximum exercise VD/VT is high, and $P(a - ET)CO_2$ and $P(A - a)O_2$ are at the borderline of abnormality *(branchpoint 5.1).* The breathing reserve is high *(branchpoint 5.3).* This suggests that the disease process is either that of pulmonary vascular or circulatory origin. Pa_{O_2} becomes slightly abnormal with exercise (Table 51-3 and Graph 9, Fig. 51-A). Other measurements listed under pulmonary vascular diseases are consistent with this diagnosis. However, the high heart rate reserve is inconsistent with pulmonary vascular disease

being the symptom limiting diagnosis. Returning to consider branchpoints 5.1, 5.2, and 5.5, we reach branchpoint 5.8. The patient has systemic hypertension, reduced arterial pulses in the legs and lower extremity pain with exercise suggesting that peripheral vascular disease is the diagnosis limiting exercise performance. Supporting this is the very low value of $\Delta\dot{V}_{O_2}/\Delta WR$ *(branchpoint 5.8).* ($\dot{V}_{O_2}$ could increase only slightly above that required for unloaded cycling).

CONCLUSION

Both peripheral and pulmonary vascular disease, with the former being the primary limiting disorder. The exercise induced arrhythmia also suggests the presence of myocardial ischemia, perhaps from the high cardiac afterload induced by systemic hypertension. The poor perfusion of the exercising muscles probably prevented the cellular metabolic acidosis from being reflected in the arterial blood. Note that while this patient has moderate airflow obstruction, it does not appear to be important in this patient's exercise limitation.

CASE 52 *Obstructive airway and pulmonary vascular disease, with a patent foramen ovale and systemic hypertension*

CLINICAL FINDINGS

This 64-year-old retired shipyard worker was evaluated because of increasing shortness of breath that began 7 years previously and had increased to become evident with walking two blocks or climbing one flight of stairs. He smoked one half of a pack of cigarettes daily from age 40 to 60. He was treated with isoniazid and ethambutol for pulmonary tuberculosis for 4 years, 2 decades ago. Prostatic carcinoma was diagnosed 8 months previously while he was having a transurethral prostatectomy. He took triamterene, hydrochlorothiazide, and methyldopa for the treatment of hypertension. Pulse was irregular without other evidence of cardiovascular disease. The chest x-ray studies revealed a single small pleural plaque on the left, evidence of old granulomatous disease in the right apex, and a flat diaphragm. Respiratory function tests done several days prior to exercise showed airway obstruction.

EXERCISE FINDINGS

The patient performed exercise on a cycle ergometer. He pedalled at 60 rpm without added load for 3 minutes. The work rate was then increased 15 watts per minute to his symptom limited maximum. Blood was sampled every second minute and intra-arterial blood pressure was recorded from a percutaneously placed brachial artery catheter. Resting ECG showed some premature atrial and premature ventricular contractions, poor R wave progression from leads V1 through V3, and left atrial enlargement. At 90 watts there were occasional pairs of premature ventricular contractions and 2 episodes of ventricular bigeminy. The patient stopped exercising because of shortness of breath. Under questioning, he also conceded that he had felt some substernal tightness at the highest work rate.

Interpretation

COMMENTS

This case is presented to illustrate the considerable amount of gas exchange abnormality that can occur during exercise, even with only mild abnormalities in spirometry.

The results of the resting respiratory function studies indicate that this patient has mild airflow obstruc-

TABLE 52-1. *Selected Respiratory Function Data*

MEASUREMENT	PREDICTED	MEASURED	
Age, yr		64	
Sex		Male	
Height, cm		178	
Weight, kg	80	82	
Hematocrit, %		47	
		BEFORE BRONCHODILATOR	AFTER BRONCHODILATOR
VC, L	3.82	4.52	4.75
IC, L	2.55	3.25	
TLC, L	5.93	8.66	
FEV_1, L	2.98	2.69	2.78
FEV_1/VC, %	78	60	58
MVV, L/min	121	90	112
DL_{CO} ml/mm Hg/min	24.8	14.0	

TABLE 52-2. *Selected Exercise Data*

MEASUREMENT	PREDICTED	MEASURED
Maximum $\dot{V}O_2$, L/min	2.15	1.42
Maximum HR, beats/min	156	159
Maximum O_2 pulse, ml/beat	13.8	8.9
$\Delta\dot{V}O_2$/ΔWR, ml/min/watt	10.3	8.1
$\dot{V}O_2$ difference, %	0.0	11.7
AT, L/min	>0.88	indeterminate
Blood pressure, mm Hg (rest, max)		185/116,263/128
Maximum $\dot{V}E$, L/min		91
Exercise breathing reserve, L/min	>15	−1
Pa_{O_2}, mm Hg (rest, max ex)		76,57
$P(A-a)_{O_2}$, mm Hg (rest, max ex)		38,65
$P(a-ET)_{CO_2}$, mm Hg (rest, max ex)		4,9
VD/VT (rest, heavy ex)		0.38,0.47
HCO_3^-, mEq/L (rest, 2 min recov)		24,17

tion, hyperinflation, and a moderately severe abnormality in diffusing capacity (Table 52-1). The resting electrocardiogram is abnormal, as evidenced by premature atrial and ventricular contractions and poor R wave progression from V1 to V3. The intra-arterial blood pressure is elevated. In such instances, one might have considered deferring the exercise test until blood pressure was under better control. The cuff-measured blood pressure is on the average 10 mmHg lower than the directly recorded blood pressure, as described in Chapter 6. Because of the blood pressure elevation, the patient was exercised especially cautiously. The objective was to determine if this patient was primarily limited by his heart or lung disorder.

TABLE 52-3.

TIME min	WORK RATE W	BP mmHg	HR min⁻¹	f	$\dot{V}E$ BTPS L/min	$\dot{V}CO_2$ STPD L/min	$\dot{V}O_2$ STPD L/min	O_2 pulse ml/beat	R	pH	HCO_3^- mEq/L	PO_2 ET mmHg	PO_2 a mmHg	PO_2 A-a mmHg	PCO_2 ET mmHg	PCO_2 a mmHg	PCO_2 a-ET mmHg	$\dfrac{\dot{V}E}{\dot{V}CO_2}$	$\dfrac{\dot{V}E}{\dot{V}O_2}$	$\dfrac{VD}{VT}$
Rest		185/116								7.42	24	76			38					
Rest			102	16	16.3	0.33	0.36	3.5	0.92			117			29			45	41	
Rest			103	12	8.6	0.15	0.15	1.5	1.00			118			29			50	50	
Rest		185/116	108	23	13.2	0.23	0.24	2.2	0.96	7.46	22	120	79	38	28	32	4	49	47	0.38
Unloaded			115	21	22.9	0.50	0.55	4.8	0.91			116			30			42	38	
Unloaded			117	19	28.5	0.64	0.65	5.6	0.98			117			30			42	41	
Unloaded		236/126	119	27	35.6	0.74	0.71	6.0	1.04	7.43	22	122	72	46	28	33	5	45	47	0.39
1.0	15		123	28	43.1	0.85	0.80	6.5	1.06			123			26			48	51	
2.0	30	236/128	128	30	50.9	0.95	0.89	7.0	1.07	7.44	21	123	68	52	26	32	6	51	54	0.45
3.0	45		133	38	49.8	0.91	0.92	6.9	0.99			121			27			51	51	
4.0	60	/	143	39	63.2	1.12	1.08	7.6	1.04	7.44	21	126	61	59	24	31	7	53	55	0.45
5.0	75		148	44	71.3	1.26	1.21	8.2	1.04			123			26			54	56	
6.0	90	/	157	52	88.2	1.49	1.34	8.5	1.11	7.42	20	128	60	61	22	31	9	56	62	0.48
6.5	105	263/128	159	47	90.8	1.59	1.42	8.9	1.12	7.41	19	128	57	65	22	31	9	55	61	0.47
Recovery			161	43	84.4	1.54	1.25	7.8	1.23			127			23			52	65	
Recovery			151	44	75.2	1.31	1.14	7.5	1.15			122			29			55	63	
Recovery		233/139								7.39	17		73			29				

FIGURE 52-A.

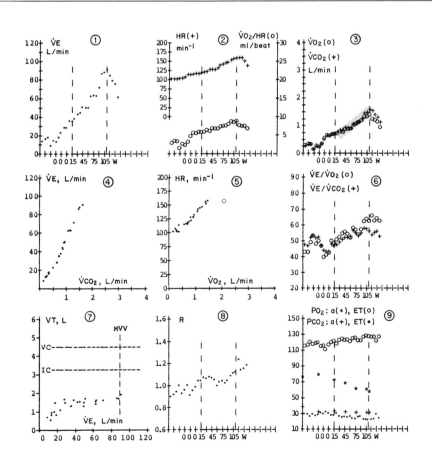

ANALYSIS

Flow Chart 1: The maximum $\dot{V}O_2$ is reduced but the anaerobic threshold cannot be reliably determined (Table 52-2). See *Flow Chart 5:* The indices of ventilation-perfusion mismatching (V_D/V_T, $P(a - ET)_{CO_2}$ and $P(A-a)_{O_2}$), are abnormal *(branchpoint 5.1)* as shown in Table 52-3 and summarized in Table 52-2. The breathing reserve is low, supporting the diagnosis of lung disease limiting this patient's exercise performance *(branchpoint 5.3)*. Breathing frequency is less than 50 at the maximum $\dot{V}O_2$ *(branchpoint 5.7)*, consistent with a diagnosis of obstructive, rather than restrictive, lung disease.

The confirmatory measurements under the heading of obstructive lung disease, however, are not found in this patient. For instance, the patient does not develop a mild respiratory acidosis and the heart rate reserve is not high. This suggests that the problem is complex. The prominent abnormalities are those that are generally seen with pulmonary vascular disease *(branchpoint 5.6)*. Referring to the pulmonary vascular diseases diagnostic box, one can find that the confirmatory data are all present, i.e., decreasing Pa_{O_2} with increasing work rate, a steep heart rate response, normal heart rate reserve, a low $\Delta\dot{V}O_2/\Delta WR$, a significant *metabolic* acidosis rather than a respiratory acidosis at maximum exercise, and a low DL_{CO}, which is disproportionately reduced compared to the degree of airflow obstruction.

Finally, it appears that this patient's abnormality in gas exchange is largely accounted for by the opening of a foramen ovale during exercise. (See the last item in the pulmonary vascular disease diagnostic box.) R is greater than 1 throughout exercise (Graph 8, Fig. A). PET_{CO_2} decreases with increasing work rate (Graph 9, Fig. 52-A) in contrast to that observed for patients with obstructive lung disease, and the calculated V_D/V_T and $P(a - ET)_{CO_2}$ not only remain abnormal but become more abnormal as work rate is increased (Table 52-3) because venous blood bypasses the lungs and mixes with arterialized blood. Decreasing PET_{CO_2} and increasing $P(a - ET)_{CO_2}$ and V_D/V_T with work rate, and a sustained high R are all characteristic of a right-to-left shunt during exercise. 100% oxygen breathing during the exercise test might have confirmed the development of the right-to-left shunt. The cardiac ectopy that became more significant as exercise progressed was probably due to myocardial ischemia consequent to systemic hypertension (documented) and pulmonary hypertension (undocumented).

The patient has a low breathing reserve, not because his ventilatory capacity is significantly reduced but rather because his ventilatory requirement is high consequent to the increasing V_D/V_T and the maintainance of a very low alveolar P_{CO_2}.

CONCLUSION

Pulmonary vascular disease, possibly secondary to obstructive lung disease, with a probable opening of a foramen ovale during exercise. Cardiac ectopy due to myocardial ischemia consequent to systemic hypertension and possible pulmonary hypertension.

Symbols and Abbreviations

Dash ($^-$) above any symbol indicates a *mean* value
Dot ($\cdot$) above any symbol indicates a *time derivative*

GASES

	PRIMARY SYMBOL		EXAMPLE
V	gas volume	V_A	volume of alveolar gas
$\dot{V}$	gas volume/unit time	$\dot{V}_{O_2}$	O_2 uptake/minute
P	gas pressure	$P_{A_{O_2}}$	alveolar O_2 pressure
$\bar{P}$	mean gas pressure	$\bar{P}_{C_{O_2}}$	mean capillary O_2 pressure
F	fractional concentration of a particular gas	$F_{I_{O_2}}$	fractional concentration of O_2 in inspired gas
f	respiratory frequency		
D	diffusing capacity	D_{CO}	diffusing capacity for co
R	respiratory exchange ratio		
RQ	respiratory quotient		
Q	gas quantity		
$\dot{Q}$	gas quantity/unit time (gas flow)	$\dot{Q}_{O_2}$	O_2 consumed/minute
STPD	standard temperature and pressure (0°C, 760 mm Hg), dry		
BTPS	body temperature and pressure, saturated with water vapor		

	SECONDARY SYMBOLS (subscripts)		EXAMPLES
I	inspired gas	$F_{I_{O_2}}$	fractional concentration of O_2 in inspired gas
E	expired gas	V_E	volume of expired gas
A	alveolar gas	$\dot{V}_A$	alveolar ventilation/minute
ET	end tidal	$P_{ET_{CO_2}}$	end-tidal CO_2 tension
T	tidal gas	V_T	tidal volume
D	dead space gas	V_D	physiological dead space volume
B	barometric	P_B	barometric pressure

235

BLOOD

PRIMARY SYMBOLS		EXAMPLES	
$\dot{Q}$	volume flow of blood/unit time	$\dot{Q}c$	blood flow through pulmonary capillaries/minute
C	concentration of gas in blood phase	Ca_{O_2}	content of O_2 in arterial blood
S	% saturation of Hb with O_2	$S\bar{v}_{O_2}$	saturation of Hb with O_2 in mixed venous blood

SECONDARY SYMBOLS (SUBSCRIPTS)		EXAMPLES	
a	arterial blood	Pa_{CO_2}	partial pressure of CO_2 in arterial blood
v	venous blood	$P\bar{v}_{O_2}$	partial pressure of O_2 in mixed venous blood
c	capillary blood	Pc_{O_2}	partial pressure of O_2 in pulmonary capillary blood

VARIABLES AND PARAMETERS

$\dot{V}_{O_2}$	oxygen uptake
$\dot{V}_{O_2}max$	maximal aerobic power
$\dot{V}_{CO_2}$	carbon dioxide output
$\dot{Q}_{O_2}$	O_2 consumption
$\dot{Q}_{CO_2}$	CO_2 production
AT	anaerobic threshold
R	gas exchange ratio
RQ	respiratory quotient
$\dot{V}_E/\dot{V}_{O_2}$	ventilatory equivalent for O_2
$\dot{V}_E/\dot{V}_{CO_2}$	ventilatory equivalent for CO_2
V_D/V_T	physiological dead space/tidal volume ratio
V_D	physiological dead space
BR	breathing reserve
HR	heart rate
HRR	heart rate reserve

LUNG VOLUMES AND FLOWS

V_T	tidal volume = volume of air inhaled or exhaled with each breath
VC	vital capacity = maximal volume that can be expired after maximal inspiration
IC	inspiratory capacity = maximal volume that can be inspired from the resting end-expiratory level
ERV	expiratory reserve volume = maximal volume that can be expired from the resting end-expiratory level
FRC	functional residual capacity = volume of gas in lungs at end-expiration
RV	residual volume = volume of gas in lungs after maximal expiration
TLC	total lung capacity = volume of gas in lungs after maximal inspiration
FEV_x	forced expired volume in x seconds, e.g. FEV_1 (one second)
MVV	maximal voluntary ventilation

Glossary

Aerobic: Having molecular oxygen present; describes metabolic process utilizing oxygen.

Alveolar to arterial P_{O_2} difference: The difference between the ideal alveolar P_{O_2} and the mean arterial P_{O_2}. This difference is considered to be an index of the lungs' inefficiency with respect to oxygen exchange.

Alveolar ventilation: This is notionally the volume of inspired gas that reaches the alveoli per minute, or the volume of gas that is evolved from the alveoli per minute. In practice, it is computed as the theoretical alveolar ventilation necessary to produce the arterial level of CO_2 tension at the current CO_2 output level.

Anaerobic: Lacking or inadequate molecular oxygen; describes any metabolic process that does not use molecular oxygen.

Anaerobic threshold *(AT)*: The highest oxygen uptake attained by a subject without a sustained increase in blood lactate concentration and lactate/pyruvate ratio. This parameter is consequently an important demarcation between work rates that are of moderate and heavy work intensity.

Analog to digital converter: This is a device for transforming continuously changing information into discrete units over some small time frame, within which the value is considered to be relatively constant. This transforms continuous biological signals to a form that can be analyzed by a digital computer.

Arterial to end-tidal P_{CO_2} difference ($P(a-ET)_{CO_2}$): The difference between the mean arterial P_{CO_2} and the end-tidal P_{CO_2}. This is positive when the arterial P_{CO_2} is higher than the end-tidal P_{CO_2}.

Arterial-mixed venous O_2 difference ($C(a-\bar{v})_{O_2}$): The difference in the O_2 content of the arterial and venous blood, usually expressed in ml of O_2 per deciliter or liter of blood.

ATPS: Gas volume conditioned to the ambient temperature and pressure, and saturated with water vapor at ambient temperature.

Breath-by-breath: The expression of a particular physiological value averaged over one entire respiratory cycle. These are usually expressed in milliliters or liters per minute, i.e. the value that would be obtained if that particular breath volume and duration were maintained over an entire minute.

Breathing reserve (BR): The difference between the maximum voluntary ventilation and the maximum exercise ventilation. Hence, this represents the body's residual potential for further increasing ventilation at maximum exercise.

BTPS: Gas volume conditioned to body temperature and the ambient atmospheric pressure, and fully saturated with water vapor at the subject's body temperature.

Carbon dioxide output ($\dot{V}CO_2$): The amount of CO_2 exhaled from the body into the atmosphere per unit time, expressed in ml or liters/min, STPD. This differs from CO_2 production rate under conditions in which additional CO_2 may be evolved from the body's stores or CO_2 is added to the body's stores. In the steady state, CO_2 output equals CO_2 production rate. In rare circumstances, significant quantities of CO_2 can be eliminated from the body as bicarbonate via the gastrointestinal tract or by hemodialysis.

Carbon dioxide production ($\dot{Q}CO_2$): The amount of carbon dioxide produced by the body's metabolic processes and in some circumstances released by buffering reactions within the body, expressed in ml or liters/min, STPD.

Cardiac output: The flow of blood from the heart in a particular period of time, usually expressed as liters per minute. It is the product of the average stroke volume per beat and the heart rate, i.e. number of beats per minute.

Constant work rate test: An exercise test in which a constant power output is required of the subject.

Dead space or physiological dead space (VD): This is the theoretical volume of gas taken into the lung that is not involved in gas exchange, assuming that the gas tensions in the alveolar volume equilibrate with those of the pulmonary capillary blood as it leaves the lung. Thus, the physiological dead space is made up of the anatomical dead space and also the volume of alveoli that are ventilated but unperfused, and a certain portion of those that are underperfused i.e., alveolar dead space.

Dead space/tidal volume ratio: The proportion of the tidal volume that is made up of the physiological dead space, i.e., this is an index of the relative inefficiency for pulmonary gas exchange.

Diffusing capacity: This is a measure of the rate of uptake of a particular gas across the alveolar-capillary bed for a specified driving pressure for that gas. It is

measured, therefore, as the volume of gas per unit time per pressure difference, e.g. ml/min/mm Hg. It is also referred to as the pulmonary gas transfer index (a term that more properly reflects the measurement).

Diffusion defect: A defect in the lungs' ability for gas diffusion. This is typically caused either by an abnormally increased diffusion path length or by conditions in which the transit time of the red cell through the pulmonary capillary bed is so fast that insufficient time is available for complete diffusion equilibrium.

Disability: A legal term that considers the effect of a functional impairment on the patient's ability to perform a specific work task, and other factors such as age, sex, education, social environment, job availability, and the energy requirements of the occupation.

End-tidal PCO_2: The PCO_2 of the respired gas determined at the end of an exhalation. This is commonly the highest PCO_2 measured during the alveolar phase of the exhalation.

End-tidal PO_2: The PO_2 determined in the respired gas at the end of an exhalation. This is typically the lowest PO_2 determined during the alveolar portion of the exhalation.

Exponential: A process in which the instantaneous rate of change of a variable is proportional to the "distance" from a steady state or required level; hence, the rate of change of the function under consideration is rapid when it is far from its steady state value and slows progressively as the function approaches its steady state. If the process is known to be, or may be reasonably estimated to be, exponential, the time to reach 63% of the final value, i.e., to approach within 37% of the final value, is termed the time constant (τ) of the response. If the process is exponential, this time constant is related to the half time (the time to reach 50% of the final value) by the equation $T\frac{1}{2} = 0.693 \times \tau$.

Fick method for cardiac output: A means of estimating cardiac output from the uptake of O_2 by the lungs and the arterial-mixed venous O_2 content difference $\dot{Q} = \dot{V}O_2/C(a - \bar{v})_{O_2}$. When the same principle is used to measure cardiac output with CO_2 as the test gas, the CO_2 output is divided by the $C(a - \bar{v})_{CO_2}$.

Frequency response: This reflects the fidelity with which a device can track rapidly changing physiological information. The frequency response of the device is usually determined by applying some rapidly changing signals of a particular amplitude, spanning a range of frequencies, and then establishing the range over which the device accurately tracks the signal.

Gas exchange ratio (R): The ratio of the carbon dioxide output to the oxygen uptake per unit time. This ratio reflects not only tissue metabolic exchange of the gases but also the influence of transient change in gas storage on O_2, and especially CO_2, exchange at the lungs, i.e., the gas exchange ratio exceeds the respiratory quotient during hyperventilation as additional CO_2 is evolved from the body's stores; the gas exchange ratio is less than the respiratory quotient during transient hypoventilation when CO_2 is retained in the body's stores.

Half time ($T\frac{1}{2}$): Unlike the time constant, which requires evidence of exponentiality for its determination, the half time of a response is a simple description of the time to reach half of the change to the final value, regardless of the function. It is, therefore, generally representative of the speed of approaching the steady state.

Heart rate reserve (HRR): The difference between the predicted highest heart rate attainable during maximum exercise and the actual highest heart rate — usually for exercise testing involving large muscle masses such as during cycle or treadmill ergometry.

Ideal alveolar P_{O_2}: A term that describes the alveolar P_{O_2} that would be obtained if the lung were an ideal gas exchanger, i.e., with ventilation being uniformly matched to perfusion.

Impairment: A medical term reflecting an abnormality of physiologic function that persists after treatment. For exercise, it could represent any defect in the ventilatory-circulatory-metabolic coupling of external to internal respiration.

Incremental exercise test: An exercise test designed to provide gradational stress to the subject. The work rate is usually increased over uniform periods of time, for example, every 4 minutes, every minute, every 15 seconds, or even continuously (e.g., ramp-pattern increment).

Laminar flow: A condition in which the flow of fluid is characterized by the uniform direction of flow of any plane sheet of the fluid, each of which flows parallel to any other in the direction of flow.

Mass spectrometer: A device that separates molecules of gas of a particular type, in a mixed gas stream, on the basis of its mass. Two types are commonly used: The fixed collector, which uses a magnetic means of separating the gases; these are then sensed at particular locations. Alternatively, a quadruple mass spectrometer utilizes shifts in an electro-magnetic field to separate the gases such that only one gas arrives at the sensing site at any discrete moment in time.

Maximum exercise heart rate: The highest obtainable heart rate during a maximum effort test.

Maximum exercise ventilation: The highest minute ventilation achieved during a maximum work rate test. This is usually determined by tests that tax large muscle masses, such as cycle or treadmill ergometry.

Maximum voluntary ventilation (MVV): The upper limit of the body's ability to ventilate. This is conventionally measured from maximal volitional effort for short periods of time, e.g. 15 seconds, and expressed in units of liters per minute, BTPS.

Minute ventilation ($\dot{V}I$ or $\dot{V}E$): The volume of air taken into or exhaled from the body in one minute. This is conventionally expressed in units of body temperature, saturated with water at atmospheric pressure (BTPS).

Mixed venous: The averaged partial pressure, or gas content, of the blood returning from all the tissues of the body and, having been properly mixed in the right heart, is normally represented by the concentration or partial pressure of a substance in the pulmonary arterial blood.

Mixing chamber: A device that mixes the dead space and alveolar gas to obtain an estimate of the average value of the mixed expired gas. This is typically achieved by exhaling into a baffled chamber that mixes several breaths. The mean value can be measured downstream from the chamber. Considerable care, however, must be taken in using such a device to align the delayed mixed expired value with the appropriate volume measurement.

O_2 content: The volume of O_2 (STPD) in a unit volume (liter, deciliter, milliliter) of blood. This includes the major component that is bound to hemoglobin and that amount physically dissolved in the blood.

O_2 debt: The additional oxygen utilized in excess of the baseline needs of the body following a bout of exercise.

O_2 deficit: The oxygen equivalent of the total energy utilized to perform the work that did not derive from reactions utilizing atmospheric oxygen taken into the body after the start of the exercise. Consequently, for moderate intensity exercise, this O_2 deficit represents the energy equivalent of the depletion of the high energy phosphate stores and the reactions that involve oxygen stored in the body at the start of the work. For heavy or severe exercise, the oxygen deficit includes, in addition, the energy equivalent of the anaerobic processes.

O_2 delivery: The amount of oxygen delivered to a tissue per unit time. It is, therefore, the product of the oxygen content of arterial blood and the blood flow to that tissue.

O_2 difference: The difference between the O_2 uptake predicted for a work rate during an incremental exercise test and the highest O_2 uptake attained.

O_2 flow: The amount of oxygen actually flowing per unit time, either from the heart or into a region of interest, such as a muscle or a muscle fiber. This, therefore, is a product of the oxygen content of the arterial blood and the blood flow.

O_2 pulse: The oxygen uptake divided by the heart rate. Hence, it is the amount of oxygen extracted by the tissues of the body over a single beat of the heart or of a stroke volume.

Oximeter: A device that uses transmission techniques to estimate the saturation of hemoglobin with oxygen. Direct oximetry is done on blood samples. For indirect oximetry, a site for measurement, such as the earlobe or pinna, is selected because blood comes close to the skin, traverses the capillary bed with little loss of oxygen and, hence, the mean capillary value will reflect arterial values.

Oxygen consumption ($\dot{Q}O_2$): The amount of oxygen utilized by the body's metabolic processes in a given time, expressed in ml or liters/min, STPD.

Oxygen uptake ($\dot{V}O_2$): The amount of oxygen extracted from the inspired gas in a given period of time, expressed in ml or liters/min, STPD. This can differ from oxygen consumption under conditions in which oxygen is being utilized from the body's stores. In the steady state, oxygen uptake equals the oxygen consumption.

Phase I: The period of time following the onset of exercise in which the mixed venous blood entering the pulmonary capillary bed has not changed its composition. This is a result of transit delays from the site of increased metabolism. Normally, this period is 15 to 20 seconds. During this phase, therefore, any increase in O_2 uptake reflects increased blood flow through the lungs and not an increased a $-$ $\bar{v}$ difference across them.

Phase II: The period of time following the onset of exercise when the mixed venous blood gas concentrations are chang*ing*. It, therefore, reflects the "ki-

netic phase" of the gas exchange that begins at the end of Phase I and continues until a steady state is obtained.

Phase III: The steady state phase of gas exchange during exercise. It reflects the period in which the mixed venous gas concentrations have become constant.

Physiological dead space: See Dead space.

Pneumotachograph: A device used to measure gas flow. It is typically composed of a screen across which the pressure drop of flowing gas may be measured. This determines the instantaneous gas flow that may be integrated over the breath to yield the volume of air.

Pulse pressure: The difference between the systolic and the diastolic blood pressures.

Respiratory quotient (RQ): The ratio of the rate of carbon dioxide production to oxygen consumption. This ratio reflects the metabolic exchange of the gases in the body's tissues and is dictated by substrate utilization.

Response time: A means of characterizing the rate at which a device or system responds to a given signal. For example, in response to a sudden application of a constant level of input, how long does the output take to become constant? This can be characterized as a time constant, τ, or the time to reach 90% of the final value.

STPD: Gas volume at standard conditions of temperature and pressure, free of water vapor. The standard conditions are zero degrees C, 760 mm Hg (i.e., a "standard" atmosphere) pressure, and dry.

Set point: This is a term used in control system theory that reflects the particular value of a regulated variable that the output of the system regulates. For example, a CO_2 set point is considered to be the operating level of arterial P_{CO_2}, which is maintained at its relatively constant (i.e., set point) value by changes in ventilation at some level of CO_2 output.

Steady state: This is a characteristic of a physiological system in which its functional demands are being met such that its output per unit time becomes constant. The time to achieve a steady state commonly differs for different physiological systems. For example, following the onset of constant load exercise, oxygen uptake rises to reach its steady state appreciably faster than that of CO_2 output or of ventilation. Hence, the steady state should be considered specific for the particular physiological function. A constant value attained by the system is not sufficient, however, to determine that the system is in a steady state. If the system reaches the limit of its output, and hence, its output becomes constant, as in the case of oxygen uptake reaching its maximum value, a steady state does not prevail. The system in this instance is in a limited, not a steady state.

Stroke volume: The volume of blood ejected from either ventricle of the heart at a single beat.

Sustainable work rate: This is a relative term that reflects the extent to which a particular work rate may be sustained for sufficient time for the successful completion of a particular occupational, recreational, or laboratory induced work rate. Therefore, at a sustainable work rate, the subject does not fatigue within the time constraints of the requirements of the test.

Thermodilution blood flow measurement: A technique in which a bolus of iced saline is injected into a vascular stream, such as the right atrium, and sampled at a mixed downstream point, such as the pulmonary artery. From the degree of cooling of the downstream blood resulting from the bolus injection of the known volume of 0°C saline, intervening flow of blood can be estimated.

Tidal volume to inspiratory capacity ratio: The ratio of the volume of air actually breathed during a breath to the air potentially available for that breath, measured from the end expiratory lung volume to the maximum inspiratory volume. Hence, it reflects the proportion of the potential inspiratory volume excursion that is actually utilized for a particular breath.

Transcutaneous gas tension: The technique for estimating the partial pressure of the gas in the capillary blood perfusing a region of skin with high flow and low metabolic rate. The intent of this measurement is to estimate arterial blood gases. To this end, it must be interpreted with caution.

Transducer: A device that transforms energy from one form to another. Consequently, a pressure transducer is a device that changes pressure into an electrical signal that can be analyzed and used for display or recording.

Turbulent flow: A condition in which the fluid flow has characteristic eddies, whorls, and diverse directional currents, such that additional energy needs to be applied to create a given fluid flow.

$\Delta\dot{V}O_2$ (6 – 3): The difference in oxygen uptake between the sixth and the third minute of a constant load exercise test. Normal subjects typically attain a steady state for constant load exercise within 3 minutes when working at or below the *AT;* hence, the $\Delta\dot{V}O_2$ (6 – 3) is zero. A positive value for this index reflects a degree of continuing nonsteady state for the work and usually signals fatiguing exercise.

$\dot{V}O_2$ max: The highest oxygen uptake obtainable for a given form of ergometry despite further work rate increases and effort by the subject. This is characterized by a plateau of oxygen uptake despite further increases in work rate.

$\Delta\dot{V}O_2/\Delta$work rate: This is the increase in oxygen uptake in response to a simultaneous increase in work rate. Under appropriate conditions (steady state aerobic work), this may be used to estimate the efficiency for muscular work.

Wasted ventilation: The difference between the computed alveolar ventilation and the measured minute ventilation. Also known as the physiological dead space ventilation. This term is meant to reflect the volume of the respired air that did not participate in alveolar capillary gas exchange, and it is equal to $V_D \times f$.

Work: A physical quantification of the force operating upon a mass that causes it to change its location. Under conditions where force is applied and no movement results (for example, during an isometric contraction), no work is performed, despite the increased metabolic energy exchange.

Work rate or power: This reflects the rate at which work is performed, i.e., work per unit time. This is usually measured in kilopond $\times$ meters per minute ($kp \cdot m/min$) or alternatively in watts (where 1W is equivalent to 6.12 $kp \cdot m/min$.).

APPENDIX C

Devices and Systems for Collecting
and Analyzing Physiological Data

Systems

THE PROPER interpretation of exercise test data depends on accurate data collection and correct calculations. A variety of systems, measuring devices, recorders, calculation devices, and other equipment have been used for these purposes. Computer techniques recently have been incorporated to facilitate data storage and calculations. However, useful information can be obtained from even very simple systems.

SYSTEM WITH "MINIMAL" EQUIPMENT

Exercise testing can be performed with little or no equipment. A measured course, stairway, or hallway provides a reproducible and functional exercise stress. Data collected can include review of symptoms, physical examination, and heart rate and blood pressure at the conclusion of exercise. Arterial blood gases may be obtained, albeit with some inconvenience, when the subject has stopped.

SYSTEM WITHOUT ANALYSIS OF EXPIRED GASES

A treadmill or cycle ergometer permits a more controlled exercise stress to be administered. Because the subject is relatively stationary, blood pressure and heart rate may be obtained repeatedly, and a continuously monitored electrocardiogram incorporating 1, 3, or 12 leads may be used. An ear oximeter would also be a useful noninvasive tool. Oxygen administration may be conveniently given during exercise for some forms of testing. While subject to potential important errors, the work rate on a cycle or treadmill can be translated into an estimate of oxygen uptake.

MANUALLY OPERATED SYSTEM FOR EXPIRED GAS ANALYSIS

Noncontinuous collection of expired gas may be performed using a manually operated system during exercise. Subjects breathe through a suitable breathing valve from which expired gas is collected in a meteorological balloon, impermeable plastic, or Douglas type bag. Timed collections of mixed expired gas may be made at intervals during exercise. While most often used during constant work rate exercise testing, this method can be used to collect repeated samples of expired gas over relatively short intervals. Thus, it may be used during some non-steady conditions. If desired, a series of bags can be connected to stopcocks for sequential sampling. After collection, bags can be emptied into a spirometer or through a gas meter to determine volume. Mixed expired CO_2 and O_2 can be determined using appropriate analyzers. Because speed of analysis is not crucial, water vapor may be removed from the expired gas prior to analysis. This may simplify calculation of O_2 uptake and CO_2 output.

Bags or balloons are generally light in weight and are hung vertically to avoid added resistance to the expired breathing circuit. Care must be taken that bags or balloons are leak-free and are "washed out" with approximately mixed expired gas prior to collection to minimize errors. In addition, changes in expired gas composition may occur from diffusion of gas through the bags if analysis is greatly delayed.

A semiautomated system using bags to collect expired gas was described by Wilmore and Costill.[1] This system used a rotating valve to deliver gas to one of three collection bags. The other two bags were simultaneously either having their contents analyzed or, after analysis, being evacuated. Ventilation could be determined by a gasmeter or pneumotachograph in series with the collection bags. Thus, sequential samples could be automatically obtained and analyzed.

SEMIAUTOMATED OR AUTOMATED SYSTEMS USING MIXING CHAMBERS

The availability of rapidly responding gas analyzers made it possible to display nearly instantaneous CO_2 and O_2 concentrations of expired gas. While these analyzers made analysis of manually collected gas easier, they also led to the development of systems for continuous determination of gas exchange during exercise, using an appropriate flow measuring device and a mixing chamber.

In this type of system, expired gas is sampled from a mixing chamber into which all expired gas is channeled. The intent of the mixing chamber is to approximate a sample of mixed expired gas from which CO_2 output and O_2 uptake can be calculated.

For an ideal mixing chamber, with instantaneous and complete mixing of gas, the introduction of a constant flow of gas Y will eventually result in the gas in the mixing chamber having the identical composition of gas Y. The time course for the concentration of gas Y can be described as approximately exponential, and for this ideal mixing chamber, the characteristics can be described by a time constant = $Vmc/\dot{V}$, where Vmc is the volume of the mixing chamber and $\dot{V}$ is the constant flow of gas into and out of the chamber. The time constant is related to the time the mixing chamber takes to reach the new gas concentration after a step-change in the input gas is introduced. The change reaches about 95% of its final value after three time constant intervals have elapsed.

A large gas flow (or minute ventilation) or a mixing chamber of small size will produce a short time constant. Under these conditions, this chamber would respond rapidly to a change in gas concentration; that is, a step-change in input would be quickly reflected in a change in concentration sampled from the chamber. When tidal volume increases a large amount relative to the volume of the mixing chamber, however, fluctuations in the gas concentration of the mixing chamber will result. On the other hand, mixing cannot be expected to be complete and instantaneous, although high gas velocities and the use of baffles in the mixing chamber contribute to gas mixing. Too large a mixing chamber volume compared to minute ventilation can result in an impractically long time to reach any new equilibrium. Thus, a compromise between stability of concentration, mixing, and equilibration time is necessary. Most authors suggest a mixing chamber volume of 5 to 6 liters for testing adults during exercise.[2,3] At rest, the time constant for a chamber of this size would be about one minute (a 95% concentration change would be reached in about 3 minutes). The time constant will decrease as ventilation increases during exercise.

These factors suggest that fixed volume mixing chambers may be satisfactory during exercise in which $\dot{V}E$, FE_{CO_2}, and FE_{O_2} are changing only slowly, but may not be satisfactory when rapid changes are expected. In the latter situation, an alteration in actual mixed expired gas concentration will not be reflected in the mixing chamber until after a new equilibrium is reached. Thus, if ventilation is being continuously measured, some time or volume adjustment must be made to match the correct mixed expired gas concentrations with the correct ventilation when calculating $\dot{V}O_2$ and $\dot{V}CO_2$.

Variables measured using such a system may include expired ventilation, mixed-expired CO_2 and O_2, heart rate, and respiratory rate. All of these can be recorded on a calibrated multichannel physiological recorder. An automated system using a mixing chamber can also be designed to record these data and calculate variables periodically during exercise.

AUTOMATED BREATH-BY-BREATH SYSTEMS

Gas exchange variables change rapidly at the onset of exercise, during exercise in which work rate changes more frequently than every 3 to 4 minutes, and at the beginning of recovery period. The ability to measure these rapidly changing values would make it possible to select certain useful work rate protocols such as 1 minute incremental increases in work rate. Because mixed expired bag collection and mixing chamber systems may not be suitable, a number of breath-by-breath systems have been designed.

Breath-by-breath systems measure air flow or volume continuously, and simultaneously determine instantaneous expired CO_2 and O_2 concentrations. The CO_2 output and O_2 uptake during each breath are calculated and the total from all breaths over a measured time period gives $\dot{V}O_2$ and $\dot{V}CO_2$. To make accurate measurements, the ventilation and gas concentrations must be determined repeatedly at short intervals. The number of different measurements and the large number of samples needed make breath-by-breath systems impractical without the aid of computer controlled data sampling and calculations.

While these systems are considerably more complicated than the noncomputerized systems, the same principles and formulae are used. The added complexity makes the detection and correction of errors more difficult. Nevertheless, both individually designed and commercially made breath-by-breath systems have proven to be accurate and reproducible, allowing tests to be completed quickly, with less discomfort to the patient and more rapid reporting. We have used breath-by-breath systems for both research applications and for evaluation of patients.[4,5] These make it possible to determine gas exchange rapidly and accurately under a wide variety of conditions.

Measurement of Volume, Flow Rate, or Ventilation

Several methods of measuring volume and flow rates during exercise can be used. Each has advantages and disadvantages that make them suitable for different types of systems. While expired ventilation or flow is usually measured, many of the physiologic variables desired can be calculated from inspired volume or flow with the appropriate adjustments. Devices for measuring volume and/or flows may be used directly as part of the breathing circuit, or may be used to measure volumes from a collecting container. If the device is used directly, then flow resistance, linearity, and frequency response may be important considerations.[6] If flow is measured rather than volume, e.g., with a pneumotachograph, then flow rate must be electrically or mathematically integrated over time to determine volume per unit time. If volume is measured directly, using a gas meter, spirometer, or volume transducer, then flow can be, but is not often, calculated by the differentiation of the instantaneous volume signal.

DRY GAS METER.   A dry gas meter, such as a Parkinson-Cowan type, can be used to measure the volume collected in Douglas bags or rubber meteorological balloons. Thus, it is suitable for a manually operated system with intermittent collection of expired gas. Alternatively, the dry gas meter can be used directly in either the inspired or expired side of a breathing valve circuit. The dry gas meter is reasonably accurate, especially if used with constant flow, but may be subject to mechanical leaks and maladjustment. Moisture in the expired gas has also been recognized as a potential cause of error.[7]

SPIROMETER.   A large spirometer, such as a Tissot type water sealed spirometer of 120, 350, or 600 liters capacity, is an extremely useful device in the exercise laboratory. It can be used to measure volumes collected into bags or relatively impermeable balloons, for calibration of other volume and flow devices, or used directly in a manually operated system. The advantages of a large spirometer include accuracy, simplicity, and ease of quality control. Disadvantages are its size and bulk, the difficulty connecting recording devices, and, if used as a direct measurement device, poor frequency response and potential resistance to breathing.

PNEUMOTACHOGRAPHS.   Pneumotachographs are devices used to measure instantaneous gas flow. The most commonly used devices consist of either a number of parallel tubes (Fleisch) or a series of fine wire mesh screens. Each device, therefore, offers a small resistance to airflow. The pressure drop across this resistance can be measured and related to the amount of airflow.

There is a linear relationship between gas flow and pressure drop given by Poiseuille's law. The linear coefficient is constant for constant dimensions of the resistive element for a given gas viscosity. This, however, holds true only during conditions of laminar flow (also called nonturbulent flow). In general, conditions approximating laminar flow in smooth walled tubes will be met if the gas velocity is low compared to the cross section of the tube. In addition, laminar flow is disrupted by changes in the size or direction of conducting tubing. The resultant turbulent flow can be restored to laminar if the gas is allowed to flow through a relatively long, straight, smooth walled tube of appropriate size.

Fleisch Pneumotachograph.   In this device, laminar flow is encouraged by using small flow channels and low velocities of gas. In the Fleisch pneumotachograph, this is accomplished by making the resistance element a bundle of parallel channels. A small flexible plastic tube is connected at each end of the resistance element and the two tubes are then connected to a differential pressure transducer. During gas flow through the pneumotachograph, the differential pressure is proportional to the flow. The electrical signal from the transducer is then further processed or displayed directly. The pressure transducer must be relatively sensitive since the approximate pressure difference at the usually recommended maximal flow rate is only 12 to 13 mm H_2O.

The pneumotachograph by definition introduces additional resistance into the breathing circuit. Because the Fleisch pneumotachograph is made in several different sizes, with larger sizes intended for measuring higher flow rates, the resistance is minimal and appears to be undetectable by the subject (on the order of 2 to 6 mm $H_2O/L/s$).

Linearity.   The size of the pneumotachograph, the upstream gas flow geometry, the range of flowrates used, and the method of measurement determine its linearity. For a given pneumotachograph, pressure drop can be shown to be a satisfactory linear function of gas flow rate until flow rate exceeds some particular value. Beyond this value, pressure drop increases nonlinearly with flow rate. The Fleisch pneumotachograph is available in six different sizes. For exercise testing in adults, flow rates encountered generally indicate that a no. 3 Fleisch pneumotachograph is appropriate. This represents a balance between linearity in the flow rates up to 5 to 10 L/s and adequate sensitivity in the low flow range.

A known constant flow of air can be generated by a vacuum cleaner, appropriate valves, and a calibrated flow meter. From this a curve of pressure drop across the pneumotachograph vs. flow can be derived.[6] Yeh et al.[8] used a weighted-averaging technique and calibrated syringe to determine the pneumotachograph pressure-flow characteristics, a method that avoids the use of a flow generator. This method should prove satisfactory for a computer-aided data acquisition system. Generally, pneumotachograph manufacturers provide data on expected pressure-flow characteristics of their products, but these should be rechecked after installation and after attachment of devices needed for actual measurements.

Finucane et al.[6] studied the influence of upstream geometry using Fleisch pneumotachographs. They found that the pressure-flow relationship was linear over the widest gas flow range when the immediate upstream geometry was a pipe of the same internal diameter as the pneumotachograph. They suggested that for a no. 3 Fleisch, 11 cm of straight pipe, and for a no. 4 Fleisch, 12 cm of straight pipe were optimal. A rough guide would be to use a straight smooth pipe with a length of 5 to 6 times the diameter of the flow meter immediately prior to the pneumotachograph in the entering air stream.

Finally, extension of the linear flow rate range can be attempted either by electrically altering the output of the differential pressure transducer as has been done by several manufacturers, or, in computer-based systems, mathematically adjusting the pressure signal. The linear flow range has been increased by as much as 50 to 100% with, generally, less than 2% deviation from linearity at full recommended maximal flow.

Frequency Response.   Rapidly changing flow rates may not be measured with perfect fidelity if the pneumotachograph is unable to respond instantaneously. Since the pneumotachograph has no moving parts, any delay is due solely to the inertia of gas movement. This inertia is the result of an additional pressure difference needed to accelerate the gas within the pneumotachograph and would appear as a greater pressure difference at a given flow rate. Finucane et al.[6] found that for Fleisch pneumotachographs flow values did lag behind pressure changes for sinusoidal flow at frequencies up to 10 Hz. However, the lag was small and in all probability is insignificant compared to the frequency response of other parts of the breathing circuit used for exercise studies. It is necessary also to consider the frequency characteristics of the differential pressure transducer and any linearizing circuit, the response of the chart recorder if used, and the sampling frequency of digital sampling if a computer-based system is used. In addition, a minimum number of interconnecting fittings should be employed.[9]

Temperature.   Pneumotachographs used for measuring flow of ambient air are usually kept at ambient temperature. Since expired gas is usually warmer and contains more water vapor than ambient air, contact of this gas with an ambient temperature pneumotachograph would result in condensation and obstruction of the pneumotachograph resistance elements. These pneumotachographs, therefore, are often used with an electric heater to warm the pneumotachograph to a temperature slightly above expired gas temperature. Too high a temperature will result in significant cooling during calibration and use, with resultant inconsistent errors.

The problem is more complicated, however, because a heated pneumotachograph not only warms the expired gas (if the gas is cooler than the pneumotachograph), but warms it by a variable amount depending on the flow of gas. Warming the gas will increase its volume and thereby alter the pressure-flow relationship. While theoretical methods can be used to estimate the degree of warming, two practical methods may eliminate the problem. Both methods make the expired gas temperature as it enters the pneumotachograph and the pneumotachograph temperature equal. Either the expired gas can be kept warm[5] prior to entering a heated pneumotachograph, or the expired gas can be allowed to cool to ambient temperature before reaching an ambient temperature pneumotachograph. In the former method, the temperature of the pneumotachograph should be only slightly warmer (0.5° C) than the temperature of the gas passing through it. If the expired gas is cooled, then the method must guarantee that even a large flow of expired gas can be quickly cooled to ambient temperature. The ease of pneumotachograph calibration is also a consideration, with the use of the ambient temperature pneumotachograph somewhat simpler.

Gas Density and Viscosity. Oxygen is significantly more viscous than nitrogen. Because viscosity is a direct factor in Poiseuille's law relating pressure difference and flow rate for a given straight tube, it follows that air and 100% oxygen would have a different pressure-flow relationship. Calibration and calculation methods need to consider this effect or unexpected errors will arise. For 100% oxygen breathing, we find that flow rates are measured approximately 11% higher for a pneumotachograph calibrated with a known flow rate of air. Although only gas viscosity is a direct factor in Poiseuille's law, gas density is a determinant of whether laminar or turbulent flow will exist at a given gas velocity in a given straight tube. A low density, high viscosity gas, such as a mixture consisting of a high proportion of helium, maintains laminar flow at higher velocities and, therefore, pressure difference and flow rate remain linear at higher flow rates.

Turbine Volume Transducer. This is a relatively new device that uses a lightweight impeller to directly measure the volume of gas flow. It has proven to be linear over a wide range of flow rates, to behave identically for air and for O_2, and to offer good frequency response characteristics. This device may have significant advantages over other volume measurement devices in breath-by-breath exercise testing. Of note is that it has been used for measuring bidirectional gas flows, i.e., both inspiratory and expiratory gas. Because of gas temperature changes, however, a correction must be used to obtain expired volume using the principle of nitrogen balance between inspired and expired gas. Also, the speed of the impeller is sensitive to water or saliva deposition.

CALIBRATION. Validation of any flow or volume device is essential for confidence in the ability of the device to measure accurately and reproducibly under testing conditions. A water-sealed spirometer is recommended as a primary standard for volume measurements and spirometer volume change over a timed period can be used as a flow standard. Secondary standards include calibrated large volume syringes of 1 to 4 liters and various gas flow meters. These secondary standards should be calibrated against a spirometer before use. If flow or volume signals are further processed by analog or digital means, the results are subject to the response characteristics and calculation methods of these instruments as well.[9]

Pneumotachographs have special calibration considerations related to the problems of temperature, water vapor, viscosity, and geometry. The simplest method is to calibrate the pneumotachograph under identical conditions to the testing process. Thus, a known volume or flow of gas of essentially identical temperature, relative humidity, and gas composition to the anticipated measured gas should be delivered to the pneumotachograph through identical upstream geometry. The flow range at which a linear pressure drop is expected should be determined rather than assumed from manufacturers' specifications. Care should be taken to calibrate and use the pneumotachograph within the linear range.

Breathing Valves

Breathing valves separate inspired from expired gas flows so that expired gas can be collected and analyzed. The ideal valve prevents contamination of either gas flow by the other. The ideal valve also has low resistance to both inspiration and expiration, low rebreathed volume (low valve dead space), and operates silently. Other advantages would include low size and weight, lack of generation of turbulence in the airstream, ease of cleaning, and low cost.

As expected, no valve design is ideal. However, for testing healthy fit exercising adults, a low resistance valve is preferred because of the high ventilation observed. These valves usually consist of 2 or 3 sets of one-way "J valves" each for inspiration and expiration. The small "J valves" allow rapid opening and closing. Examples include triple J valves, double J valves, and Otis-McKerrow type valves. All of these have dead-space volumes of 100 to 320 ml that should be considered if calculation of V_D/V_T is intended. A high capacity Rudolph valve may also be suitable for high flow applications. At lower flow rates, Koegel and Hans-Rudolph valves with smaller dead space volumes and slightly higher flow resistances may be used. The Koegel valve, for example, has a specified dead space of 64 ml, exclusive of the mouthpiece. We find this valve as well as the Hans-Rudolph valve to be satisfactory for clinical purposes.

While manufacturers' specifications are helpful, some characteristics of valves should be estimated in the laboratory prior to use. Dead-space could be determined for the valve plus attached mouthpiece by measuring the amount of water it can contain. Valve resistance is usually determined during constant airflow using a vacuum cleaner and flow meter, and is expressed as cm H_2O/L/sec. This value may be different between inspiration and expiration. Commonly, dry gas or room air is used for calibration. This can cause underestimation of valve resistance during exercise testing, as the valve flaps can require additional pressure to open when wet and gas flow is pulsatile. Some valves, even if they have low resistance to constant airflow, may appear to subjects to "stick" closed temporarily, perhaps altering their pattern of breathing. Finally, valves may have or develop backleaks, especially when subjected to high flows and pressures during heavy exercise. These leaks should be suspected for any valve, but especially after prolonged use, infrequent cleaning, excessive secretions, or damage to component parts. Errors in ventilation or gas exchange measurements may be important clues to a leaking breathing valve. If a leak is suspected, simultaneous recording of inspiratory and expiratory flow during exercise may reveal the presence and location of the leak.

Gas Analyzers

Details of Scholander and Haldane analysis of expired gases can be found in standard references.[10] These methods are very accurate but time consuming and tedious, making them impractical for large numbers of repeated measurements. Nevertheless, they are useful for calibration of other gas analyzers and primary analysis of stored gases used for calibration.

Carbon dioxide analyzers measure absorption by CO_2 of characteristic wavelengths of infrared light. Thus, infrared light is passed through a cell containing the gas to be measured, and the amount of light transmitted is compared to a known constant value. The absorption is proportional to the CO_2 fraction. The measurement cell must be kept clean and free from water condensation.

Oxygen analyzers operate using several different principles. Two types are commonly used. The Paul-

ing type or paramagnetic analyzer measures the change in a given magnetic field introduced by changes in oxygen quantity in a chamber located within the magnetic field. As other respiratory gases have little paramagnetic susceptibility, these will not have an effect on the magnetic field. Electrochemical O_2 analyzers depend on chemical reactions between O_2 and a reusable substrate that result in the generation of an electrical current. This current is proportional to the quantity of O_2 molecules reacting with the substrate. Because a current is produced, these analyzers are sometimes called fuel cell O_2 analyzers.

Both of these types of devices measure partial pressure and therefore are affected by water vapor, pressure in the sampling systems, and changes in barometric pressure and altitude. Thus, for a given fractional concentration of O_2, changes in any of these conditions at the sensor location will erroneously result in different measured O_2 fractions. Because the sample flow rate delivering gas to the analyzer is generally held constant, a change in sampling system pressure may result from changes in resistance of the delivery tubing. Care must be taken to insure that: (1) resistance is identical during calibration and measurement; and (2) water condensation, saliva, or foreign bodies are not trapped in the delivery tubing.

While CO_2 analyzers are sensitive to pressure but less sensitive to flow or resistance changes, both CO_2 and O_2 analyzers report the fraction of CO_2 or O_2 of the total gas, including any water vapor present. This is important during calibration because ambient air usually contains some water vapor, resulting in a measured O_2 concentration below that of dry air, i.e., less than the 20.93% of dry air. Carbon dioxide would be affected in the same way. Expired gas, if water is not removed prior to analysis, is saturated with water vapor at the lowest temperature that it reaches prior to being analyzed. Because temperature determines the partial pressure of water in a saturated gas, this temperature must be accurately known or estimated if expired CO_2 and O_2 are to be accurately determined using these analyzers. An alternative is to pass the gas over anhydrous calcium sulfate. This substance removes water vapor and allows determination of CO_2 and O_2 concentrations as if the gas were dry. Additional consideration of the significance of water vapor in calculating $\dot{V}_{O_2}$ can be found in Appendix D.

In a mass spectrometer of the fixed collector type, sampled gases are ionized to positively charged ions by an electron beam. Then, in a near vacuum, the ions are accelerated by an electric field and subjected to a magnetic field. The directions the ions take in the magnetic field are dependent on their mass/

charge ratios without the additional effects of interactions between molecules. The different ions representing different gases then are detected by appropriately located detectors that produce a voltage output proportional to the number of ions detected. The individual detector voltages can be electronically divided by the total voltage. This quotient is the fractional concentration of each gas. Note that, because the total is dependent on the sum of the individual detectors, any gas for which there is no detector does not contribute to the total. For respiratory mass spectrometry, detectors for O_2, CO_2, and N_2 are typically used; ordinarily there are no detectors for water vapor, argon, or other inert gases present in trace amounts in air. Thus, the O_2 or CO_2 concentrations given by a mass spectrometer are concentrations relative to a dry gas containing no water vapor, regardless of whether the originally sampled gas contained water or not.

Gas analyzers, including mass spectrometers, should be checked for linearity within the range of needed values. This can be done by analyzing gases of known concentration of O_2 and CO_2. If an analyzer is nonlinear, a calibration curve at several concentrations can be drawn, or alternatively a continuous curve can be developed.[11]

Calibration should be performed with gases of known concentration. The analyzers should be warmed up for sufficient time to insure against electrical drift, an identical sampling arrangement to that used during testing should be used, and the sample cells should be cleaned if necessary. A device for drying gas prior to analysis may or may not be used during calibration procedures. Most often a two point calibration can be used if the analyzer is sufficiently linear. It is convenient to use dry room air as one calibration point, assuming an O_2 of 20.93% and CO_2 of 0.0004% (essentially zero). A calibration gas of approximately 15% O_2, 5% CO_2, and balance N_2 (but whose actual values are accurately known) is appropriate for the second point since these concentrations are in the middle of the anticipated range of expired gas concentrations. The concentrations of the calibration gas mixture should not be assumed to be accurate as stated by the supplier, but should be analyzed independently by Haldane or Scholander techniques or by a carefully calibrated mass spectrometer. A useful procedure is to keep for long term use a tank of gas for which O_2 and CO_2 are very accurately known, then using this gas to calibrate the mass spectrometer. Subsequently, the mass spectrometer can be used to measure concentrations of tanks used for day to day calibration.

The gas transport delay time and the response time of each analyzer to the introduction of a new gas is an important aspect of breath-by-breath exercise systems. This is further addressed in Appendix D. For manual analysis of mixed expired gases, delay and response times are not critical.

Arterial Blood Gases and Arterial Catheters

Arterial blood gases may be obtained by arterial puncture or drawn through indwelling arterial catheters. Arterial punctures may be difficult to perform if the subject is moving, usually cannot be obtained repeatedly, and, if uncomfortable, may affect the subject's response to exercise and the results of the blood gases. Arterial punctures may be particularly difficult at or near a subject's exhaustion. Frequently, arterial punctures are performed just after the completion of exercise. These results may be significantly different than immediately prior to cessation of work,[12] especially for Pa_{O_2} and $P(A-a)_{O_2}$. Nevertheless, arterial punctures are useful if the exercise protocol permits and if only several blood samples are needed.

Indwelling arterial catheters make the repeated sampling of arterial blood for blood gases simpler, faster, and painless, and they permit continuous monitoring of blood pressure during exercise as well. A description of the insertion of a brachial artery catheter is included in Appendix E.

Arterial punctures and catheterization are rarely complicated by pain or other discomfort, bleeding, arterial spasm, distal arterial thromboembolism, thrombosis, and infection. Most frequently, subjects will complain of mild discomfort and hematoma formation following puncture. Sufficient pressure for an adequate amount of time after puncture or removal of the catheter and an elastic pressure dressing can help avoid this problem. Arterial catheters should be generally used with special care in patients with known peripheral vascular disease.

Noninvasive Measurement of Blood Gases

EAR OXIMETRY

Ear oximetry is used to measure ear capillary oxygen saturation, generally considered to be equal to arterial blood saturation. Instruments analyze the transmission of several (up to eight) wavelengths of light through the antihelix or ear lobe. Some devices incorporate a heater in the ear probe to augment and maintain ear perfusion. Oxygen saturation with these instruments is calculated with automatic adjustment for ear thickness and skin pigmentation and can be displayed digitally or the results sent to a recorder or computer. Procedures for calibration and validation are unique to each device, as well as characteristics such as response time and sensitivity to movement, stray light, and other artifacts. The weight of the device and ease of attachment to the exercising subject are also important considerations.

The major disadvantage of ear oximetry is that saturation rather than P_{O_2} is measured. Thus, while there is good correlation between measured arterial O_2 saturation and ear O_2 saturation for several types of oximeters,[13-15] decreases in arterial P_{O_2} in the range of $P_{O_2} > 60$ mm Hg result in only small decreases in O_2 saturation. For patients with arterial $P_{O_2} < 60$ mm Hg or whose Pa_{O_2} decreases to below 60 during exercise, ear oximetry proves to be quite useful. For other patients whose resting and exercise Pa_{O_2} is > 60 mm Hg but who are suspected of significant decreases in PaO_2 during exercise, one approach is to use ear oximetry during a preliminary test. If arterial oxygen saturation decreases by more than 3 to 5%, then an arterial catheter is placed for direct measurement of Pa_{O_2} and $P(A-a)_{O_2}$ during a repeat exercise study. Nevertheless, clinically important decreases in Pa_{O_2} may occur that could be undetectable by saturation measurement alone.

TRANSCUTANEOUS P_{O_2}

Transcutaneous P_{O_2} (Pt_{CO_2}) is measured using a Clark electrode attached to the skin. A current proportional to the number of oxygen molecules diffusing out of the skin beneath the electrode is produced. This current is determined and reported as partial pressure in mm Hg. The Pt_{CO_2} reflects arterial P_{O_2}, the blood flow to the skin under the electrode, the hemoglobin concentration and oxyhemoglobin dissociation curve, and the number of and distance from the epidermal capillaries. To improve blood flow, the electrodes in use heat the skin under the sensor to 43 to 45° C. This necessitates correction of the Pt_{CO_2} for the rightward shift of the oxyhemoglobin dissociation curve. This is done automatically by the instruments. Reports by Schonfeld et al.[16] and McDowell and Theide[17] on normal subjects and patients suggest that transcutaneous P_{O_2} might be a reasonable estimate of arterial P_{O_2} during exercise. The reader is referred to these papers for additional details.

Pulmonary Artery Catheters

A pulmonary artery catheter can add valuable information during exercise testing in some kinds of patients. Measurements that can be made with it include pulmonary artery pressure, pulmonary artery wedge pressure, mixed venous blood gases, and cardiac output by thermal indicator dilution. The Swan-Ganz catheter is balloon-tipped and flow-directed, and a physician can pass it through a large vein in the arm through the right atrium, right ventricle, and into the pulmonary artery with or without fluoroscopic guidance. Since arrhythmias and heart block potentially occur during placement, this should be done only with ECG monitoring and appropriate resuscitation equipment and medications standing by. For pressure measurements, a calibrated transducer and recorder are needed for continuous recordings. Samples of blood can be drawn from the catheter tip for mixed venous blood gases needed for the calculation of cardiac output using the Fick equation (see Appendix D) or precise calculation of venous admixture.

The thermodilution method introduces a bolus of physiological fluid (usually isotonic saline) of known volume, temperature (usually 0° C), and specific heat and specific gravity into a blood vessel transporting the total cardiac output. The temperature change downstream reflects the volume of dilution of the bolus and cardiac output can be calculated from this. The injection site is in the right atrium and the temperature sensor is in the pulmonary artery. The product of time and temperature change is inversely proportional to cardiac output. While this calculation can be done manually, a dedicated computer unit is most often used.

Stetz et al.[18] reviewed a number of studies and concluded that thermodilution cardiac outputs in catheterization laboratories and intensive care units were of comparable accuracy to Fick or dye-dilution methods. They suggested, however, that a 20 to 26% difference in cardiac output should be found before concluding that two single determinations were different. Advantages of thermodilution include safety, lack of recirculation, speed, and repeatability.

The disadvantages of a pulmonary artery catheter include increased risks, costs, and preparation time. Complications can include arrhythmias, heart block, bleeding, perforation of the right ventricle or pulmonary artery, and infections. However, under specific circumstances, the information obtained from these catheters may outweigh the risks.

Treadmill and Cycle Ergometers

Treadmills allow subjects to perform familiar walking and running exercise at measured speeds and grades of incline. A variety of protocols for increasing work performed have been reported, and both very low work rates and very high work rates may be obtained.

Subjects performing on treadmills have maximum oxygen uptakes approximately 5 to 10% higher than on cycle ergometers. In addition, some subjects and patients are simply not able to cycle due to problems of coordination.

On the other hand, treadmills require more space than a cycle ergometer, demand extra caution during testing, and may introduce movement artifacts in measurement of ventilation and oxygen uptake. Subjects must not hold on tightly to any part of the treadmill, such as a railing, because this will affect measured oxygen uptake. Because work rate can only be approximated from body weight, speed, and grade, oxygen uptake measurements are highly desirable during exercise. Work efficiency during treadmill walking cannot be precisely determined because of the difficulty in estimating work rate.

Treadmill speed and grade should be routinely checked. Grade may be determined by measurement using a plumb line and tape measure. Speed can be accurately determined by using a stopwatch to time the movement of a mark made on the treadmill belt. These speed and grade values permit comparisons of subjects between different tests.

Cycle ergometers permit very good estimation of the work rate by knowing the resistance to cycling. Leg cycling may be performed sitting or supine. Advantages of the cycle ergometer over the treadmill include the ability to quickly vary the work rate in step, incremental, or ramp fashion; ability to determine work efficiency; smaller size; potentially greater safety since the subject is supported at all times; and, less movement artifact during exercise on measurements. Some subjects and patients, however, may not be able to pedal the cycle due to lack of coordination and experience. The seat may become uncomfortable during a prolonged exercise study.

In the upright position, seat height is important and should be carefully adjusted. When seated, the subject's foot at the lowest point of the pedalling cycle should be such that the knee is almost but not completely straight. It is useful to record the seat height in the subject's records so that future studies may be done identically. Subjects should be asked to wear tennis shoes suitable for the types of pedals on the cycle. Toe clips may or may not be used as desired.

Two types of cycle ergometers are in general use. Mechanically-braked devices use an adjustable brake to provide resistance to pedalling. The adjustment is made by increasing or decreasing contact of a braking device on a moving flywheel attached to the pedals. The work rate achieved is related to the cycling frequency or speed of the flywheel. As such, a particular work rate is only achieved if the subject cycles within a very narrow range of speed. Electrically-braked cycle ergometers on the other hand use a magnetic field to produce a resistance to pedalling that can be easily made to vary appropriately with flywheel speed, varying the resistance to cycling. Thus, a given work rate is present for a range of cycling speeds. In addition, the work rate on the electrically-braked devices may be set by a remote controller or may be adjusted automatically by a digital computer controller.

When subjects must pedal at a particular rate, metronomes and/or tachometers can be used to assist subjects' performance.

Calibration of the cycle is highly desirable both when used initially and periodically thereafter. Manufacturers' specifications and calibration procedures should be followed. Commercially-available or specially built devices that generate known amounts of power can act as standards for calibration and verification.[19] In addition, because oxygen uptake in an individual maintains a very constant relationship to work rate, a number of readily available subjects may be used for rough checks on cycle work rate accuracy.

When a subject pedals on the cycle with "no resistance added," work is obviously being performed. The work rate may be as much as 20 to 30 watts for some cycle ergometers and may vary considerably with pedalling rate. This work rate may exceed the maximal capacity of some severely limited patients. Manufacturer specifications may provide information on the work rate of "unloaded cycling," but users should make this determination themselves.

WORK AND POWER

During exercise, the muscles require delivery of oxygen appropriate for the work being performed. The rate of oxygen utilization is related to the physical energy required to perform exercise. In basic physical units, force ($kg \cdot m \cdot s^{-2}$ or newton) = mass (kg) × acceleration ($m \cdot s^{-2}$). When this force is applied over a distance, work is performed. Thus, work ($kg \cdot m^2 \cdot s^{-2}$ or newton-m or joule) = force ($kg \cdot m \cdot s^{-2}$ or newton) × distance (m). However, we are most often interested in the rate of work or power = work ($kg \cdot m^2 \cdot s^{-2}$ or newton-m or joule)/ unit time (s). The unit of power is the watt. A watt is equal to 1 joule $s^{-1} = 1$ newton $\cdot m \cdot s^{-1} = 1$ kg $\cdot m^2 \cdot s^{-3}$.

For a cycle ergometer, a rotating flywheel is restrained by a friction belt or electromagnet. The work rate is then the distance traveled by a point on the circumference of the wheel times the rotational frequency of the flywheel times the restraining force.

This force can be expressed as newtons or, commonly, as kiloponds, where 1 kilopond (kp) = 1 kg $\times$ 9.81 m $\cdot$ s^{-2}. Thus, the work rate or power can be expressed as joules/sec = watts = 6.12 kp $\cdot$ m $\cdot$ min^{-1}. To convert from kp $\cdot$ m $\cdot$ min^{-1} to watts, divide by 6.12. Thus, a work rate of 612 kp $\cdot$ m $\cdot$ min^{-1} is equal to 100 watts.

Calculator and Computer Systems

There is a potential for tremendous amounts of information to be obtained during exercise testing, depending of course on the types and numbers of variables measured. Because of this large amount of information, computers have found great usefulness in many exercise laboratories.

For manually operated systems the volume and complexity of data are manageable using a hand-held or desktop calculator. Programmable calculators and microcomputers nevertheless can make calculations less tedious and less subject to error.[20] These may be programmed using readily available programming languages with little attention to speed or memory capacity.

Semiautomated and automated systems, whether using mixing chambers or breath-by-breath analysis, can require rapid sampling, calculation, and reporting of data. The rapidity of data collection naturally leads to large volumes of data that quickly become difficult to manage without a computer system. Computers can be programmed to collect data at desired rates, match signals over time, calculate derived variables, perform numerical integration, incorporate correction and calibration factors, store data, and subsequently report data in convenient tables or graphs. In addition, programs can direct the operator through calibration of the exercise system and provide checks on quality control and reproducibility.

The state-of-the-art in computers for exercise physiology laboratories is constantly changing and recommendations based on current technology may become quickly obsolete. Nevertheless, certain criteria may be used to suggest whether a computer based system is suitable. Data sampling is under the direction of an analog-to-digital converter. This device should have adequate sampling rate and the computer should be able to accept these data at this rate. The analog-to-digital converter also must have sufficient resolution of conversion from the voltage output of the anaylzer to the digital number sent to the computer. A 10– or 12–bit or more conversion is usually adequate. Sufficient computer memory is needed for both programs and data. The size of most exercise physiology computation programs, however, will not exceed moderate size computer memo-

ries. Finally, the speed of calculation may be a limiting factor for some breath-by-breath systems that must perform large numbers of calculations. The type of computer language and the speed of the computer may be relevant here.

A commercially available exercise testing system with a computer should meet criteria of sufficient memory, sampling rate, and speed for its purposes, and possibly versatility for other applications. In addition, the programs should be easily modified to fit the needs of a particular laboratory or to correct potential errors in the originally written programs. Optimally, it should provide a graphical and tabular report of the patient's results ready for the medical record, requiring only the physician's interpretation.

Because most computers are general-purpose devices that can manipulate numbers and other information in a similar way, any number of computers may be adaptable for the exercise physiology laboratory. However, because an exercise testing system may be complicated, discussions and critiques of the methods, programs, sampling rate and systems, data analysis, and data display should involve the physician, physiologist, technician, and programmer.

References

1. Wilmore, J. H., Costill, D. L.: Semiautomated systems approach to the assessment of oxygen uptake during exercise. J. Appl. Physiol., 36:618–620, 1974.
2. Poole, G. W., Maskell, R. C.: Validation of continuous determination of respired gases during steady-state exercise. J. Appl. Physiol., 38:736–738, 1975.
3. Spiro, S. G., Juniper, E., Bowman, P., Edwards, R. H. T.: An increasing work rate test for assessing the physiological strain of submaximal exercise. Clin. Sci. Molec. Med., 46:191–206, 1974.
4. Beaver, W. L., Wasserman, K., Whipp, B. J.: On-line computer analysis and breath-by-breath graphical display of exercise function tests. J. Appl. Physiol., 34:128–132, 1973.
5. Sue, D. Y., Hansen, J. E., Blais, M., Wasserman, K.: Measurement and analysis of gas exchange during exercise using a programmable calculator. J. Appl. Physiol., 49:456–461, 1980.
6. Finucane, K. E., Egan, B. A., Dawson, S. V.: Linearity and frequency response of pneumotachographs. J. Appl. Physiol., 32:121–126, 1972.
7. Wilmore, J. H., Davis, J. A., Norton, A. C.: An automated system for assessing metabolic and respiratory function during exercise. J. Appl. Physiol., 40:619–624, 1976.
8. Yeh, M. P., Gardner, R. M., Adams, T. D., Yanowitz, F. G.: Computerized determination of pneumotachometer characteristics using a calibrated syringe. J. Appl. Physiol., 53:280–285, 1982.
9. Jackson, A. C., Vinegar, A.: A technique for measuring frequency response of pressure, volume, and flow transducers. J. Appl. Physiol., 47:462–467, 1979.
10. Consolazio, C. F., Johnson, R. E., Pecora, L. J.: Physiological Measurements of Metabolic Function in Man. New York: McGraw-Hill, 1963.
11. Gabel, R. A.: Calibration of nonlinear gas analyzers using exponential washout and polynomial curve fitting. J. Appl. Physiol., 34:400–401, 1973.
12. Ries, A. L., Fedullo, P. F., Clausen, J. L.: Rapid changes in arterial

blood gas levels after exercise in pulmonary patients. Chest, 83:454–456, 1983.

13. Burki, N. K., Albert, R. K.: Non-invasive monitoring of arterial blood gases. A report of the ACCP section on respiratory pathophysiology. Chest, 83:666–670, 1983.

14. Chapman, K. R., D'Urzo, A., Rebuck, A. S.: The accuracy and response characteristics of a simplified ear oximeter. Chest, 83:860–864, 1983.

15. Chaudhary, B. A., Burki, N. K.: Ear oximetry in clinical practice. Am. Rev. Respir. Dis., 117:173–175, 1978.

16. Schonfeld, T., Sargent, C. W., Bautista, D., Walters, M. A., O'Neal, M. H., Platzker, A. C. G., Keens, T. G.: Transcutaneous oxygen monitoring during exercise stress testing. Am. Rev. Respir. Dis., 121:457–462, 1980.

17. McDowell, J. W., Thiede, W. H.: Usefulness of the transcutaneous P_{O_2} monitor during exercise testing in adults. Chest, 78:853–855, 1980.

18. Stetz, C. W., Miller, R. G., Kelly, G. E., Raffin, T. A.: Reliability of the thermodilution method in the determination of cardiac output in clinical practice. Am. Rev. Respir. Dis., 126:1001–1004, 1982.

19. Clark, J. H., Greenleaf, J. E.: Electronic bicycle ergometer: A simple calibration procedure. J. Appl. Physiol., 30:440–442, 1971.

20. Powles, A. C. P., Jones, N. L.: A pocket calculator program for noninvasive assessment of cardiorespiratory function. Comput. Biol. Med., 12:163–173, 1982.

Calculations — Formulae and Examples

T HIS APPENDIX presents the most essential formulae for calculating gas exchange and other related variables during exercise. An example accompanies the formula for each variable, using typical data acquired during exercise testing. While the calculation of these variables uses well-defined and tested formulae, several areas deserve particularly close attention. Thus, at the end of this Appendix, we address the specific problems of water vapor in the calculation of $\dot{V}O_2$; the problem of making corrections for the dead space of the breathing valve; aspects of breath-by-breath gas exchange analysis; and, a particular method of determining the *AT*, the V-slope method.

Formulae and Example of Gas Exchange Calculation

The formula for calculating each variable must take into account the conditions under which measurements are made and certain conventions that are followed. For the example calculation, we assume that expired gas is collected for two minutes into, for example, a meteorological balloon or Douglas bag. Volume is measured in a large spirometer; fractional concentrations of O_2 and CO_2 are measured to within 0.04% using gas analyzers or a mass spectrometer. For the gas analyzers, the gas is passed through a column of calcium sulfate to remove water vapor prior to analysis. An arterial blood sample is obtained during the collection of expired gas.

The measurements used for the example calculation are given in Table D-1, page 262.

MINUTE VENTILATION ($\dot{V}E$)

The volume of gas exhaled is divided by the time of exhalation in minutes to determine minute ventilation ($\dot{V}E$). By convention, $\dot{V}E$ is reported at body temperature saturated with water vapor at ambient pressure (BTPS), as in formula 1. It may be necessary during calculation to obtain $\dot{V}E$ (STPD) using formula 2, or from the appropriate tables (Appendix F).

A. Most commonly, ventilation is measured at ambient temperature and gas is fully saturated with water vapor at that temperature (ATPS). Formula 1 is used to adjust volume from ATPS to BTPS. The temperature and water vapor correction factors can also be found in Appendix F.

$$\dot{V}E \ (L/min,BTPS) = \dot{V}E \ (L/min,ATPS) \times \frac{(273 + 37)}{273 + T}$$

$$\times \frac{P_B - P_{H_2O} \ (at \ T)}{P_B - 47} \quad (1)$$

where T is ambient temperature, body temperature is 37° C, P_{H_2O} at 37° is 47 mm Hg, and P_B is barometric pressure.

B. Once $\dot{V}E$ (BTPS) is found, $\dot{V}E$ (STPD) can be obtained using formula 2. This converts $\dot{V}E$ (BTPS) to STPD (273°K, barometric pressure = 760 mm Hg, and no water vapor present) for $\dot{V}_{CO_2}$ and $\dot{V}_{O_2}$ calculations.

$$\dot{V}E \ (L/min,STPD) = \dot{V}E \ (L/min,BTPS) \times \frac{273}{(273 + 37)}$$

$$\times \frac{(P_B - 47)}{760}$$

which becomes,

$$\dot{V}E \ (L/min,STPD) = \dot{V}E \ (L/min,BTPS) \times 0.826, \ if \ P_B$$
$$= 760 \ mm \ Hg. \quad (2)$$

Example:

$$\dot{V}E \ (L/min,ATPS) = \frac{Total \ Volume \ (ATPS)}{Total \ Collection \ Time}$$

$$= \frac{54.2}{2 \ min} = 27.1$$

then, from formula 1

$$\dot{V}E \ (L/min,BTPS) = 27.1 \times \frac{310}{(273 + 22)}$$

$$\times \frac{(760 - 19)}{(760 - 47)} = 29.6$$

and, from formula 2,

$$\dot{V}E \ (L/min,STPD) = 29.6 \times 0.826 = 24.3$$

RESPIRATORY FREQUENCY (f)

$$f \ (min^{-1}) = \frac{number \ of \ complete \ breaths}{total \ time \ for \ complete \ breaths} \quad (3)$$

Example:

$$f \ (min^{-1}) = \frac{41 \ breaths}{2 \ min} = 20.5$$

TIDAL VOLUME (VT)

$$V_T \ (L,BTPS) = \frac{\dot{V}E \ (L/min,BTPS)}{f} \quad (4)$$

Example:

$$V_T \ (L,BTPS) = \frac{29.6}{20.5} = 1.44$$

CO$_2$ OUTPUT ($\dot{V}_{CO_2}$)

The CO_2 output and O_2 uptake are reported under STPD conditions. If $\dot{V}E$ and $\dot{V}I$ are measured at or converted to STPD conditions, $F_{E_{CO_2}}$ is the fraction of dry gas volume, and $F_{I_{CO_2}}$ is zero or negligible:

$$\dot{V}_{CO_2} \ (L/min,STPD) = \dot{V}E \ (L/min,STPD) \times F_{E_{CO_2}} \quad (5)$$

or, for P_B = 760 mm Hg,

$$\dot{V}_{CO_2} \ (L/min,STPD) = \dot{V}E \ (L/min,BTPS)$$
$$\times 0.826 \times F_{E_{CO_2}} \quad (6)$$

Example: Substituting $\dot{V}E$ and $F_{E_{CO_2}}$ (Table D–1) into formula 5,

$$\dot{V}_{CO_2} \ (L/min,STPD) = 24.3 \times 0.041 = 0.997$$

O$_2$ UPTAKE ($\dot{V}_{O_2}$)

For the derivation of the formula for $\dot{V}_{O_2}$ and consideration of water vapor, see Appendix D, Special Considerations. Formula 7 below should be used only after drying expired gas (if an electrochemical O_2 analyzer is used) or with a mass spectrometer.

If $\dot{V}E$ is measured at or converted to STPD, $F_{I_{O_2}}$ is 0.2093 (dry room air), $F_{E_{CO_2}}$ and $F_{E_{O_2}}$ are fractions of CO_2 and O_2 in dry gas, and $F_{I_{CO_2}}$ = 0, then:

$$\dot{V}_{O_2} \ (L/min,STPD) = \dot{V}E \ (L/min,STPD)$$
$$\times (\Delta F_{O_2})true,dry \quad (7)$$

where $(\Delta F_{O_2})true,dry = 0.265 - 1.265 \times F_{E_{O_2}} - 0.265 \times F_{E_{CO_2}}$ for a person breathing room air. The $(\Delta F_{O_2})true$ can also be obtained from the nomogram in Appendix F.

Example: Substituting from Table D–1 into Formula 7:

$$(\Delta F_{O_2})true,dry = 0.265 - 0.205 - 0.0108 = 0.049$$
$$\dot{V}_{O_2} \ (L/min, STPD) = 24.3 \times 0.049 = 1.19$$

GAS EXCHANGE RATIO (R)

$$R = \frac{\dot{V}_{CO_2} \ (L/min,STPD)}{\dot{V}_{O_2} \ (L/min,STPD)} \quad (8)$$

Example:

$$R = \frac{0.997}{1.19} = 0.84$$

VENTILATORY EQUIVALENT FOR CO_2 AND O_2 ($\dot{V}E/\dot{V}CO_2$, $\dot{V}E/\dot{V}O_2$)

The ventilatory equivalent for CO_2 and O_2 are measurements of ventilatory requirement for a given metabolic rate. Thus, by convention they are expressed as $\dot{V}E$ (L/min,BTPS) divided by $\dot{V}CO_2$ or $\dot{V}O_2$ (L/min,STPD). In this calculation, the valve deadspace (VDm) per breath is subtracted from the total $\dot{V}E$:

$$\dot{V}E/\dot{V}CO_2 =$$

$$\frac{\dot{V}E \ (\text{L/min,BTPS}) - [f \ \text{min}^{-1} \times VDm \ (\text{L})]}{\dot{V}CO_2 \ (\text{L/min,STPD})} \quad (9)$$

$$\dot{V}E/\dot{V}O_2 =$$

$$\frac{\dot{V}E \ (\text{L/min,BTPS}) - [f \ \text{min}^{-1} \times VDm \ (\text{L})]}{\dot{V}O_2 \ (\text{L/min,STPD})} \quad (10)$$

Example:

$$\dot{V}E/\dot{V}CO_2 = \frac{29.6 - [20.5 \times 0.064]}{0.997} = 28.4$$

$$\dot{V}E/\dot{V}O_2 = \frac{29.6 - [20.5 \times 0.064]}{1.19} = 23.8$$

OXYGEN PULSE ($\dot{V}O_2$/HR)

$\dot{V}O_2$/HR (ml,STPD/beat)

$$= \frac{\dot{V}O_2 \ (\text{L/min,STPD}) \times 1000 \ \text{ml/l}}{\text{HR (beats/min)}} \quad (11)$$

Example:

$$\dot{V}O_2/\text{HR (ml,STPD/beat)} = \frac{1.19 \times 1000}{120} = 9.9$$

ALVEOLAR PO_2 (PA_{O_2})

PA_{O_2} (mm Hg) = $FI_{O_2} \times (PB-47)$

$$- \frac{PA_{CO_2}}{R} (1 + FI_{O_2} (1 - R)) \quad (12)$$

where PB is barometric pressure in mm Hg, PA_{CO_2} is ideal alveolar PCO_2 in mm Hg, R is the gas exchange ratio, and FI_{O_2} is the fraction of inspired O_2, dry. Usually the assumption that $PA_{CO_2} = Pa_{CO_2}$ is used and the term $FI_{O_2} \times (1 - R)$ may be dropped be-

cause it is so small that it has an insignificant effect on the calculated PA_{O_2}, especially during air breathing. This simplifies the formula to:

$$PA_{O_2} \ (\text{mm Hg}) = FI_{O_2} \times (PB-47) - \frac{Pa_{CO_2}}{R} \quad (13)$$

While R is often assumed to be 0.8 at rest, this assumption may be incorrect; it should certainly be measured during exercise.

Example: Substituting into formula 13,

$$PA_{O_2} \ (\text{mm Hg}) = (0.2093 \times 713) - \frac{36}{0.84} = 106$$

ALVEOLAR-ARTERIAL PO_2 DIFFERENCE ($P[A-a]O_2$)

$$P(A - a)_{O_2} \ (\text{mm Hg}) = PA_{O_2} - Pa_{O_2} \quad (14)$$

where PA_{O_2} is determined as above and Pa_{O_2} is arterial PO_2.

Example:

$$P(A - a)_{O_2} \ (\text{mm Hg}) = 106 - 91 = 15$$

ARTERIAL-END TIDAL PCO_2 DIFFERENCE ($P[a - ET]CO_2$)

$$P(a - ET)_{CO_2} = Pa_{CO_2} - PET_{CO_2} \quad (15)$$

where Pa_{CO_2} is arterial PCO_2 and PET_{CO_2} is end-tidal PCO_2.

Example:

$$P(a - ET)_{CO_2} = 36 - 38 = -2$$

PHYSIOLOGICAL DEAD SPACE (VD)

$$VD \ (\text{L}) = VT \ (\text{L}) \times \frac{(Pa_{CO_2} - P\bar{E}_{CO_2})}{Pa_{CO_2}} - VDm \ (\text{L}) \quad (16)$$

where VT is tidal volume; Pa_{CO_2} is arterial PCO_2; $P\bar{E}_{CO_2}$ is mixed expired PCO_2; and VDm is mechanical dead space (valve). Mixed expired PCO_2 can be calculated from:

$$P\bar{E}_{CO_2} = \frac{\dot{V}CO_2 \ (\text{L/min,STPD})}{\dot{V}E \ (\text{L/min,STPD})} \times (PB - 47 \ \text{mm Hg})$$

Example:

$$P\bar{E}_{CO_2} = \frac{0.997 \times 713}{24.3} = 29$$

$$V_D \text{ (L)} = 1.44 \times \frac{36 - 29}{36} - 0.064 = 0.22$$

PHYSIOLOGICAL DEAD SPACE/TIDAL VOLUME RATIO (V_D/V_T)

$$\frac{V_D}{V_T} = \frac{(Pa_{CO_2} - P\bar{E}_{CO_2})}{Pa_{CO_2}} - \frac{V_{Dm} \text{ (L)}}{V_T \text{ (L)}} \quad (17)$$

Example:

$$\frac{V_D}{V_T} = \frac{36 - 29}{36} - \frac{0.064}{1.44} = 0.15$$

CARDIAC OUTPUT

The cardiac output ($\dot{Q}$) can be determined by thermal indicator dilution (see Appendix C) or by the Fick method using $\dot{V}_{O_2}$ and arterial-mixed venous O_2 content difference:

$$\dot{Q} \text{ (L/min)} = \frac{\dot{V}_{O_2} \text{ (ml/min,STPD)}}{(Ca_{O_2} - C\bar{v}_{O_2}) \text{ ml } O_2/\text{L blood}} \quad (18)$$

where Ca_{O_2} is O_2 content in arterial and $C\bar{v}_{O_2}$ is O_2 content in mixed venous blood. These can be calculated from:

$$C_{O_2} \text{ (ml } O_2/100 \text{ ml)} = (S_{O_2} \times 0.01 \times 1.34 \text{ ml } O_2/\text{g Hb} \\ \times [\text{Hb}]) + (0.003 \text{ ml } O_2/\text{mm Hg}/100 \text{ ml} \times P_{O_2}) \quad (19)$$

where [Hb] is hemoglobin concentration in g/100 ml blood and S_{O_2} is the oxyhemoglobin saturation.

Example:

$$Ca_{O_2} \text{ (ml } O_2/100 \text{ ml)} = (95\% \times 0.01 \times 1.34 \times 15) \\ + (0.003 \times 91) = 19.4$$

$$C\bar{v}_{O_2} \text{ (ml } O_2/100 \text{ ml)} = (50\% \times 0.01 \times 1.34 \times 15) \\ + (0.003 \times 27) = 10.1$$

$$(Ca_{O_2} - C\bar{v}_{O_2}) = 19.4 - 10.1 = \\ 9.3 \text{ ml } O_2/100 \text{ ml} = 93 \text{ ml } O_2/\text{L}$$

$$\dot{Q} \text{ (L/min)} = \frac{1190 \text{ (ml/min,STPD)}}{93 \text{ ml } O_2/\text{L blood}} = 12.8$$

The above method of cardiac output measurement requires a sample of mixed venous blood. A noninvasive determination of cardiac output can be made, however, using an analogous formula for CO_2 and an estimate of mixed venous CO_2 content (indirect Fick).

The mixed venous P_{CO_2} can be approximated by several techniques, for example, single-exhalation[1] and rebreathing.[2] With the rebreathing method, a mixture of CO_2 and high inspired O_2 is rebreathed, and the P_{CO_2} of the rebreathed gas rapidly approaches that of mixed venous blood. The content of CO_2 ($C\bar{v}_{CO_2}$) can then be determined using hemoglobin concentration and the CO_2 dissociation curve adjusted for estimated oxygen saturation.[3] The arterial P_{CO_2} is used to determine arterial CO_2 content (Ca_{CO_2}) and, using $\dot{V}_{CO_2}$, cardiac output is:

$$\dot{Q} \text{ (L/min)} = \frac{\dot{V}_{CO_2} \text{ (ml/min,STPD)}}{(C\bar{v}_{CO_2} - Ca_{CO_2}) \text{ ml } CO_2/\text{L blood}} \quad (20)$$

The arterial P_{CO_2} must be used in this calculation rather than the end-tidal P_{CO_2}. This is because the CO_2 content vs. P_{CO_2} curve (CO_2 dissociation curve) is steep, and a small error in P_{CO_2} results in a large error in CO_2 content. In addition, the $P_{ET_{CO_2}}$ is higher than Pa_{CO_2} in normal subjects but lower than Pa_{CO_2} in patients with $\dot{V}_A/\dot{Q}$ unevenness during exercise. The accuracy of the cardiac output also depends on an extremely accurate blood gas analysis for both arterial and mixed venous P_{CO_2} values. In addition, the oxygen content of the blood greatly affects the CO_2 content (Haldane effect), and the mixed venous oxygen is not known using these estimates. Because of these reasons, cardiac output measurements by this indirect, noninvasive method should be considered very approximate and used with caution.

Calculations at Maximum Exercise

BREATHING RESERVE (BR)

$$BR \text{ (L/min)} = \\ MVV \text{ (L/min)} - \dot{V}_E \text{ (L/min)} \text{ at maximum exercise} \quad (21)$$

$$BR \text{ (\%)} = \\ \frac{MVV \text{ (L/min)} - \dot{V}_E \text{ (L/min)} \text{ at maximum exercise}}{MVV \text{ (L/min)}} \times \\ 100 \quad (22)$$

where MVV is maximum voluntary ventilation at rest.

Example: If MVV is 82 L/min and $\dot{V}_E$ at maximum exercise is 65 L/min, then:

$$BR \text{ (L/min)} = 82 - 65 = 17$$

$$BR \text{ (\%)} = \frac{82 - 65}{82} \times 100 = 21\%$$

Heart Rate Reserve (HRR)

$$\text{HRR (beats/min)} = \text{Predicted maximum HR} \\ - \text{HR at maximum exercise} \qquad (23)$$

$$\text{HRR (\%)} =$$

$$\frac{\text{Predicted maximum HR} - \text{HR at maximum exercise}}{\text{Predicted maximum HR}} \times \\ 100 \qquad (24)$$

where predicted maximum HR (adults) = 220 − age (years).

Example: For a 60-year-old man, predicted maximum HR = 220 − 60 = 160. If HR at maximum exercise is 145 beats/min, then:

$$\text{HRR (beats/min)} = 160 - 145 = 15$$

$$\text{HRR (\%)} = \frac{160 - 145}{160} \times 100 = 9\%$$

Special Considerations of Calculation of Gas Exchange Variables

Water Vapor and Oxygen Uptake ($\dot{V}_{O_2}$)

Oxygen uptake ($\dot{V}_{O_2}$) is most often determined by collection and analysis of expired gas. The usual calculation method determines $\dot{V}_{O_2}$ using expired ventilation, expired CO_2 fraction, and expired O_2 fraction, and is based on the assumption that the volumes of nitrogen (and other inert gases) inspired and expired are not different overall. During rest and exercise, this method has been found to be satisfactory.[4,5] Nevertheless, errors may be introduced if careful attention to methods and calculations is not taken. This is especially true of water vapor because it can greatly affect the end result.

If the Scholander or Haldane methods of gas analysis or a mass spectrometer is used, or water vapor is removed prior to measurement, then measured gas concentration is the fraction of total gas excluding the volume of water vapor. Thus, the dilution of the concentration of each gas caused by water vapor can be ignored and calculations are relatively simple:

$$\dot{V}_{O_2} \text{ (L/min,STPD)} = (F_{I_{O_2}} \times \dot{V}_I \text{ [L/min,STPD])} \\ - (F_{E_{O_2}} \times \dot{V}_E \text{ [L/min,STPD])}$$

where $F_{I_{O_2}}$ and $F_{E_{O_2}}$ are the O_2 fractions of dry gas volume. If, overall, the volumes of inspired and expired nitrogen (and other inert gases) are equal during breathing, then:

$$\dot{V}_I \times F_{I_{N_2}} = \dot{V}_E \times F_{E_{N_2}}, \text{ and } \dot{V}_I = (F_{E_{N_2}}/F_{I_{N_2}}) \times \dot{V}_E$$

where $F_{I_{N_2}}$ and $F_{E_{N_2}}$ are the fractional concentrations of nitrogen and other inert gases.

Because $(F_{I_{N_2}} + F_{I_{O_2}} + F_{I_{CO_2}}) = 1$ and $(F_{E_{N_2}} + F_{E_{O_2}} + F_{E_{CO_2}}) = 1$, then:

$$\dot{V}_I = \frac{(1 - F_{E_{O_2}} - F_{E_{CO_2}})}{(1 - F_{I_{O_2}} - F_{I_{CO_2}})} \times \dot{V}_E$$

and

$$\dot{V}_{O_2} \text{ (L/min,STPD)} =$$

$$\left[\frac{F_{I_{O_2}} \times (1 - F_{E_{O_2}} - F_{E_{CO_2}})}{(1 - F_{I_{O_2}} - F_{I_{CO_2}})} - F_{E_{O_2}} \right] \times \\ \dot{V}_E \text{ (L/min,STPD)}$$

The quantity in brackets is called the true O_2 difference, (ΔF_{O_2})true.

If we assume that $F_{I_{CO_2}} = 0$ or is negligible, then:

$$(\Delta F_{O_2})\text{true} = \frac{(F_{I_{O_2}} - F_{E_{O_2}} - F_{I_{O_2}} \times F_{E_{CO_2}})}{(1 - F_{I_{O_2}})}$$

and

$$\dot{V}_{O_2} \text{ (L/min,STPD)} = \dot{V}_E \text{ (L/min,STPD)} \times (\Delta F_{O_2})\text{true}$$

For room air inspired gas, $F_{I_{O_2}}$ (dry) = 0.2093, and:

$$\dot{V}_{O_2} \text{ (L/min,STPD)} = \dot{V}_E \text{ (L/min,STPD)} \\ \times (0.265 - 1.265 \times F_{E_{O_2}} - 0.265 \times F_{E_{CO_2}}) \qquad (25)$$

If water vapor is not removed from the gas and the method of gas analysis measures gas fraction of the total gas volume including water vapor, such is the case for most O_2 analyzers, then the water vapor reduces each dry gas fraction by the factor:

$$\frac{(P_B - P_{H_2O})}{P_B} \text{ or } (1 - F_{H_2O})$$

In this case, the determination of $\dot{V}_{O_2}$ is affected by water vapor as follows. First, $\dot{V}_{O_2}$ can be expressed using $\dot{V}_I$ and $\dot{V}_E$ measured under the conditions of measurement, i.e., at temperature T and containing some water vapor:

$$\dot{V}_{O_2} \text{ (L/min,STPD)} = \frac{273}{273 + T} \times \frac{P_B}{760} \\ \times (\dot{V}_I \times F_{I_{O_2}} - \dot{V}_E \times F_{E_{O_2}}) \qquad (26)$$

where $\dot{V}_I$ and $\dot{V}_E$ are L/min at temperature T, and $F_{I_{O_2}}$ and $F_{E_{O_2}}$ are fractions of $\dot{V}_I$ and $\dot{V}_E$ respectively, including the volume of water vapor.

Because $\dot{V}_I = (F_{E_{N_2}}/F_{I_{N_2}}) \times \dot{V}_E$, and

$$F_{E_{N_2}} + F_{E_{O_2}} + F_{E_{CO_2}} + F_{E_{H_2O}}) = 1 \text{ and} \\ (F_{I_{N_2}} + F_{I_{O_2}} + F_{I_{CO_2}} + F_{I_{H_2O}}) = 1,$$

then substituting into equation 26 gives:

$$\dot{V}_{O_2} \text{ (L/min,STPD)} = \dot{V}_E \text{ (L/min at T)} \times k(T,P_{H_2O})$$
$$\times (\Delta F_{O_2})true \quad (27)$$

where

$$k(T,P_{H_2O}) = \frac{273}{273 + T} \times \frac{P_B}{760}$$

and

$(\Delta F_{O_2})true$

$$= \frac{F_{I_{O_2}} \times (1 - F_{E_{CO_2}} - F_{E_{H_2O}}) - F_{E_{O_2}} \times (1 - F_{I_{H_2O}})}{(1 - F_{I_{O_2}} - F_{I_{H_2O}})}$$

The calculation of $\dot{V}_{O_2}$ is simpler if the expired gas is dried prior to analysis for O_2 and CO_2. Beaver[6] provides a nomogram for calculation of oxygen uptake in the presence of water vapor, however, that can be used to determine $\dot{V}_{O_2}$ and R from a sample of mixed expired gas assumed to be fully saturated with water vapor at a known temperature (Appendix F). The subject is assumed to be breathing room air and the O_2 and CO_2 analyzers display the fractions of total expired gas including water vapor. Significant errors would result if water vapor is not taken into account. Again, the correction is not needed if gas fractions are measured as fractions of dry gas.

Breath-by-breath measurement systems must deal with this problem as well. Here, rapidly responding gas analyzers and mass spectrometers are used. A mass spectrometer may be adjusted to "ignore" water vapor if the sum of ion voltages is made up of only those measuring N_2, O_2, CO_2, and argon, with water vapor ignored in both inspired and expired gases. If this method is used, then the volume multiplied by true O_2 fraction should be adjusted to the dry volume.

Rapidly responding electrochemical and paramagnetic O_2 analyzers and infrared CO_2 analyzers read fractions of total gas volume and therefore read lower concentrations than if the same gas were measured after being dried. As shown in equation 27, the values can be used in a breath-by-breath system if $F_{E_{H_2O}}$ and $F_{I_{H_2O}}$ are known.[7] The assumption that expired gas is fully saturated at some known temperature is the starting point for three other approaches to dealing with this in breath-by-breath systems.

First, the expired gas sample can be kept warm to prevent condensation. If gas is fully saturated at a known temperature, the $F_{E_{H_2O}}$ can be estimated. A heated sampling tube is necessary and the temperature must be accurately known. For example, assuming a value of $37°$ C when actual expired gas temperature is $32°$ C can result in a 7 to 8% error in $\dot{V}_{O_2}$. During exercise, expired gas rapidly cools in the mouthpiece and breathing valve to as low as $32°$ C. Because gas for analysis is most often sampled at this

location in breath-by-breath systems then, even if the gas is rewarmed, there will have been some unknown loss of water vapor to condensation.

A second approach is to allow the sampled gas to cool to a known temperature. This avoids the problem of indeterminate loss of water vapor from cooling followed by rewarming. Auchincloss et al.[8] described a water bath that cooled expired gas to $15°$ C prior to rewarming and analysis. If a small diameter sampling tube and low flow rate can be used, then gas may be allowed to cool to ambient temperature. This latter method is convenient and simple, but care should be taken that water droplets do not alter resistance and flow characteristics of the sampler and do not affect the linearity and response of the analyzer.

Finally, Deno and Kamon described a dryer for use in on-line breath-by-breath systems.[9] Removing water vapor by passing gas through a tube containing calcium sulfate is generally unsuitable for breath-by-breath methods because it introduces unacceptable delay times, may distort the gas concentration profile, and cannot meet the challenge of large gas sample flows. Deno and Kamon used a copper condenser tube and separator immersed in an ice bath at $1°$ C. Even at flow rates of saturated $38°$ air up to 1 L/min, P_{H_2O} was maintained at 5 mm Hg. Response times were compatible with those reported for breath-by-breath systems albeit at moderately high sample flow rates (1 L/min).

The use of the above equations during breathing of oxygen-enriched inspired gas mixtures has potential problems. The relationship of $\dot{V}_I$ to $\dot{V}_E$ is subject to large differences for small measurement errors when $F_{I_{O_2}}$ and $F_{E_{O_2}}$ are high and $F_{I_{N_2}}$ and $F_{E_{N_2}}$ are low. In addition, the assumption that $\dot{V}_I \times F_{I_{N_2}} = \dot{V}_E \times F_{E_{N_2}}$ is not valid for a transient washout period during which hyperoxic gas is inspired and more nitrogen is removed during expiration than is added during inspiration. Also, while breathing 100% oxygen, the equations given above cannot be used because there is no inspired or expired nitrogen after the washout period.

VALVE DEAD SPACE AND PHYSIOLOGICAL DEAD SPACE/TIDAL VOLUME RATIO

The physiological dead space consists of the anatomic dead space and the alveolar dead space. During measurement, the volume of the breathing valve and mouthpiece apparatus is considered to be in series with the anatomic dead space. This apparatus dead space is usually subtracted from the V_D calculated by the Engoff modification of the Bohr equation:

$$V_D = V_T \, (L) \times \frac{Pa_{CO_2} - P\bar{E}_{CO_2}}{Pa_{CO_2}} - V_{Dm} \, (L)$$

Where V_D is subject dead space, V_T is tidal volume, and V_{Dm} is the volume of the apparatus (or mechanical valve dead space).

Bradley and Younes,[10] Suwa and Bendixen,[11] and Singleton et al.[12] all report that the effective dead space of the valve (the correction term [V_{Dm}]) may be different than the measured mechanical deadspace. The reader is referred to their thorough analyses of the "proper" correction value under various conditions.

In practice, most reports of V_D during exercise have corrected for apparatus dead space by subtracting the entire mechanical dead space. Any potential error can be minimized if the valve dead space is small and the subject's tidal volume is relatively large compared to V_{Dm}. Valves with large dead spaces may be necessary, however, because they usually offer smaller breathing resistances at high inspiratory and expiratory flows. These high flows would be encountered when studying healthy normal subjects with large tidal volumes during exercise. On the other hand, patients with small tidal volumes will usually not generate high flows during exercise and the small dead space valves will be satisfactory.

Calculations for Breath-By-Breath Analysis

Breath-by-breath methods use the same formulae as for mixed-expired gas collections. Conceptually, the expired volume is divided into small sequential samples. The volume of each is determined and, when multiplied by the gas concentrations appropriate for that sample adjusted for the time difference between the flow and gas concentration signals, gives the volume of CO_2 eliminated or O_2 taken up for that sample. The results are summed mathematically and then reported either per breath or per unit time. Thus, the term "breath-by-breath" applies to the method of expired gas analysis and data reduction and does not necessarily mean that each breath is individually reported.

If V_E is the sum of all volume exhaled between time 0 and time T, then:

$$V_E = \sum_{t=0}^{T} V_{exp}(t + \Delta t)$$

where $V_{exp}(t + \Delta t)$ is the volume expired between time t and $t + \Delta t$, Δt is a time interval, and T is the total time of expiration for single or multiple breaths.

This is satisfactory if volume is directly measured over small time intervals. If expired flow rather than volume is measured, then:

$$V_E = \int_0^T \dot{V}exp(t) dt$$

where $\dot{V}exp(t)$ is the expired flow over the infinitesimally small time interval dt. The volume exhaled over that time is the product $\dot{V}exp(t)dt$. In practice, a small constant Δt is substituted for dt and the mean flow during the time interval $(t + \Delta t)$ is used as $\dot{V}exp(t)$:

$$V_E = \sum_{t=0}^{T} \dot{V}exp(t + \Delta t) \times \Delta t$$

where $\dot{V}exp(t + \Delta t)$ is the mean flow rate during the time interval $t + \Delta t$. The minute ventilation ($\dot{V}_E$) is the V_E/T or the volume per unit time.

In a breath-by-breath system, the $\dot{V}_{CO_2}$ is calculated by multiplying the nearly instantaneous $F_{E_{CO_2}}$ for each small time interval by the simultaneous expired volume during that interval. These products are then integrated:

$$V_{CO_2} = \int_{t=0}^{T} \dot{V}exp(t) dt \times F_{E_{CO_2}}(t)$$

where $\dot{V}exp(t)dt$ is the instantaneous expired volume and $F_{E_{CO_2}}(t)$ is the instantaneous expired CO_2 concentration at time t, adjusted for the delay between when the gas is sampled and when the analyzer reads the appropriate concentration. In practice, the small time interval Δt is substituted for dt:

$$V_{CO_2} = \sum_{t=0}^{T} \dot{V}exp(t + \Delta t) \times \Delta t \times F_{E_{CO_2}}(t)$$

where $\dot{V}exp(t + \Delta t)$ is the mean flow for the time period t to $t + \Delta t$, $F_{E_{CO_2}}(t)$ is the mean expired CO_2 during this time period, and Δt is a small time interval. For the volume of O_2 taken up during expiration, substitute the true O_2 difference [(ΔF_{O_2})true] for $F_{E_{CO_2}}$ in this equation. The $\dot{V}_{CO_2}$ and $\dot{V}_{O_2}$ are equal to the volume of CO_2 or O_2 divided by the time during exhalation, whether expressed per breath or per minute or other time unit.

An analog integrator or analog-to-digital converter and digital computer can perform the necessary multiplication and summation. The respired gas is not, strictly speaking, measured and analyzed continuously, but instead is rapidly sampled, e.g., every 0.02

sec. The resultant expired flow vs. time curve is, therefore, made up of sequential points sampled at intervals Δt or at a frequency $f = 1/\Delta t$. The rate of sampling is important because rapid and large changes in expired flow (or gas concentration) may occur during exercise and could be missed if the data are sampled at too slow a rate. Bernard,[13] using generalized simulated curves of expired flow and expired CO_2, found that a sample rate of 30 Hz was adequate during exercise, and that rates of 40, 50, and 100 Hz achieved little improvement in fidelity. Beaver et al.[14] in their analysis suggested that a sampling frequency equal to twice the highest frequency occurring in the signal to be measured should be used. They suggested that for human exercise testing a frequency of 50 Hz is satisfactory to record flow and mass spectrometer signals.

A minor consideration is the method of summation or numerical integration. Bernard[13] suggested that a trapezoidal rule was adequate for integration of respiratory signals. This is identical to assuming, as above, that the mean expired flow and gas concentrations during the time period between t and t + Δt was equal to the average of the values measured at the beginning and end of the time period.

A more serious potential problem deals with time-matching of the appropriate expired flow (or volume) and expired gas concentration because of delay in the transport to and measurement by most gas analyzers. For manual analysis of mixed expired gases, delay and response times are not crucial. Especially when flow rate and/or gas concentration are rapidly changing, it is essential that the appropriate instantaneous flow rate be multiplied by the proper time-matched expired gas concentration. While flow rates can be determined accurately and nearly instantaneously with good fidelity, gas analyzer measurements cannot usually be made without some delay and distortion inherent to the transport of gas to the analyzer and the intrinsic characteristics of the analyzer. The accuracy of a breath-by-breath system is dependent on the ability of the system to match flow rate and appropriate gas concentration prior to integration. Thus, each sampled flow rate must be stored in some way until the appropriate expired gas concentration value has been determined. This matching process is usually performed as part of the computer program for on-line exercise systems.

Bernard[13] used simulated curves of expired CO_2 and expired flow to estimate potential error caused by the time delay between measurements of these two variables. Using perfectly time-matched hypothetical curves as standard, less than a 5% difference in calculated $\dot{V}CO_2$ was found if the time difference was less than 25 msec. Of importance is that the theoretical sampling rate was 100 Hz, the signals were given random noise, and the product of flow and CO_2 was integrated using the trapezoid rule.

In practice, there are two components contributing to the time difference between simultaneous gas concentration with respect to instantaneous flow. Most systems use a capillary tube with a pump to draw a continuous expired gas sample into the analyzer. The gas transport time is dependent on the dimensions of the tube and the pump flow rate, but the time is typically on the order of 200 ms. Secondly, the gas analyzer output itself has an intrinsic response time that further adds to the delay. For infrared CO_2 analyzers, electrochemical O_2 analyzers, and respiratory mass spectrometers the time constants for response are in the range of 50 to 100 ms. The net result is that an instantaneous change in gas concentration at the sampling end of the tubing is accurately measured but only after introducing corrections to account for these delays. The mixing and diffusion of gas within the sampling tubing may further distort the result. These must also be accounted for in these corrections.

In most solutions to this problem, an instantaneous or step change in gas concentration is compared to the gas analyzer measurement over time. Attempts are then made to determine optimal methods of compensating for the gas transport and gas analyzer delays.

Although the gas analyzer response time component is certainly important, matching of flow and gas concentration signals for gas transport delay, i.e., the time simply to reach the analyzer, alone considerably improves results. Using this method, Bates et al.[15] found a tenfold reduction in error from the uncorrected value and suggested that this simple adjustment might be sufficient.

To account for the gas analyzer response time, an additional correction function is usually used. This function is derived from analysis of the total response of the gas analyzer system. Beaver et al.[14] indicated that the most significant wave shape distortion is removed by a total delay correction equal to transport delay plus one time constant and analyzed the magnitude of potential errors. Investigators have used various functions to describe the response characteristics of their gas analyzers or mass spectrometers.[15–18] We[19] have found that an equal area method for analyzer delay time gives a one time constant delay if the analyzer response curve is exponential and an empirically determined longer delay time if the curve is sigmoid. Factors that affect selection of an optimal method included the level of noise in the measured signal, the sampling rate, and the type of calculation desired.

The importance of matching flow rate and appropriate gas concentration cannot be overly stressed for a breath-by-breath system. While there is not universal agreement on the optimal way of dealing with gas analyzer response time, a satisfactory balance between degree of accuracy, speed, and reproducibility can be reached. We believe that our relatively simple method[19] is adequate and does not justify a more complex calculation.

V-Slope Method for Determining the Anaerobic Threshold (*AT*)

Because of the physiological significance of the *AT*, it is highly desirable to make this measurement whenever possible. Ordinarily the *AT* is selected by examining certain records simultaneously, such as ventilatory equivalents for O_2, CO_2, PET_{CO_2}, PET_{O_2}, and R. However, for the following reasons it might be very difficult for even an experienced examiner to delineate the *AT* by gas exchange methods: (1) the patient's breathing pattern might be too irregular to identify the work rate or $\dot{V}_{O_2}$ at which $\dot{V}_E/\dot{V}_{O_2}$ or PET_{O_2} start to increase; (2) some patients, particularly those with lung disease, may not have the normal ventilatory response to the metabolic acidosis of exercise; and, (3) the exercise test protocol work rate may not be increased rapidly enough for the metabolic acidosis to develop at a rapid enough rate. In addition, sometimes the examiner may select the respiratory compensation point rather than the *AT* because the increase in hyperventilation in response to metabolic acidosis is more apparent than the increase in ventilation at the *AT*.

To obviate these problems, Beaver et al.[20] selected a more basic measurement to determine the $\dot{V}_{O_2}$ above which metabolic acidosis occurs. This is based upon the fact that CO_2 is released when lactic acid is buffered by bicarbonate in the cells, and that this CO_2 is rapidly transferred to the lungs. This additional CO_2 (i.e., evolved by buffering) can be detected by an increase in CO_2 output over and above the CO_2 produced from aerobic energy-generating mechanisms. Thus, these investigators plotted breath-by-breath $\dot{V}_{CO_2}$ against $\dot{V}_{O_2}$ during an incremental exercise test so as to identify the point at which $\dot{V}_{CO_2}$ increases out of proportion to aerobic metabolism. They call this the V-slope method.

With the V-slope method, the first minute or two of data collected at the start of the period of increasing work rates are not analyzed because of nonlinearities related to CO_2 solubility in tissues. Also, data at heavy exercise levels above which respiratory compensation for the metabolic acidosis and hyperventilation for CO_2 occurs (PET_{CO_2} decreases) are deliberately excluded from analysis. The intervening data demonstrate a transition at approximately the middle work rate range at which the plot of $\dot{V}_{CO_2}$ against $\dot{V}_{O_2}$ becomes more steep as shown in Figure 3-7. The V-slope method analyzes the lower and upper linear components of the $\dot{V}_{CO_2}$-$\dot{V}_{O_2}$ relationship by least square linear regression. The computer selects the upper and lower slopes, and finds the point of intersection between them. This point is the *AT*. The *AT* derived by this method has a coefficient of variation that is much less than that determined by former methods and agrees very well with the point at which standard bicarbonate starts to decrease and at which arterial lactate increases to values above 1 mEq/L.[20]

Beaver et al.[20] described a two-step method for smoothing the data. This process reduces the noise without compromising accuracy in order to make the analysis easier. First, all the breath-by-breath data points are transformed by interpolation into data points of regular time intervals so that the analysis is not biased by an irregular distribution of points. A 9-second moving average filter is used to smooth the breath-by-breath fluctuations further. These fluctuations are primarily in $\dot{V}_{CO_2}$ rather than $\dot{V}_{O_2}$ since irregular breathing patterns do not load or unload substantially more or less oxygen into the pulmonary capillary blood but can affect the rate at which CO_2 leaves the blood. Second, to compensate for these irregularities, breath-by-breath corrections are made in $\dot{V}_{CO_2}$. These corrections are derived from changes in PET_{CO_2}, the solubility coefficient of CO_2 in blood, and pulmonary blood flow estimated from the heart rate change as described in the original report.[20] While PET_{CO_2} does not equal Pa_{CO_2}, changes in PET_{CO_2} do parallel those for Pa_{CO_2}.

Beaver et al.[20] were able to determine the anaerobic threshold from exercise gas exchange data in 10 out of 10 subjects by the V-slope method. These correlated closely with the *AT* determined from bicarbonate and lactate measurements. In contrast, it was not possible even for very experienced examiners to estimate the *AT* as reliably for all 10 subjects.

References

1. Kim, T. S., Rahn, H., Farhi, L. E.: Estimation of the true venous and arterial P_{CO_2} by gas analysis of a single-breath. J. Appl. Physiol. *21*:1338–1344, 1966.
2. Jones, N. L., Campbell, E. J. M., McHardy, G. J. R., Higgs, B. E., Clode, M.: The estimation of carbon dioxide pressure of mixed venous blood during exercise. Clin. Sci. *32*:311–327, 1967.
3. McHardy, G. J. R.: The relationship between the differences in pressure and content of carbon dioxide in arterial and venous blood. Clin. Sci. *32*:299–309, 1967.
4. Wagner, J. A., Horvath, S. M., Dahms, T. E., Reed, S.: Validation of open-circuit for the determination of oxygen consumption. J. Appl. Physiol. *34*:859–863, 1973.

5. Wilmore, J. H., Costill, D. L.: Adequacy of the Haldane transformation in the computation of exercise $\dot{V}_{O_2}$ in man. J. Appl. Physiol. *35*:85–89, 1973.

6. Beaver, W. L., Wasserman, K., Whipp, B. J.: On-line computer analysis and breath-by-breath graphical display of exercise function tests. J. Appl. Physiol. *34*:128–132, 1973.

7. Beaver, W. L.: Water vapor corrections in oxygen consumption calculations. J. Appl. Physiol. *35*:928–931, 1973.

8. Auchincloss, J. H., Gilbert, R., Baule, G. H.: Control of water vapor during rapid analysis of respiratory gases in expired air. J. Appl. Physiol. *28*:245–247, 1970.

9. Deno, N. S., Kamon, E.: A dryer for rapid response on-line expired gas measurements. J. Appl. Physiol. *46*:1196–1199, 1979.

10. Bradley, P. W., Younes, M.: Relation between respiratory valve dead space and tidal volume. J. Appl. Physiol. *49*:528–532, 1980.

11. Suwa, K., Bendixen, H. H.: Change in Pa_{CO_2} with mechanical dead space during artificial ventilation. J. Appl. Physiol. *24*:556–563, 1968.

12. Singleton, G. J., Olsen, C. R., Smith, R. L.: Correction for mechanical dead space in the calculation of physiological dead space. J. Clin. Invest. *51*:2768–2772, 1972.

13. Bernard, T. E.: Aspects of on-line digital integration of pulmonary gas transfer. J. Appl. Physiol. *43*:375–378, 1977.

14. Beaver, W. L., Lamarra, N., Wasserman, K.: Breath-by-breath measurement of true alveolar gas exchange. J. Appl. Physiol. *51*:1662–1675, 1981.

15. Bates, J. H. T., Prisk, G. K., Tanner, T. E., McKinnon, A. E.: Correcting for the dynamic response of a respiratory mass spectrometer. J. Appl. Physiol. *55*:1015–1022, 1983.

16. Noguchi, H., Ogushi, Y., Yoshiya, I., Itakura, N., Yambayashi, H.: Breath-by-breath $\dot{V}_{CO_2}$ and $\dot{V}_{O_2}$ require compensation for transport delay and dynamic response. J. Appl. Physiol. *52*:79–84, 1982.

17. Mitchell, R. R.: Incorporating the gas analyzer response time in gas exchange computations. J. Appl. Physiol. *47*:1118–1122, 1979.

18. Arieli, R., Van Liew, H. D.: Corrections for the response time and delay of mass spectrometers. J. Appl. Physiol. *51*:1417–1422, 1981.

19. Sue, D. Y., Hansen, J. E., Blais, M., Wasserman, K.: Measurement and analysis of gas exchange during exercise using a programmable calculator. J. Appl. Physiol. *49*:456–461, 1980.

20. Beaver, W. L., Wasserman, K., Whipp, B. J.: A new method for detecting the anaerobic threshold by gas exchange. J. Appl. Physiol. (in press), 1986.

TABLE D-1. *Measurements Used for Example of Calculation of Gas Exchange*

measured volume: 54.2 (L, ATPS)	valve dead space = 64 ml
collection time: 2 min	ambient temperature (T) = 22° C
number of breaths: 41 in 2 min	barometric pressure (PB) = 760 mm Hg
heart rate (HR) = 120/min	partial pressure of water,
	saturated at 22° C (P_{H_2O}) = 19 mm Hg
body temperature = 37° C.	
$F_{I_{O_2}}$ = 0.2093 (20.93%)	Pa_{O_2} = 91 mm Hg
$F_{I_{CO_2}}$ = 0.0004 (0.04%)	Pa_{CO_2} = 36 mm Hg
$F_{E_{O_2}}$ = 0.162 (16.2%)	pH = 7.44
$F_{E_{CO_2}}$ = 0.041 (4.1%)	Sa_{O_2} = 95%
(Fractions of dry gas volume)	
	$P_{ET_{CO_2}}$ = 38 mm Hg
Hemoglobin 15 g/100 ml	$P\bar{v}_{O_2}$ = 27 mm Hg; $S\bar{v}_{O_2}$ = 50%

Preparation for the Exercise Test

Requesting the Test

We use a request form for exercise studies. On this form the referring physician gives us:

a. patient name, address, telephone number
b. patient weight, height, sex, age
c. tentative diagnosis and reason for study
d. type of test and special requirements

Most often, the exercise test should be discussed with the referring physician so that the type of test and reason for doing it are already known. In addition, the discussion helps select whether the cycle or treadmill is the preferable form of ergometry, whether an arterial catheter or ear oximeter is desired, and whether 12-lead electrocardiograms are needed during exercise. This is also a time at which the patient's medications, previous studies, special needs or limitations, and other details can be brought out.

Preparing the Patient

We give the patient an appointment slip on which we remind the patient of the date and time of the procedure. We have also found it useful to include:

a. A brief explanation of the procedure;
b. A reminder to wear loose-fitting comfortable clothes and shoes suitable for exercise;
c. A suggestion to avoid eating a heavy meal before the exercise test.

Physician Preparation

The physician in attendance during the test obtains a brief history of the patient's medical problems and the specific symptoms limiting exercise. The history should include a list of medications, an idea of physical activity status, and some estimate of the safety of exercising the patient. A brief physical examination should include blood pressure and pulse, cardiopulmonary examination, peripheral pulses, and upper and lower extremity muscles and joints. Prior to exercise, the physician should obtain and evaluate pertinent resting studies such as the chest roentgenogram, electrocardiogram, arterial blood gases, and pulmonary function. Then, the physician is in position to inform the patient of the risks and benefits of the exercise study and obtain consent.

Preparation of the Laboratory

The laboratory should be air-conditioned and regulated at a comfortable temperature and humidity. The patient's view should be pleasant and not cluttered with tubing, wires or a bulletin board with distracting papers hanging from it. If blood is to be sampled, the syringes should be prepared and placed in a convenient location so that there is no confusion or extra motion during the time of the study. The number of people in the laboratory should be minimal — those needed for making the measurements and for safety. Finally, extra sounds should be kept to a minimum. Soft background music helps dampen noise but will not interfere with communication between the examiner and the technician. In summary, a pleasant, professional environment is needed in order to get the maximum confidence and therefore performance by the patient.

ECG Lead Placement

The ECG leads should be placed on appropriate, stable areas of the body. We use adhesive silver/silver-chloride gel ECG patches like those used in intensive care units. The skin is shaved if necessary and wiped with rubbing alcohol before the patches are applied.

The site of the three leads for monitoring heart rate and rhythm is shown in Figure 5-1. However, we do not hesitate to move the site of the leads as necessary to get an optimal tracing.

We use 12-lead ECG in addition for patients in whom we suspect myocardial ischemia. The positions of the leads are shown in Figure 5-1. The arm leads are placed close to the monitoring lead patches above the scapulae; the leg leads are placed on the low back above the iliac crests. These locations minimize movement artifact. The chest (V-leads) are positioned in standard locations on the anterolateral chest wall. Again, adhesive ECG patches are used. A technician obtains an ECG at rest, approximately every other minute during exercise, and more often if an arrhythmia is noted or complaints of chest pain are offered.

Arterial Catheter Placement

EQUIPMENT

1. Appropriate catheter.
2. Cournand-type needle with sharp, hollow stylus.
3. 2 cc syringe with 26 gauge needle for local anesthesia.
4. Sterile saline suitable for intravascular injection.
5. Heparinized saline, 50 unit/cc, for catheter flushing.

SELECTION OF CATHETER

We use a polyethylene catheter that is 25 cm long and has a diameter of 1.37 mm. The tip is tapered to fit a guide wire (50 cm × 0.63 mm) that fits through a 19-gauge thin-walled Cournand needle. The catheter is long enough so that the end used for collection can be brought around to the back of the arm and sampling can be done without the subject altering the position of his arm or being aware when blood is sampled.

ARTERY SELECTION AND ARM POSITIONING

The brachial or radial artery is generally used. Complications such as thrombosis are exceedingly rare when the appropriate precautions are taken. We find the brachial artery to be preferable, however, because it is larger and the catheter has less effect on compromising its lumen. Also, the arm need not be secured to a board and sliding of the catheter in and out of the artery with movement is not a problem. The radial pulse should be palpated to assure continued patency.

Positioning the arm is very important.
a. Extend arm; place a rolled towel or cushion under elbow for maximum extension.
b. Pronate hand.
c. Palpate brachial artery on medial side of antecubital fossa.

ANESTHESIA

If the patient is not allergic, anesthetize the skin and area around the artery. It is more humane and the likelihood of the artery going into spasm is reduced. We use 1 to 2% lidocaine without epinephrine. After positioning the arm, inject local anesthetic: a) intradermally above the artery, b) subcutaneously just above the artery, and, c) subcutaneously on either side of the artery. Total amount should be about 1 to 2 ml.

ARTERIAL PUNCTURE AND CATHETER INSERTION

a. Use a 19-gauge Cournand needle.

b. Locate artery between fingers in area of anesthesia.

c. Insert sharp, hollow stylus in needle.

d. Holding needle by shield, while keeping stylus in needle with thumb (be sure not to cover hole in stylus), penetrate the skin over the artery. Position the tip of the needle above the artery. Then abruptly insert the stylus and needle tip into artery.

e. When the tip of the stylus enters the artery, blood may flow out of the stylus.

f. Insert the needle another 2 to 3 mm to be sure that tip of needle is in artery (the stylus protrudes a little beyond the tip of the needle).

g. Remove the stylus. Blood should shoot out of needle with arterial pressure. If it does not, withdraw needle slightly (it might have gone into the posterior wall of artery). Once a clear stream of arterial blood is evident, it is safe to advance the needle further into the lumen of the artery using the continuous stream of blood to document the needle's position. The needle advance may be facilitated by depressing the hub slightly to reduce the possibility of impaling the posterior wall of the artery with the needle tip. DO NOT ADVANCE THE NEEDLE WITHOUT THE STYLUS IN PLACE IF THERE IS NO FLOW OF BLOOD. It may damage the artery. If there is no blood flow, slowly withdraw the needle without the stylus as the needle tip may have passed through the inner wall of the artery. If there is still no blood flow, withdraw the tip of the needle to the skin.

h. If unsuccessful, clear the needle and stylus of any blood or clot, then try again.

i. With the needle tip in the lumen of the artery, documented by freely flowing blood, thread the guide wire for the catheter through the needle and slide it about 3 inches into the lumen of the artery. If the guidewire does not slip EASILY past the needle tip, the needle lumen is not centered in the lumen of the artery, and the needle must be repositioned.

j. Remove the needle, leaving the guide wire in place. Compress for hemostasis over the site at which the needle was inserted because the guide wire is narrow relative to the withdrawn needle.

k. Slide the smoothly tapered end of the catheter over the wire. When the catheter reaches the skin, slide it through the skin and arterial wall using a gently rotating motion.

l. When the catheter position is well established several inches into the artery, remove guide wire. Blood should flow out of the end of the catheter.

m. Attach Luer-lock stopcock to the end of catheter and flush with heparinized saline.

n. Cover site of insertion with sterile gauze and fix with tape. Tape catheter to skin. Now catheter is ready for use.

FOR DIFFICULT PUNCTURES

Limit yourself to 15 minutes of effort. If you are not successful by the end of that time, stop trying and ask someone with more experience to help, or just rely on noninvasive measurements. The latter will provide a considerable amount of information.

Blood Pressure

It is most accurate to measure blood pressure directly from an indwelling arterial catheter, The reason for this is that the background noise of the cycling or treadmill (especially) can make hearing of the Korotkoff sounds difficult. The swinging arm during walking also makes the measurement of blood pressure by the cuff method difficult. Direct arterial blood pressure recording is convenient when an arterial catheter is in place. A pressure transducer should be located at the level of the left atrium (approximately the fourth intercostal space with the patient upright) and the transducer should be carefully calibrated. Cuff-measured systolic and diastolic blood pressures average about 10 mm Hg less than directly recorded brachial artery pressures during cycle ergometry (Table 6-3.).

Tables and Nomogram

TABLE F-1. *Partial Pressure of Water of Saturated Gas at Centigrade Temperature T.*

T	PH$_2$O	T	PH$_2$O	T	PH$_2$O
10	9.20	20	17.53	30	31.83
11	9.84	21	18.65	31	33.70
12	10.51	22	19.82	32	35.67
13	11.23	23	21.07	33	37.73
14	11.98	24	22.38	34	39.90
15	12.78	25	23.76	35	42.18
16	13.63	26	25.21	36	44.57
17	14.53	27	26.74	37	47.08
18	15.47	28	28.35	38	49.70
19	16.47	29	30.04	39	52.45
20	17.53	30	31.83	40	55.34

TABLE F-2. *Factors for Conversion from ATPS to BTPS (37°C)*

	T°C.	16	17	18	19	20	21	22	23	24	25	26	27	28	29	30
	600	1.138	1.132	1.126	1.120	1.115	1.109	1.103	1.097	1.090	1.084	1.078	1.071	1.065	1.058	1.051
	610	1.136	1.131	1.125	1.119	1.114	1.108	1.102	1.096	1.090	1.083	1.077	1.071	1.064	1.058	1.051
	620	1.135	1.130	1.124	1.118	1.113	1.107	1.101	1.095	1.089	1.083	1.076	1.070	1.064	1.057	1.050
	630	1.134	1.129	1.123	1.117	1.112	1.106	1.100	1.094	1.088	1.082	1.076	1.069	1.063	1.056	1.050
	640	1.133	1.128	1.122	1.116	1.111	1.105	1.099	1.093	1.087	1.081	1.075	1.069	1.062	1.056	1.049
	650	1.132	1.127	1.121	1.116	1.110	1.104	1.098	1.092	1.087	1.081	1.074	1.068	1.062	1.056	1.049
	660	1.131	1.126	1.120	1.115	1.109	1.103	1.098	1.092	1.086	1.080	1.074	1.068	1.061	1.055	1.049
	670	1.130	1.125	1.119	1.114	1.108	1.103	1.097	1.091	1.085	1.079	1.073	1.067	1.061	1.055	1.048
	680	1.129	1.124	1.118	1.113	1.107	1.102	1.096	1.090	1.085	1.079	1.073	1.067	1.060	1.054	1.048
Pʙ	690	1.128	1.123	1.118	1.112	1.107	1.101	1.095	1.090	1.084	1.078	1.072	1.066	1.060	1.054	1.047
	700	1.128	1.122	1.117	1.111	1.106	1.100	1.095	1.089	1.083	1.077	1.072	1.066	1.059	1.053	1.047
	710	1.127	1.121	1.116	1.111	1.105	1.100	1.094	1.088	1.083	1.077	1.071	1.065	1.059	1.053	1.047
	720	1.126	1.121	1.115	1.110	1.104	1.099	1.093	1.088	1.082	1.076	1.070	1.065	1.059	1.052	1.046
	730	1.125	1.120	1.115	1.109	1.104	1.098	1.093	1.087	1.082	1.076	1.070	1.064	1.058	1.052	1.046
	740	1.124	1.119	1.114	1.109	1.103	1.098	1.092	1.087	1.081	1.075	1.070	1.064	1.058	1.052	1.046
	750	1.124	1.118	1.113	1.108	1.102	1.097	1.092	1.086	1.080	1.075	1.069	1.063	1.057	1.051	1.045
	760	1.123	1.118	1.113	1.107	1.102	1.096	1.091	1.086	1.080	1.074	1.069	1.063	1.057	1.051	1.045
	770	1.122	1.117	1.112	1.107	1.101	1.096	1.090	1.085	1.079	1.074	1.068	1.062	1.057	1.051	1.045
	780	1.122	1.116	1.111	1.106	1.101	1.095	1.090	1.084	1.079	1.073	1.068	1.062	1.056	1.050	1.044

T°C. is ambient temperature in degrees Centigrade; Pʙ is barometric pressure.

TABLE F-3. *Factors for Conversion from ATPS to STPD*

T°C.	16	17	18	19	20	21	22	23	24	25	26	27	28	29	30
600	0.729	0.725	0.722	0.718	0.714	0.710	0.706	0.703	0.699	0.695	0.691	0.686	0.682	0.678	0.674
610	0.741	0.738	0.734	0.730	0.726	0.723	0.719	0.715	0.711	0.707	0.703	0.698	0.694	0.690	0.685
620	0.754	0.750	0.746	0.742	0.739	0.735	0.731	0.727	0.723	0.719	0.715	0.710	0.706	0.702	0.697
630	0.766	0.762	0.759	0.755	0.751	0.747	0.743	0.739	0.735	0.731	0.727	0.722	0.718	0.714	0.709
640	0.779	0.775	0.771	0.767	0.763	0.759	0.755	0.751	0.747	0.743	0.739	0.734	0.730	0.726	0.721
650	0.791	0.787	0.783	0.779	0.775	0.771	0.767	0.763	0.759	0.755	0.751	0.746	0.742	0.737	0.733
660	0.803	0.800	0.796	0.792	0.788	0.784	0.780	0.775	0.771	0.767	0.763	0.758	0.754	0.749	0.745
670	0.816	0.812	0.808	0.804	0.800	0.796	0.792	0.788	0.783	0.779	0.775	0.770	0.766	0.761	0.757
680	0.828	0.824	0.820	0.816	0.812	0.808	0.804	0.800	0.795	0.791	0.787	0.782	0.778	0.773	0.768
PB 690	0.841	0.837	0.833	0.829	0.824	0.820	0.816	0.812	0.807	0.803	0.799	0.794	0.790	0.785	0.780
700	0.853	0.849	0.845	0.841	0.837	0.832	0.828	0.824	0.820	0.815	0.811	0.806	0.802	0.797	0.792
710	0.866	0.861	0.857	0.853	0.849	0.845	0.840	0.836	0.832	0.827	0.823	0.818	0.813	0.809	0.804
720	0.878	0.874	0.870	0.865	0.861	0.857	0.853	0.848	0.844	0.839	0.835	0.830	0.825	0.821	0.816
730	0.890	0.886	0.882	0.878	0.873	0.869	0.865	0.860	0.856	0.851	0.847	0.842	0.837	0.833	0.828
740	0.903	0.899	0.894	0.890	0.886	0.881	0.877	0.872	0.868	0.863	0.859	0.854	0.849	0.844	0.840
750	0.915	0.911	0.907	0.902	0.898	0.894	0.889	0.885	0.880	0.875	0.871	0.866	0.861	0.856	0.851
760	0.928	0.923	0.919	0.915	0.910	0.906	0.901	0.897	0.892	0.887	0.883	0.878	0.873	0.868	0.863
770	0.940	0.936	0.931	0.927	0.923	0.918	0.913	0.909	0.904	0.900	0.895	0.890	0.885	0.880	0.875
780	0.953	0.948	0.944	0.939	0.935	0.930	0.926	0.921	0.916	0.912	0.907	0.902	0.897	0.892	0.887

T°C is ambient temperature in degrees Centigrade; PB is barometric pressure.

TABLE F-4. *Estimated $\dot{V}O_2$ for Various Activities**

ACTIVITY	ESTIMATED $\dot{V}O_2$ (ml/kg/min)	ACTIVITY	ESTIMATED $\dot{V}O_2$ (ml/kg/min)
Basic postures		Hitching trailers, operating jacks or heavy levers	12.25
Sitting only (desk work, writing, calculating)	4.25	Masonry, painting, paperhanging	14.0
Standing only (bartending)	8.75	*Walking: moderate work*	
Walking 3.0 mph	10.5	Carrying trays, dishes	14.70
3.5 mph	14.0	Gas station mechanical work (changing tires, etc.)	15.75
Sitting: light or moderate work		*Heavy arm work*	
Driving a car	4.25	Lifting and carrying	
Driving a truck	5.30	(a) 20–44 lbs	15.75
Hand tools, light assembly	5.30	(b) 45–64 lbs	21.0
Working heavy levers	7.0	(c) 65–84 lbs	26.25
Riding mower	8.75	(d) 85–100 lbs	29.75
Crane operator	8.75	*Heavy tools*	
Driving heavy truck (including frequent on and off with some arm work)	10.5	Jackhammers, pneumatic drills	21.0
		Shovel, pick	28.0
Standing: moderate work		*Carpentry*	
Light assembly at slow pace	8.75	Light interior repair (tile laying)	14.0
Gas station operator	9.45	Building and finishing interior	15.75
Scrubbing, waxing, polishing (floors, walls)	9.45	Putting in sidewalk	17.5
Heavy assembly (farm machinery, plumbing)	10.5	Exterior remodeling (hammering, sawing)	21.0
Light welding	10.5	*Miscellaneous*	
Stocking shelves (light objects)	10.5	Pushing objects of 75 lbs or more (desks, file cabinets)	28.0
Janitorial work	10.5	Laying railroad track	24.5
Assembly line with light or medium parts at moderate pace	12.25	Cutting trees—chopping wood	
Assembly line with brief lifting every 5 minutes (45 lbs or less)	12.25	Hand saw	19.25
Same as above (parts >45 lbs)	14.0	Automatic	10.5

*From Tennessee Heart Association: Physician's Handbook for Evaluation of Cardiovascular and Physical Fitness. Nashville, Tennessee Heart Association, 1972; reprinted with permission.

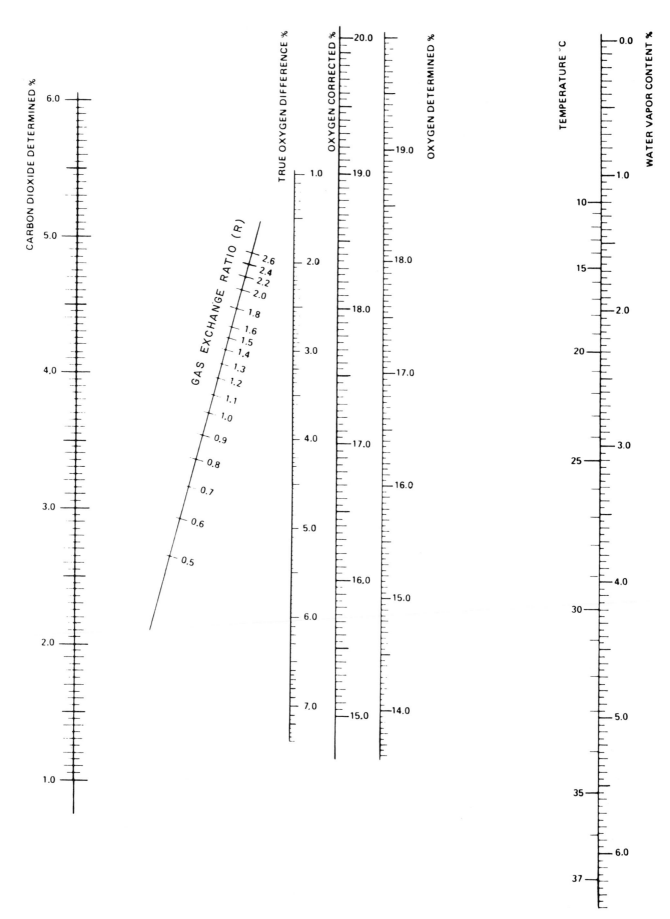

Fig. F-1. Nomogram for computing true O_2 difference ($[\Delta F_{O_2}]$ true) and gas exchange ratio (R) from a sample of expired gas, using values of expired CO_2 ($F_{E_{CO_2}}$) and expired O_2 ($F_{E_{O_2}}$) present in a wet sample whose water vapor content is known, or, if the sample is saturated with water, whose temperature is known. *Modified from* Beaver, W.L.: Water vapor corrections in oxygen consumption calculations. J. Appl. Physiol. *35*:928–931, 1973.

Index